Cell, Tissue and Disease

THE BASIS OF PATHOLOGY

Cell, Tissue and Disease

THE BASIS OF PATHOLOGY

Neville Woolf

PhD, MMed(Path), FRCPath
Bland-Sutton Professor of Histopathology,
The Middlesex Hospital Medical School
and University College, London

SECOND EDITION

Baillière Tindall
London Philadelphia Toronto
Sydney Tokyo

Baillière Tindall 24–28 Oval Road,
W.B. Saunders London NW1 7DX

The Curtis Center,
Independence Square West,
Philadelphia, PA 19106-3399, USA

55 Horner Avenue,
Toronto, Ontario M8Z 4X6, Canada

Harcourt Brace Jovanovich Group
(Australia) Pty Ltd.,
30–52 Smidmore Street,
Marrickville, NSW 2204, Australia

Harcourt Brace Jovanovich (Japan) Inc.,
Ichibancho Central Building
22–1 Ichibancho,
Chiyoda-ku, Tokyo 102, Japan

First published 1977
Second edition 1986
Reprinted 1990 and 1991

Typeset by Scribe Design, Gillingham, Kent
Printed and bound in Great Britain at the University Press, Cambridge

British Library Cataloguing in Publication Data

Woolf, Neville
  Cell, tissue and disease: the basis of pathology.
  —2nd ed.
  1. Pathology
  I. Title
  616.07   RB111

  ISBN 0 7020 1125 8

Contents

Preface to the Second Edition

Nearly nine years have passed since the first edition of this book saw the light of day. In this time there have been many interesting and exciting developments in a number of fields of study and these have cast new light in some previously obscure areas. As a result I thought it correct to rewrite virtually the whole text, and comparatively little from the first edition remains unaltered.

A justifiable criticism of the previous edition was the paucity of illustrations and an attempt has been made to remedy this deficiency. However, since this book is primarily about 'how diseases happen' rather than 'what they look like', the majority of the figures have been devised to illustrate processes and concepts rather than histopathological appearances.

Some of the material has been the subject of extensive consultation with various colleagues. In this connection, I should like particularly to acknowledge the help I have received from Dr Bill Whimster of King's College, London. Dr Geoffrey Smaldon of Baillière Tindall has been consistently helpful, understanding and forbearing during the gestation period of this edition which, I have little doubt, was rather longer than he would have wished; I am very grateful to him.

November 1985 *Neville Woolf*

Acknowledgements

Several of the figures in this book are based on illustrations published elsewhere. The sources are as follows:

Fig. 4.4: Wilhelm DL (1971) Inflammation and healing. In Anderson WA (ed.) *Pathology*, p.30, Fig. 2-18. St Louis, Missouri: CV Mosby.

Fig. 15.1: Mackaness GB (1970) Cell mediated immunity to infection. *Hospital Practice* 5: 9, and Good RA & Fisher DW (eds) *Immunobiology*. Sunderland, Massachusetts: Sinauer Associates.

Fig. 21.4: Woolf N (1975) Atherosclerosis. In Pomerance A & Davies MJ (eds) *The Pathology of the Heart*, Fig. 4.6. Oxford: Blackwell Scientific.

Fig. 30.4: Hicks RM (1983) Pathological and biochemical aspects of tumour promotion. *Carcinogenesis* 4: 1209.

Fig. 30.10: Bishop JM (1982) Oncogenes. *Scientific American* 246: 80.

Preface to the First Edition

For the student of medicine pathology is, or should be, a bridge between the basic sciences taught largely in the preclinical part of most curricula and the practice of clinical medicine.

This book has been written primarily to emphasize this bridging role and to show the applicability of the basic biological sciences to the study of the processes involved in disease.

For this reason there is relatively little emphasis on abnormal morphology per se and, where possible, the relationship between altered function and altered structure is stressed. Frequent reference is made to the experimental foundations upon which much of current knowledge rests, since enquiring students should learn not to accept their teacher's dicta too readily, unless these can be shown to be soundly based. In addition they should, even at this early stage of training, be encouraged to experience the keen pleasure of seeing the precise and elegant techniques of the more exact sciences applied to the study of problems with important clinical implications.

The basis for the text is the series of lectures given to students in the second year of the Basic Medical Sciences course at the Middlesex Hospital Medical School. Although the text was written primarily with the undergraduate in mind, it should also be of value to postgraduates preparing for the primary examinations of the Royal Colleges of Surgeons and Pathologists. Some difficult decisions involving the selection of material for inclusion have had to be made in order to keep the text reasonably brief and at the same time to avoid too great a degree of superficiality. Thus, the general pathology of injuries to cell and tissue caused by ionizing radiation and of the disorders of heredity and development have not been dealt with. It might be said that in some sections unnecessary emphasis has been given to rare conditions. I make no apology for this since not infrequently it is the rare disease which sheds new light on hitherto unexplored areas of normal function or, as in the case of 'slow viruses', opens new avenues for biological research.

It is a pleasure to acknowledge the assistance I have received from Dr Martin Israel of the Royal College of Surgeons in allowing me to draw on certain material from his excellent textbook on general pathology and in discussing various aspects of my own text with him.

April 1977

Neville Woolf

Chapter 1

The Nature of General Pathology

Pathology can justly be regarded as the bridge between the basic biological sciences and the practice of medicine. It is the study of the changes in structure and function which are produced by injury, in its broadest sense, or by inborn errors.

It is important to realize that the reactions of cells and tissues are finite. This means that identical structural features may be found in both physiological and pathological situations and that morphology per se may be an unreliable guide to the cause of some particular change. For instance, the smooth muscle cells of the uterus increase enormously in size during pregnancy — a perfectly physiological state of affairs. However, if, for example, some obstruction to the normal outflow of urine were to occur, the smooth muscle cells of the bladder wall would also increase very greatly in size — a clear indication of some dysfunction in the lower urinary tract.

Even damage to and death of cells can be physiological as well as pathological phenomena and may excite the same local tissue responses. For example, the structural changes characteristic of acute inflammation are the inevitable consequences of a wide range of injuries, and yet these same histological changes may occur in association with perfectly physiological events such as the shedding of the endometrial lining of the uterus at the end of a menstrual cycle.

The Concept of Disease

What is **disease**? Some have defined it as the condition in which the normal function of some part or organ of the body is disturbed. Others have maintained that disease does not exist except as a reaction to injury. These definitions are in no way mutually exclusive. An individual disease can usefully be regarded, in terms of simple set theory, as the common set of a number of sets, most notably type of injury, type of reaction and the location of injury (Fig. 1.1).

Viewed from a pathophysiological standpoint, one can expand this simple concept to cover situations in which cells, tissues or organs are

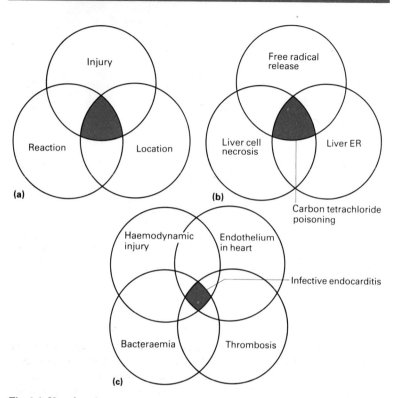

Fig. 1.1 Use of set theory to categorize disease. The chosen sets in this instance are shown in (a) and are the type of injury, its location and the type of local reaction. In example (b), carbon tetrachloride initiates free radical release in the endoplasmic reticulum (ER) of the liver cells and this leads to lipid peroxidation and liver cell necrosis. In example (c), a haemodynamic injury to the endothelium within the heart, such as might occur with a scarred mitral or aortic valve, will, in the presence of micro-organisms in the blood, give rise to infected thrombi on the heart valve surface (infective endocarditis).

acted upon unfavourably either by injurious agents or, less often, by inborn errors acting alone or in conjunction with environmental circumstances. The sequence of events which follows may be dominated by the direct effects of the injurious agent upon the cell (as in certain chemical injuries), or may be a combination of these direct effects and the local and general cell and tissue reactions which may be elicited.

The functional disturbances produced by injury to cells are often mirrored by structural changes, just as, in turn, structural damage may be followed by loss or alteration of some normal function. The sum of these effects finds its expression in the **symptoms** which the patient experiences and the **signs** which the physician observes (Fig. 1.2).

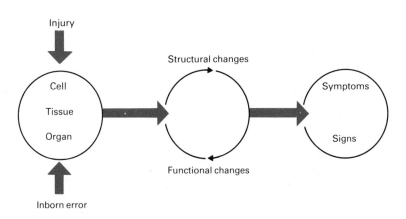

Fig. 1.2 Injury or inborn error may lead to functional and then structural disturbances within cells and tissues. These are expressed as the 'symptoms' experienced by the patient and the 'signs' observed by the physician.

Severe functional disturbances need not be accompanied by significant structural changes

A direct relationship between disordered function and disordered structure is not always present and there may be very severe functional disturbances without any significant structural changes being present. A striking example of this is to be found in **cholera.** In historical terms this has been one of the worst scourges of mankind, yet it is caused by an organism, *Vibrio cholerae,* that cannot either destroy the lining cells of the gut wall or even penetrate between them. There is no microscopic evidence that the organism damages any tissue. However, if untreated, more than half of the infected people will die of the dehydration and electrolyte disturbances which are the consequence of the profuse watery diarrhoea which *Vibrio cholerae* causes. This diarrhoea occurs because the epithelial lining cells of the intestine respond to a **toxin,** secreted by the organism, which behaves in the same way as a normal hormonal regulatory signal. When food is delivered to the small intestine a peptide binds to a receptor site on the luminal membrane of the small intestinal epithelial cell and stimulates the adenylate cyclase system, with the result that about two litres of alkaline fluid are pumped into the small intestine.

Cholera toxin. The cholera toxin consists of two parts. One portion binds to a ganglioside (GM_1) receptor site on the epithelial cell and the other is thought to pass through the cell membrane and has the effect of promoting the synthesis of cyclic adenosine monophosphate (cAMP) at

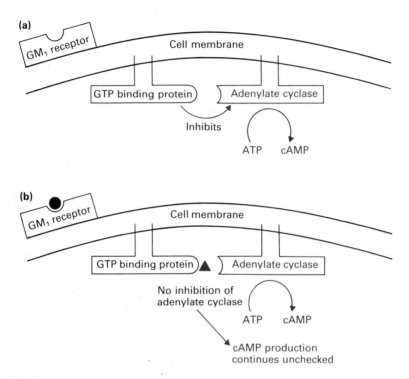

Fig. 1.3 The action of cholera toxin on small intestinal epithelial cells. (a) Normal inhibition of adenylate cyclase. (b) The B portion (●) of the toxin binds to the GM_1 receptor on the epithelial cell membrane. The A portion (▲) passes through the membrane and ribosylates the GTP binding protein which normally inhibits adenylate cyclase activity.

a maximal rate and for an unusually extended period of time, probably by suppressing a natural inhibitory mechanism which normally 'turns off' the adenylate cyclase (Fig. 1.3). This degree of overactivity results in the extrusion of anions followed by the osmotic loss of more than 10 litres of water per day into the small intestine. Since such large amounts of fluid cannot be reabsorbed, this water is lost through diarrhoea and vomiting, and the loss of fluid and electrolyte account for the deaths which occur in this disease.

Morphological change can occur without significant functional disturbance

In other situations a considerable degree of morphological alteration may be present, as, for instance, in the case of some large benign neoplasms, but functional disturbance may be slight or absent.

General Pathology

General pathology is the study of the changes which occur in cells and tissues either as a result of direct damage by, or reactions to, a wide range of unfavourable circumstances. At any given time our knowledge of these is circumscribed by the techniques which we can use for studying these processes. Despite this caveat, it is probably true to say that the number of responses of the mammalian cell is finite. These responses represent, on the whole, either (a) an increase or (b) a reduction or loss of some of the components of a large but not infinite number of normal cell processes.

This general principle only holds good so long as no change has taken place in the genome of the target cell or in the transcription of its genetic information. If such changes have occurred, then a new range of phenotypic characteristics and new responses, not characteristic of this cell, at least in its adult or fully differentiated form, may be acquired. The words 'adult or fully differentiated' should be stressed because the acquisition of apparently new functions (such as the secretion of fetal antigens by the cells of some tumours) may be the expression of functions which were normal and appropriate at an earlier stage of the organism's embryological development.

The Characteristics of a Disease

How one regards any individual disease process depends largely on one's point of view. The patient will wish to know whether he will recover or not, i.e. the **prognosis**; the clinician will wish to know the diagnostic features and the best mode of treatment, and the histopathologist will tend to classify the disease on the basis of its morphological features. All groups should want to know the basic cause (or **aetiology**) if possible, since only in the light of this knowledge is it conceivable that the disease can be avoided. Another concept of importance is the **pathogenesis** of a disease. Many people tend to confuse the terms aetiology and pathogenesis. The term pathogenesis refers not to the actual first cause of the disease but to the sequence of events which occurs from the time of the first injury to the time when the disease expresses itself in functional and structural terms.

An example of the pathogenesis of a common and serious disease may be found in the natural history of coronary artery atherosclerosis, the complications of which are responsible for approximately 25% of adult male deaths in the U.K. In morphological terms it is a disorder characterized by the presence of focally distributed thickenings of the intima of large elastic and muscular arteries. These thickenings consist

(a)

Hyperlipidaemia   Hypertension   Diabetes   Cigarette smoking

Aetiological factors

Normal artery

Intimal smooth muscle proliferation +
accumulation of lipid in intima

Necrosis at base of intimal plaque

Plaque softens with rupture of
connective tissue cap

Superimposed occlusive thrombosis

Regional myocardial underperfusion

(b)

Pain

Arrhythmogenic focus

Local failure of
contraction

Coagulative necrosis

Organization

Aneurysm at site
of scar

of an admixture of proliferated connective tissue which forms a 'cap' to the lesion and a basal accumulation of lipid and tissue debris. As these plaque-like foci increase in thickness they may cause a significant degree of narrowing of the vessel lumen. This may lead to regional underperfusion of the heart muscle, and the patient may experience chest pain provoked by exercise or cold and relieved by rest or vasodilators. Not infrequently the plaque softens as its constituents undergo necrosis and this may be followed by splitting of the connective tissue cap and exposure of the subendothelial elements of the plaque. This leads to adherence and aggregation of platelets and within a very short time this mass of platelets and fibrin (a **thrombus**) may block the lumen of the artery. The segment of ventricular wall supplied by this artery will thus be deprived totally of its arterial blood supply. In clinical terms this may be expressed as the onset of severe central chest pain or serious ventricular arrhythmias which may prove fatal within a few minutes, as low output accompanied by peripheral vasoconstriction (cardiogenic shock), or as cardiac failure. In structural terms the morphological features of death of the underperfused muscle will develop over the next 24 hours or so. In most instances, if the patient lives, the dead muscle will be replaced by a scar. This, of course, lacks the contractile properties of muscle and may eventually stretch permanently, leading to the formation of a bulge or **aneurysm** on the wall of the left ventricle (Fig. 1.4). If death of the patient has occurred within a few minutes of the cutting off of the arterial blood supply, the structural changes which indicate cell injury or cell death do not occur.

Fig. 1.4 The pathogenesis of a disease is the sequence of events which follows from the application of some injurious factor and which culminates in a full-blown pathological and clinical picture. The example shown here presents a simplified scheme of the events (a) in the coronary arteries and (b) in the heart which may result from some or all of the causal factors listed.

Chapter 2

Cell Injury and its Manifestations

Under most circumstances cells try to maintain a **steady state.** If their milieu is altered in some way they will adapt to the change in circumstances without their function being significantly impaired. Obvious examples of this are to be found in situations where there is an alteration in the **functional demands** made on cells. An increase in demand usually leads to an increase in **size** of individual cells (hypertrophy), an increase in **number** of cells (hyperplasia) or both. An example of such cellular adaptation is the marked increase in size of the cardiac muscle fibres which occurs when there is overload of cardiac muscle due to high pressure in the left ventricular outflow tract as, for example, in aortic valve stenosis or in systemic hypertension. The increase in size of the individual cells leads to a significant increase in the thickness of the left ventricular wall. Conversely, when the demand for a function is reduced this may be mirrored by a marked **decrease** in cell size (atrophy). An example of this is the very rapid muscle wasting which may follow immobilization of a limb in plaster following a fracture.

If the degree of change is so great that the cell becomes unable to adjust to its changed milieu, then some **loss** in its normal range of functions is likely to occur. This degree of loss may be so great as to involve vital cellular functions and thus lead to the **death** of the cell.

Maintenance of the steady state

The maintenance of a steady state within a cell involves its continuing to perform a range of basic functions. These include:

1. Synthesis of nucleic acids, proteins, lipids and carbohydrates requires normality of the DNA templates, and subsumed within this must be the ability to excise and repair abnormal base linkages within the DNA molecule.
2. Enzymes are required of both normal type and amount for the assembly and reproduction of the cell's own organelles and membranes and for the carrying out of a variety of other functions such as the degradation of a wide range of compounds.
3. The transport of metabolites via energy-dependent transport systems

8

requires intact membranes if osmotic and fluid homeostasis are to be preserved.

4. Aerobic energy production via oxidative phosphorylation and the production of high energy phosphate bonds requires adequate oxygenation and normal amounts of suitable substrate. Hypoxia, often mediated via ischaemia (a reduction in the perfusion of a part relative to its needs), is one of the commonest and most important causes of both sub-lethal and lethal cell injury.

These systems are intimately related to each other. As Robbins has said 'the metabolic functions and structural elements are so intricately woven in the cells that whatever the precise point of attack, derangements fan out in ever widening ripples to affect other functions and elements'. Because of this it is not easy to identify precisely the targets of cell injury in terms of function rather than in terms of the cell's anatomy. Occasional exceptions exist where it is possible to identify the functional target. This is seen in cyanide poisoning in which cytochrome oxidase is inactivated leading to a block in aerobic respiration.

Despite these reservations, it is reasonable to consider the question of cell injury either in terms of the portion of the cell which is affected primarily, or in terms of the type of injury applied. Where possible, these two approaches should be combined.

The Nucleus

The nucleus, and hence the genetic constitution of the cell, may be altered in a number of ways. The abnormality may be inherited and may involve a single gene only, as in sickle cell disease, in which case there will be no obvious morphological abnormality in the nucleus or its constituent chromosomes. However, distinct chromosomal abnormalities may be present which may be expressed in alterations of the normal diploid number, as in Down's syndrome or one of the other trisomy syndromes which, as a whole, lead to a large number of congenital abnormalities. Abnormalities may also occur in the form of chromosomal breakages, producing syndromes such as ataxia-telangiectasia or Fanconi's anaemia. In the former there is progressive cerebellar ataxia, telangiectasia (complex intertwined bundles of abnormally and permanently dilated blood vessels) in the eyes and skin, a severe immunological deficiency, and extreme radiosensitivity of such a high degree that even diagnostic x-rays have been reported to be followed by leukaemia in affected patients. There appears to be a very close link between such chromosomal breakage syndromes and an increased risk of developing leukaemia or other malignant conditions involving the lymphoid system. The greatest care should be exercised to prevent exposure of these, fortunately rare, patients to chemical or physical agents, such as irradiation, which are known to damage DNA.

Toxic nuclear damage occurs in the treatment of malignant disease with cytotoxic drugs. This may come about in a number of different ways depending on the chemotherapeutic agent used. Some drugs, such as the alkylating agents (e.g. cyclophosphamide), combine directly with DNA, while others such as vincristine (the periwinkle alkaloid) damage the mitotic spindle. Others act as analogues of normal metabolites and block some of the enzyme-controlled steps in nucleic acid synthesis.

Nutritional damage to the nucleus may be seen in the cells of patients with either folic acid deficiency or vitamin B_{12} deficiency, as is seen in pernicious anaemia. The nuclei in these cells are larger than normal, but contain less DNA than is optimal for mitosis. These changes are present in many tissues but are most prominent among the red cell precursors in the bone marrow.

The Cell Membrane

Many functions are mediated via the cell membrane. These range from such vital matters as the maintenance of normal osmotic relationships between the intracellular and extracellular environments, to a variety of receptor and transduction functions.

Some inherited defects of membrane structure and function have been identified. These include such entities as lack of the ability to transport the dibasic amino acids lysine and ornithine across the luminal membrane of the renal tubular epithelial cell, so that these amino acids appear in the urine in significant amounts. A similar inherited transport defect operates in Hartnup disease, where there is a reduction in the ability to transport tryptophan from the gut across the small intestinal epithelium. Since tryptophan is an important source of nicotinic acid, a deficiency of the latter develops and leads to the appearance of the clinical signs of pellagra.

Inherited receptor defects

A paradigm of inherited receptor defects in cell membranes is to be found in **familial type IIa hypercholesterolaemia** in which peripheral cells lack high affinity receptors for low density lipoprotein (LDL). Failure to endocytose the LDL at these receptor sites leads to a failure to control the cell synthesis of cholesterol via its rate-limiting enzyme 3-hydroxy-3-methylglutaryl coenzyme A reductase (HMG CoA reductase). The consequence is a grossly elevated plasma concentration of LDL, this being associated with abnormally early development of

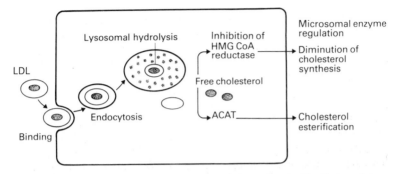

Fig. 2.1 The cell biology of familial type IIa hypercholesterolaemia. The diagram shows the course of events in normal cells which bind LDL at specific high affinity receptor sites on the plasma membrane. This LDL is then endocytosed and broken down within phagolysosomes, with the consequent release of free cholesterol in the cytoplasm. The intracellular concentration of free cholesterol controls the level of activity of HMG CoA reductase. As intracellular free cholesterol rises the enzyme is inhibited and cholesterol synthesis by the cell diminishes. The free cholesterol in the cytoplasm is esterified under the influence of acyl coenzyme A transferase (ACAT). Patients with type IIa hypercholesterolaemia either lack receptors or have receptors which do not function adequately.

atherosclerosis and ischaemic heart disease (Fig. 2.1).

Complement-related membrane injury

If complement becomes bound to a cell surface its activation leads to lysis of the cell membrane and escape of the cell contents into the extracellular environment. An example of this is the lysis of red blood cells which follows incompatible blood transfusions or other immune-mediated forms of haemolysis. Electron micrographs of cell membranes following activation of complement bound to antigen/antibody complexes on the cell surface show the presence of rather uniform dark areas. These were at one time thought to be holes, but are now believed to be areas in which there is a local piling up of the lipid moieties of the cell membrane at sites where the C8 component of complement has become inserted into the membrane. Each 'hole' is a single complex containing one molecule each of complement components 5–8 and six molecules of C9. C8 opens and shuts a trans-membrane channel; if this channel remains open then lysis of the cell will occur. The binding of C9 serves to jam this channel open.

Free radicals and membrane injury

It has become increasingly clear that the formation of free radicals is the common effector pathway for a number of different types of cell injury, including ischaemic injury, certain drug-induced haemolytic anaemias, paraquat poisoning, carbon tetrachloride poisoning, radiation injury, certain cellular correlates of ageing, and oxygen toxicity.

A free radical is an atom or molecule which has a single unpaired electron in its outer orbital. Such chemical species are very active and not only react with molecules within the cell membrane, but often convert these to free radicals as well, thus forming a positive amplification system. Free radicals can arise in a number of ways. One of these is through the absorption of radiant energy. The cell damage which occurs in the course of therapeutic irradiation is, to a very considerable extent, brought about by the generation of these radicals. In a number of situations the reduction of molecular oxygen results in the gain of one rather than two electrons, with the formation of a highly reactive anion O_2^- known as the superoxide anion. The generation of superoxide is an important part of the body's defences against bacterial infection, and bacterial killing by neutrophile leucocytes and by macrophages cannot take place effectively without the formation of oxygen free radicals. This subject is dealt with in more detail in Chapter 5. Another interesting model of free radical mediated injury is carbon tetrachloride poisoning. Carbon tetrachloride is changed by mixed function oxidases into the free radical CCl_3^- in the smooth endoplasmic reticulum of liver cells. This leads to peroxidation of the phospholipids of the liver cell membranes, first in the smooth endoplasmic reticulum, where the transformation of CCl_4 has taken place, and later in all the intracellular membranes. If the P450 enzyme system has been induced by previous administration of barbiturates, the amount of free radical formation will be increased and the amount of cell damage will be greater than would be expected for that dose of CCl_4.

The presence of scavenging mechanisms both within cells and in the extracellular environment suggests that generation of free radicals is a regular accompaniment of redox reactions within the cells and tissues and is not merely an occasional event associated with such abnormal circumstances as irradiation or poisoning. One of the most important scavenging mechanisms is a group of enzymes, the superoxide dismutases, whose function is the catalytic dismutation of the superoxide anion to hydrogen peroxide and molecular oxygen. The superoxide dismutases are so widely distributed as to suggest that the superoxide anion is an important by-product of oxidative metabolism. The hydrogen peroxide formed in the course of the dismutation reaction is further detoxified to water by catalases and peroxidase. The peroxidation of unsaturated lipids in the cell membranes is normally inhibited by hydrophobic scavengers such as vitamin E and glutathione peroxidase.

The free radicals can also react with molecules in the ionic or water compartments of the cell. Molecules which have scavenging potential in ionic environments include such compounds as reduced glutathione, ascorbic acid and cysteine. In ex vivo circumstances the importance of these scavengers can be demonstrated by depleting their concentration within isolated cells. When this is done the functional and morphological changes that follow lipid peroxidation within membranes are reproduced precisely, even though no measures have been taken to increase the generation of free radicals (Fig. 2.2a and b).

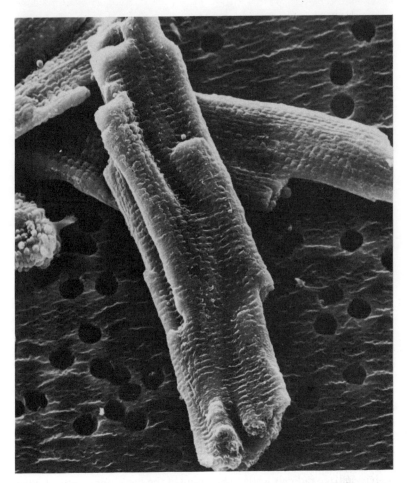

Fig. 2.2a Scanning electron micrograph of normal, mature heart muscle cells from a rat. The well-marked transverse ridges on the plasma membranes represent the T tube system. × 3400.

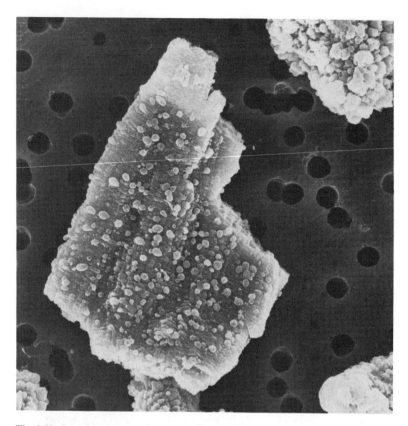

Fig. 2.2b Scanning electron micrograph of isolated heart muscle cells from a rat. These cells have been treated with diamide, a compound which decreases the intracellular content of reduced glutathione and thus renders the cell more susceptible to free radical induced damage. The cells are contracted and have numerous blebs on the plasma membrane. This morphological feature appears to be a common result of lipid peroxidation of cell membranes following free radical initiation. × 5300.

The type of injury induced by the action of free radicals depends not only on the activity of the radicals generated, but also on the structural and biochemical environment. For instance, in the extracellular space the glycosoaminoglycans of the ground substance may be degraded by free radicals; this might well be important in relation to some of the destructive processes which occur in the joints (e.g. rheumatoid arthritis). So far as plasma membranes are concerned, uncontrolled activity of free radicals leads to blebbing of the membranes and a failure to maintain the normal fluid and ionic relationships between the intra- and extracellular compartments.

Lysosomes and Cell Injury

Lysosomes are involved in disease in three main ways. The first of these arises as a result of an inherited deficiency of one of the lysosomal enzymes which are responsible for the normal degradation and turnover of a wide range of molecules. The substrates which cannot be degraded accumulate in the lysosomes, mainly within phagocytic cells but also in liver parenchymal cells, neurones, fibroblasts and renal tubular epithelial cells. This group of disorders is known as the **storage diseases**. Carbohydrates, such as glycogen, complex mucopolysaccharides and a wide variety of sphingolipids are some of the molecules which may accumulate in this way and an equally wide range of clinical and pathological syndromes has been described. Cultured cells from affected patients usually show the same metabolic abnormalities. In some instances (e.g. Hurler's syndrome, one of the mucopolysaccharidoses) the inexorable advance of the disease has been halted by transplanting bone marrow from unaffected and histocompatible donors to the affected children.

The second way in which lysosomes are involved in cell and tissue injury is when there is release of intra-lysosomal enzymes into the cell cytoplasm. Lysosomal membrane rupture, mediated by a single mechanism, occurs in two apparently widely disparate diseases: gout and silicosis. In the first of these the neutrophile is the cell affected; in the second, the macrophage is the source of the released enzymes. In both of these, phagocytosis of crystalline material is followed by lysosomal fusion and the formation of abnormal hydrogen bonds between the particle surface and the lysosomal membrane. The resulting perturbation of the lysosomal membrane leads to rupture, with spillage of the enzyme content both into the cytoplasm of the cell and into the surrounding area (Fig. 2.3). The third way in which lysosomes may be involved in a disease process is by secretion of lysosomal enzymes (usually from macrophages) into the immediate environment of these cells. The possibility that such events might be associated with the development of some forms of arthritis was mooted after the observations of Fell and her colleagues that if articular cartilage was incubated with an excess of vitamin A, the glycosaminoglycan of the matrix was destroyed, though the cartilage cells themselves appeared to be viable. In vivo, injections of large doses of vitamin A or papain, both of which render lysosomal membranes unstable, into rabbits led to a loss of the rabbits' ability to prick up their ears; the histological correlate of this was once again a loss of the complex carbohydrate in the cartilage matrix. If lysosomal enzymes are injected into the joints of small animals the tissue response resembles that seen in rheumatoid disease and, in humans, joint fluid from

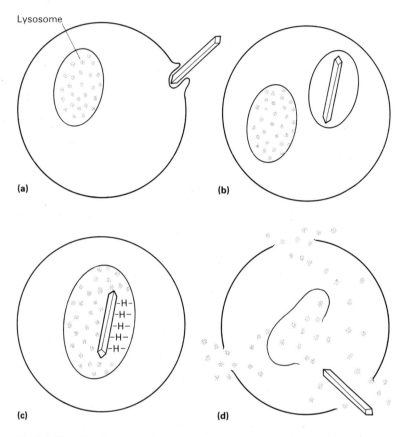

Lysosome

(a)

(b)

(c)

(d)

Fig. 2.3 Tissue injury resulting from intracytoplasmic release of lysosomal enzymes following the formation of abnormal hydrogen bonds between the lysosomal membrane and the surface of an ingested particle, as seen in gout and silicosis. (a) Phagocytosis of crystal. (b) The primary lysosome fuses with the phagosome. (c) Hydrogen bonds form between the crystal surface and the lysosomal membrane. This leads to immobilization of the affected area of the normally mobile lysosomal membrane. (d) As a result of this 'adhesion' between the crystal and part of the lysosomal membrane, the latter ruptures and spills its content of hydrolytic enzymes.

patients with rheumatoid arthritis contains lysosomal enzymes. These data have been interpreted as suggesting that the effector pathway for damage to the articular cartilage in the destructive arthritides is the inappropriate release of lysosomal enzymes. Clearly the instability of the lysosomal membranes in this situation is not due to either vitamin A intoxication or the presence of papain and, for the present, the pathogenesis of the lysosomal change remains obscure.

Some Morphological Expressions of Cell Injury

The presence of cell injury of varying degrees of severity can often be correlated with morphological changes within the cells. The pathological literature of the nineteenth and early twentieth centuries abounds with more or less graphic, but more or less meaningless, descriptive terms such as **cloudy swelling** or **hyaline (glassy) degeneration.**

Two of the commonest ways in which **sub-lethal** cell injury is manifested are by alterations in **cell volume** and by the accumulation of excess triglyceride (**fatty change**).

Changes in cell volume (acute cellular oedema)

The control of the volume of a cell within fairly narrow limits is one of the outstanding characteristics of mammalian cells. This control is exerted largely by sodium and potassium transport mechanisms which are energy dependent and linked with membrane-bound enzymes.

If these control mechanisms break down, a large amount of isotonic fluid collects within the cell and the cell volume increases. The mitochondria also become swollen; it is for this reason that, on light microscopic examination, the cell cytoplasm appears granular. This increase in intracellular fluid content or **acute cellular oedema** particularly occurs if the cells become hypoxic, but may occur also in the course of fever or cell injury by certain bacterial toxins and chemical poisons.

The normal cell has a higher potassium concentration and a lower sodium content than is present in the extracellular fluid. This differential in respect of sodium and potassium is maintained by the ATP energy-dependent membrane transport system known as the **sodium pump**; part of this system is the ouabain-sensitive ATPase situated in the plasma membrane of the cell.

Hypoxia and the other forms of cell injury mentioned above cause a fall in the production of ATP and the ratio of ATP to ADP (adenosine diphosphate) falls significantly. This leads to a partial failure of the sodium pump. Potassium ions diffuse out of the cell into the extracellular fluid, and the reverse applies to sodium ions, which enter the cell in large amounts. Since the hydration shell of sodium is greater than that of potassium, water enters the cells from the extracellular fluid as well and this will, of course, lead to an increase in cell volume.

Trump and his colleagues have studied the effects of hypoxia on the cell in detail and have outlined the following sequence of events (Fig. 2.4). As the oxygen tension falls, mitochondrial phosphorylation decreases rapidly with a consequent fall in ATP. This drop in ATP stimulates the activity of the enzyme **phosphofructokinase** and this

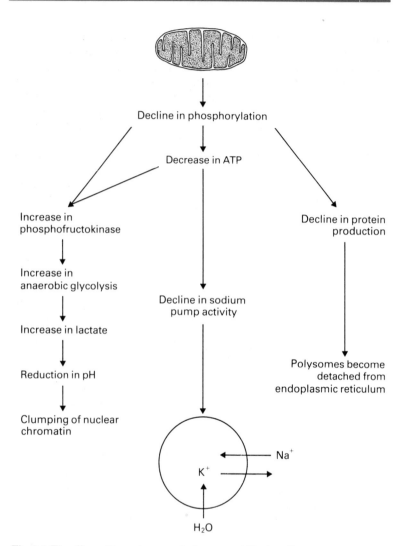

Fig. 2.4 The effects of hypoxia on metabolic events within the cells.

leads to an increase in the rate of anaerobic glycolysis. This, in its turn, causes an accumulation of lactate, which, together with the increase in inorganic phosphate, lowers the intracellular pH. Morphologically this is believed to be reflected in the appearance of clumping of the nuclear chromatin.

At this point the decline in ATP will have produced its effect on the sodium pump and the accumulation of sodium and water mentioned above takes place. Protein production is also adversely affected at this stage and this is expressed in morphological terms by **detachment of polysomes** from the membranes of the endoplasmic reticulum and the scattering of both free and bound polysomes into monomeric ribosomes. At this stage the process is still reversible: both the function and the structure of the protein-secreting apparatus can be restored to normal if the cell's oxygen supply is brought back to normal levels. At this stage the cytoskeleton also appears to have been affected and the plasma membrane of the cells may show blebs or the appearance of microvilli.

If the hypoxia continues beyond this point, the degree of cell damage may reach a point at which restoration of normal structure and function cannot now occur and the cell will die. The mitochondria become markedly swollen and accumulate dense flocculent material (probably

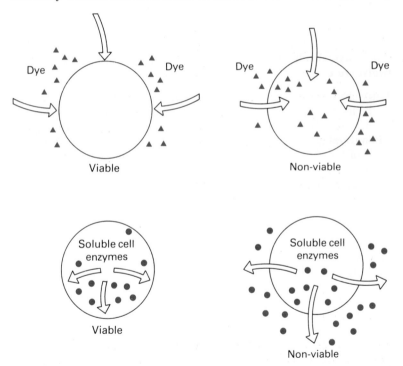

Fig. 2.5 Lethal damage to cells is associated with change in permeability of the cell plasma membrane. The viable cell normally excludes dye molecules in the incubating medium. Lethal injury is associated with staining of the cells. Similarly, water-soluble intracellular enzymes do not leak out of a viable cell, but lethal cell damage is associated with escape of such enzymes into the intracellular fluid. The concentration of these enzymes can be monitored in samples of plasma.

calcium and lipid), and the intracellular membranes become fragmented. Nuclear chromatin starts to undergo attack by enzymes (presumably of lysosomal origin) and as this proceeds the nucleus becomes digested away (this is known as **karyolysis**). At this stage not only is there equilibration between extra- and intracellular ionic concentrations, but other molecules begin to move freely across the plasma membrane so that dyes in the ECF can move into the cell, while the cell's own enzymes leak out (Fig. 2.5). This alteration in plasma membrane permeability can constitute a valuable marker of cell injury in the patient. For example, death of cardiac muscle cells is associated with the release into the ECF, and then into the plasma, of intracellular enzymes such as creatine kinase and β-hydroxybutyric acid dehydrogenase. The plasma concentrations of these enzymes can be monitored in patients with a suspected diagnosis of ischaemic damage to the myocardium and can provide an additional method for assessing whether the degree of ischaemic damage is increasing.

Parenchymal cell fatty change — the accumulation of excess triglyceride

Fatty change is the term applied when parenchymal cells, notably those of the **liver, heart** and **kidney**, contain stainable triglyceride. When the tissues are examined microscopically the fat may be seen in the form of small droplets or, if these coalesce, as large single drops which occupy most of the cell area and push the remaining cytoplasmic contents and the nucleus to the edge of the cell. In conventionally prepared tissue sections, which must be dehydrated in alcohol and 'cleared' in various organic solvents before being embedded in paraffin wax, the fat droplets are dissolved away leaving intra-cytoplasmic spaces. Therefore, the presence of triglyceride cannot be confirmed by appropriate staining methods. The fat can, however, be demonstrated by cutting sections from blocks of tissue which have been very rapidly frozen and then staining these sections with dyes which dissolve preferentially in triglyceride, such as mixtures of Sudan III and IV or Oil-Red O, both of which stain the fat-containing droplets a bright orange-red.

Macroscopically, organs affected by severe fatty change have a pale yellowish-brown colour and may feel greasy. Rarely, the degree of fat accumulation in the liver may be so great that blocks of tissue float in water or fixative solutions. In the liver the distribution of fat is usually diffuse in the organ as a whole, though not necessarily in individual liver acini. However, in the kidney, fatty change shows up as a series of yellowish streaks in the cortex, since the accumulation of fat is non-uniform and tends to be confined to the epithelial cells lining the convoluted tubules. In the heart, severe fatty change is commonly seen as a pale and rather flabby myocardium. However, the fatty change seen sometimes in patients suffering from chronic anaemia produces a curious striped appearance which is most obvious in the subendocardial layer of the interventricular septum and in the papillary muscles. In a rare departure from the well-known tendency of morbid anatomists to characterize morphological alterations in terms of food, this appearance has been called '**tabby cat**' or '**thrush-breast**' striation.

Origin of the excess intracellular triglyceride

The excess fat which accumulates in affected cells is largely derived from the fat stored in adipose tissue and does not appear as a result of some 'unmasking' phenomenon of fat already present within the cell. A variety of experimental models can be used to demonstrate this. For example, if an animal is poisoned with phosphorus it develops acute liver damage associated with severe fatty change. Starving the animal before the administration of the phosphorus, with resulting depletion of its adipose tissue fat stores, prevents the development of the fatty change, even though the liver cell damage occurs as before. Similarly cells grown in culture can accumulate triglyceride only if triglyceride is present in the culture medium.

The causes of triglyceride accumulation within liver cells

The liver cell occupies a central place in fat metabolism, and the disorders (including various types of poisoning) which result in hepatic fatty change can be understood most easily in terms of disturbance of the various processes related to fat metabolism (Fig. 2.6).

The liver cell normally receives fat in two forms and from two sources. The first form is non-esterified **free fatty acid** (FFA), which is derived from the peripheral adipose tissue stores and is released from the adipocytes when lipolysis occurs. The second form of fat is the **chylomicron**, which is a large molecule synthesized within the small intestinal epithelium and which consists of triglyceride (90%), phospholipid and apoprotein B. If this apoprotein cannot be synthesized, then chylomicrons cannot be assembled and the triglyceride derived from the diet accumulates within the intestinal epithelium.

Within the liver cell, hydrolysis of the chylomicrons takes place, liberating free fatty acids and glycerol. Acetate, from which additional free fatty acids can be synthesized, is also present within the liver cell. Irrespective of their origin, most of the FFA are esterified to form triglyceride, some are incorporated into phospholipid, and others are converted into cholesterol. The triglyceride within the liver cell, which

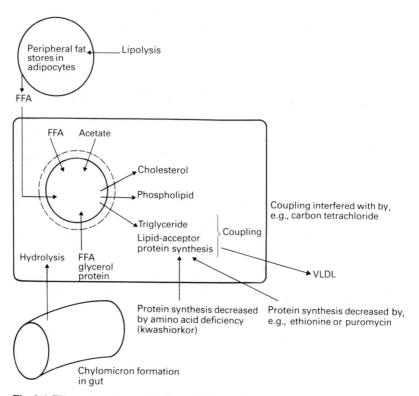

Fig. 2.6 The processes involved in fat metabolism within the liver cell.

is kept in the form of a micelle by phospholipid, is then coupled to a lipid-acceptor protein or apoprotein and secreted from the liver in the form of very low density lipoprotein (VLDL).

It should be clear therefore that accumulation of excess triglyceride may reflect either an increase in the amount of lipid being brought to the liver, particularly in the form of non-esterified fatty acids (NEFA), or an inability of the liver cell to carry out the functions outlined above in respect of the delivery of a normal amount of lipid.

High NEFA levels in the presence of normal liver cells. High plasma concentrations of non-esterified fatty acids in the presence of normal liver cells are seen when there is a decrease in the energy normally supplied by carbohydrates. Increased fat catabolism is needed to make up for the energy shortfall and this leads to lipolysis of the fat in adipose tissue stores and a rise in the plasma concentration of free fatty acids. This occurs in starvation or where there is some block in normal carbohydrate metabolism such as in **uncontrolled diabetes mellitus, galactosaemia** and some forms of **glycogen storage disease.**

Normal plasma NEFA levels in the presence of injury or abnormality of liver cells. Since the number of functions carried out by the liver cells in respect of the free fatty acids delivered to it is large, the number of ways in which liver cell injury can be reflected by fatty change is correspondingly great. Liver cell injury affecting (amongst others) these particular functions includes:

Anoxia due to severe congestive cardiac failure. The cells first affected are those in the centrilobular zone. This gives the affected organ a mottled red and yellow appearance. The red areas represent the congested central veins and the dilated and congested sinusoids around them, and the yellow areas represent the central and intermediate parts of the lobule in which fatty change is present. This is known as **'nutmeg' liver.**

Severe protein and calorie undernutrition. In severe protein and calorie undernutrition (known as **kwashiorkor** when seen in children), the liver cell (because of a shortage of the necessary amino acid substrates) is not able to synthesize the lipid-acceptor proteins needed for the export of triglyceride in the form of VLDL. A very marked degree of triglyceride accumulation may occur under these circumstances, so much so that the liver, when removed at post-mortem examination, may float in water or aqueous fixatives. Sequential liver biopsy studies have shown that hepatic fatty change of this type that is occurring by itself and not as part of some process likely to cause destruction of the affected cells (e.g. carbon tetrachloride poisoning) is completely reversible if patients suffering from kwashiorkor are given a diet containing adequate amounts of protein.

Chronic alcoholism. Chronic alcoholism is one of the commonest causes of significant hepatic fatty change in over-privileged Western communities. The metabolic effects on the liver cell of ingestion of excess amounts of alcohol are complex. It used to be believed that fatty change occurred as a consequence of malnutrition, especially in respect of the protein intake, but this is now deemed to be unlikely. The substitution of large amounts of alcohol for part of the diet in healthy non-alcoholic volunteers by Rubin and Lieber produced fatty change in their livers very rapidly; similar results have been obtained in baboons who were given large amounts of alcohol while being kept on an adequate diet. Interference with oxidation of fatty acids is likely to be the most important cause of intracellular triglyceride accumulation in alcoholics, but there may also be an associated hyperlipidaemia (Frederickson type V) characterized by a rise in plasma triglyceride concentrations.

Other chemical and bacterial toxins. Many chemicals have been shown to be capable of inducing hepatic fatty change both in humans and in experimental animals. These include carbon tetrachloride, puromycin, ethionine and phosphorus, to name only a few. The fact that carbon tetrachloride can damage liver cells through the generation of free radicals has been mentioned earlier. There is some evidence that the metabolic events associated with this, which lead to the death of liver cells, are different from those which result in the accumulation of fat within the liver cell. Carbon tetrachloride reduces the secretion of protein by the liver cell, and the suggestion has therefore been made that the fat accumulates because of lack of secretion of adequate amounts of lipid-acceptor protein. However, work with other models such as **orotic acid** poisoning has shown that inhibition of protein secretion is *not* a prerequisite for intracellular fat accumulation and that the fault may be, at least in the early stages, a **failure of coupling** between triglyceride and the lipid-acceptor protein.

The **decline in protein synthesis** which appears to be associated with some examples of both toxic and non-toxic hepatic fatty change may be brought about in a number of ways. For example, **puromycin**, an antibiotic which has a structure resembling the terminal portion of transfer RNA, is a powerful inhibitor of protein synthesis in the rat. This is accomplished by a decrease in the rate of **transcription** of ribosomal RNA, this being associated with a later effect on RNA maturation. **Ethionine**, on the other hand, decreases protein secretion by acting as a drain on hepatic ATP. This is because ethionine, which is the ethyl analogue of the amino acid methionine, competes successfully with the latter for ATP and combines with the ATP to form S-adenosyl-ethionine plus inorganic orthophosphate. S-adenosyl-ethionine is inactive in so far as transfers of methyl groups is concerned and simply acts as an adenosyl trap. Hepatic ATP is thus drained and there is a consequent reduction in messenger RNA synthesis, a break-up of polyribosomes and a decline in protein synthesis.

So-called lipotropic factors. When rodents are fed on diets which are deficient in choline, methionine, betaine and inositol they develop fatty livers. Choline has been called a lipotropic factor because without it phospholipids are not formed; the other substances mentioned provide a source of labile methyl groups. Such dietary deficiencies in small rodents decrease lipoprotein synthesis and this leads to intracellular accumulation of fat. If the intracellular stores of labile methyl groups are exhausted (as can be achieved by giving rats excess amounts of nicotinic acid, which is excreted in the urine as its N-methylated derivative trigonelline), phospholipid synthesis declines and fat accumulates within the liver cell. There is, however, *no* evidence that such deficiencies have a significant role in the causation of fatty liver in humans.

Chapter 3

Cell and Tissue Death

If changes in the environment are such that cells cannot achieve a new steady state, these cells die: i.e. the energy-dependent, organized interactions between DNA templates, membranes and enzyme systems break down and all the functions of the cells cease. Cell death occurs regularly under physiological as well as pathological conditions; for example, there is a high turnover of epithelial cells in the skin and in the small intestine. In many **diseases**, cell death is responsible for producing the symptoms and signs characteristic of that disease and the extent of such cell death may well determine the outcome. The character of a given disease is often determined by the **type** of cell which dies. For example, in poliomyelitis the anterior horn cells of the spinal cord are the prime targets for destruction by the polio virus. The patient thus develops a lower motor neurone type of paralysis in those muscles whose motor nerve supply is related to the affected neurones. Many such examples could be given. The effect of differences in the **extent** of cell death on the natural history of certain pathological states is well shown in myocardial infarction. If the amount of cardiac muscle which undergoes irreversible damage is great, failure of the pumping function of the heart is likely to ensue and there may be a sudden and severe fall in cardiac output. It may not be possible to compensate for this by using inotropic drugs, and it may be necessary for a balloon pump to be inserted into the patient's ascending aorta for output to be restored to near normal.

Morphological Changes in Cell Death

Cell death may be defined, in physiological terms, as the **irreversible breakdown of the energy-dependent functions of the cell.** For the histopathologist, cell death means the series of **morphological changes** which occur in relation to a cell or group of cells following lethal injury. It is the element of time and the unfettered action of **enzymatic degradation** and **protein denaturation** which determine the differences between functional cell death and cell death as morphologically defined. The cells of a piece of tissue removed at operation or biopsy and placed immediately in fixative are dead but show *no* morphological abnormalities indicative of cell death.

25

The morphological features seen in dead cells vary depending on which of the two processes — enzymatic digestion or protein denaturation — is dominant. Some degree of enzymatic degradation is nearly always present and this is manifested by various nuclear and cytoplasmic changes.

Autolysis

If enzymatic degradation is the dominant element then dead cells are likely to be completely removed. This process may be accomplished by the activation of enzymes which are normally present within the affected cell. This process of **self-digestion** is known as **autolysis**. The enzymes are derived largely from lysosomes. The precise sequence of events leading to the activation and release of lysosomal enzymes is not known, but it is likely that a decrease in the intracellular pH is an important factor. Release of lysosomal enzymes in cell death can be inferred from the following:

1. Ultracentrifugal fractionation of dead cells shows that lysosomal enzymes are no longer particle-bound but appear in the supernatant.
2. There is evidence of enzymatic digestion of cell components in the loss of both DNA and RNA protein and glycogen.

Cytoplasmic changes

The cytoplasm shows a decrease in basophilia (indicating a loss of RNA protein) and an increased affinity for acid dyes such as eosin. This increased eosinophilia is due to denaturation of some of the cytoplasmic proteins with exposure of basic groups which bind the eosin. When appropriate special stains such as the periodic acid-Schiff method are used, loss of glycogen is noted and there may be some fragmentation and clumping of the cytoplasmic contents.

Nuclear changes

Irreversible damage to the nucleus shows itself in one of three patterns:

1. **Karyolysis.** There is a gradual fading away of the basophilic nuclear material, presumably as a result of the activity of DNases.
2. **Karyorrhexis.** Here the nucleus undergoes fragmentation and the debris is either phagocytosed by other cells or just disappears.

3. **Pyknosis.** The nucleus shrinks and becomes intensely basophilic. This stage is often followed by karyorrhexis.

The immediate result of these changes (as seen in a section stained with haematoxylin and eosin) is a highly eosinophilic cell which has lost its nucleus. Its survival or not in this form depends on whether further enzymatic digestion takes place.

Heterolysis

If enzymatic digestion is accomplished by enzymes derived from cells other than the dead or dying ones, the process is termed **heterolysis**. Here the enzymes are derived from the lysosomes of cells such as neutrophil polymorphonuclear leucocytes or mononuclear phagocytes (macrophages). Heterolysis may occur as a result of **endocytosis**, in the course of which phagocytes ingest portions of dead or dying cells and segregate them into phagocytic vacuoles (**phagosomes**). The lysosomes of the phagocyte then fuse with the phagosomes to form secondary lysosomes in which enzymatic digestion of all or part of the ingested cell debris takes place. However, phagocytosis is not an absolute prerequisite for heterolysis and the latter can take place as a result of the local release of lysosomal enzymes by phagocytes.

Apoptosis

Normal cell **turnover** implies that all the fully differentiated cells populating a given tissue must die and be replaced in a controlled and 'programmed' manner. The term **apoptosis** (literally a 'dropping off' as in relation to petals or leaves) has been suggested for this controlled type of cell deletion which appears to play an opposite role to mitosis in the regulation of the size of animal cell populations. In structural terms, the process appears to take place in two stages. First, the cell separates from its neighbours and both the nucleus and the cytoplasm become condensed. The cell then breaks up into a number of membrane-bound, ultrastructurally well-preserved fragments. These fragments are then either shed from epithelium-lined surfaces or are phagocytosed by other cells, where they undergo a series of changes resembling in vitro autolysis within phagosomes. Apoptosis appears to be involved in the turnover of cells in many healthy adult tissues and is also responsible for the focal elimination of certain cells during normal embryonic development. It occurs spontaneously in some untreated malignant neoplasms and also occurs in some types of therapeutically induced regression of malignant tumours. It is implicated in both physiological involution and atrophy of various tissues and organs.

Necrosis

Necrosis is the term commonly applied when cell death occurs in part of an organ or tissue and where continuity with neighbouring viable tissue is preserved. Various morphological forms exist. The differences between them, in some instances, mirror the dominance of one of the processes which have been described above. The morphological type may, as in the case of **caseation necrosis**, provide a clue to the cause of the tissue injury.

Coagulative necrosis

In coagulative necrosis, denaturation of intra-cytoplasmic protein is the dominant process. The dead tissue becomes firm and slightly swollen. The protein molecules within the cytoplasm become unfolded and this renders the tissue both more opaque than normal and more reactive to certain dyes such as eosin. Microscopically, the cells show the signs of nuclear death described above, but the most noteworthy feature is the **retention of the general architectural pattern of the tissue**, despite the death of its constituent elements. Coagulative necrosis occurs typically in ischaemic injury, such as may occur in the heart or kidney. However, for reasons which are not clear, ischaemic injury in the central nervous system leads to necrosis dominated by enzymatic digestion and liquefaction of the dead tissue.

Caseation necrosis

Caseation necrosis is found characteristically in **tuberculosis.** It is a form of coagulative necrosis, in that no liquefaction has occurred, but microscopically the affected tissue appears completely **structureless** under the microscope and exhibits a greater than usual affinity for acidic dyes such as eosin. It owes its somewhat unfortunate name (**caseous = cheese-like**) to its macroscopic appearance, large areas of caseous necrosis bearing some resemblance to white, crumbly goat cheese. On chemical analysis, large amounts of lipid are found to be present in these necrotic areas in addition to the coagulated protein.

Liquefaction (or colliquative) necrosis

In liquefaction necrosis the dominant factor is the effect of hydrolytic lysosomal enzymes. The end result is a local accumulation of protein-rich, semi-fluid material. It is not particularly common as a primary event except, as mentioned above, in the brain. However, if necrotic tissue becomes secondarily infected by pus-forming organisms, liquefaction commonly takes place.

Traumatic fat necrosis

This is almost exclusively seen in the female breast, especially if the breast is heavy and pendulous. Essentially it results from the rupture of adipocytes with release of their contents. The released fat undergoes lipolysis and is converted to fatty acids and glycerol. Clinically the lesion appears as a hard lump in the breast, which may give the impression that a malignant neoplasm is present. On slicing the excised specimen one may see a small central cystic area in which some oily droplets are present. At the periphery the adipose tissue is much firmer and also more opaque than usual. Histological examination of conventionally prepared material shows the presence of numerous granular macrophages which contain phagocytosed lipid. Fatty acid crystals are also often present and these excite a foreign body giant cell reaction (multinucleate cells formed as a result of the fusion of macrophages).

Another type of fat necrosis is seen in the peritoneal cavity as a consequence of **acute haemorrhagic pancreatitis.** In pancreatitis the enzymes secreted by the exocrine pancreas are released from the acini and ducts and thus reach the interstitial tissues. The proteolytic and lipolytic enzymes damage the cell membranes and convert the intracellular triglyceride into glycerol and fatty acids. These latter combine with calcium in the interstitial fluid to form **soaps** which appear as small, intensely white and opaque patches on the adipose tissue of the pancreas, omentum and other areas of the peritoneum.

Gangrene

Strictly speaking the term **gangrene** should be limited to necrosis of tissues associated with a superadded infection by putrefactive microorganisms. The organisms concerned are often clostridia (gram-positive, spore-forming bacilli) derived from the gut or soil, but may also be anaerobic streptococci or members of the family Bacteroidaceae. Clinically, the term gangrene is often used to describe any black, foul-smelling area which is in continuity with living tissues. This state of affairs can be brought about primarily through the actions of bacterial toxins, or secondarily through a combination of ischaemia and superadded infection. True gangrene may occur, for example, in the gastrointestinal tract, most commonly as a result of cutting off of the blood supply which can lead to extensive necrosis. The presence of a resident population of potentially putrefactive organisms provides an ideal source for superadded infection. Another example of true gangrene is so-called **gas gangrene**, which is a rapidly spreading form of tissue necrosis, often involving muscle, which is due to infection by saccharolytic and proteolytic clostridia. These organisms make a wide range of toxins which are destructive to cell membranes and to the macromolecules of the interstitial ground substance. It is these toxins that constitute the basis for the spreading which is so menacing a feature of gas gangrene. Clostridial infection of this type not infrequently complicates deep penetrating injuries, but may also occur as a rare complication of acute suppurative appendicitis, in strangulation of the gut and in the puerperium. The presence of dead tissue as a result of injury and the additional factor that the oxygen supply may be very poor is a combination which favours the multiplication of these anaerobic organisms. The affected muscles and the adjacent soft tissues are oedematous and often very painful. They may feel **crepitant** (crackly) on palpation because of the formation of gas bubbles in the tissue as a result of the fermentation of sugars by the bacterial toxins. The infection may remain localized or may become generalized (septicaemia). Evidence of such spread may be seen at post-mortem examination in the form of bubbles in some of the solid viscera (most notably the liver) and also in the form of signs of haemolysis such as haemoglobin staining of the aortic intima.

Gangrene brought about by ischaemia may occur, as already stated, in the gut and is also not uncommonly found in the lower limb. The background to this is usually severe atherosclerosis of the large and medium-sized arteries of the limb. The stenosing lesions, which are composed partly of proliferated fibromuscular tissue and partly of lipid accumulations derived mainly from the plasma, then become complicated by superimposed thrombosis. Diabetic patients and cigarette smokers are particularly at risk. In younger patients ischaemic necrosis of the lower limbs may occur as a result of **thrombo-angiitis obliterans** (Buerger's disease). This is a condition in which an inflammatory process involving the whole vascular bundle (veins as well as arteries) occurs, leading to arterial occlusion.

If the limb is oedematous and a fairly thick layer of adipose tissue is present, the ischaemic necrosis may well be associated with infection by putrefactive organisms. In this case the typical appearances of **wet gangrene**, with large blebs on the skin surface, occasionally accompanied by gas production, may be seen. Where these do not occur, and where the arterial narrowing has progressed slowly over a long period, the appearances of so-called **dry gangrene** are seen. Starting at the most distal extremities the tissues become dessicated and black. The affected areas are very cold; there is no unpleasant smell and no bleb or gas formation. The black discoloration of the skin is due to staining by haemoglobin which diffuses from the small vessels into the extravascular compartment. Not infrequently a line of demarcation forms at the junction between the living and dead tissues and the latter may actually separate off (so-called spontaneous amputation).

Chapter 4

Acute Inflammation I: Introduction

When living tissue is injured the surrounding areas undergo a series of changes which result in phagocytic cells and elements of circulating plasma entering the damaged area. This process is known as **acute inflammation** and usually continues as long as the tissue injury persists. Such reactions to injury are, in phylogenetic terms, very ancient indeed, and many of the processes now recognized as being involved in inflammation such as chemotaxis and phagocytosis are present in simple unicellular and multicellular organisms. The acquisition of a complicated circulatory system added very significantly to the complexities of the inflammatory response, and it is the changes which occur in the calibre and permeability of the arterioles, capillaries and venules, which make up the microcirculation, which dictate the most prominent of the symptoms and signs of acute inflammation.

Is the inflammatory process helpful or harmful? John Hunter, the famous London surgeon, stated in 1794 that 'inflammation in itself is not to be regarded as a disease but as a salutary operation consequent upon some violence or disease.' This is true, but not the whole truth. It is certainly fair to say that the overall biological significance of inflammation is, indeed, that of a defence mechanism, but it is equally true that some inflammatory reactions can have crippling or life-threatening consequences.

In general terms, any process which injures cells may cause an inflammatory reaction. Because acute inflammation associated with invasion of the tissues by pathogenic microorganisms such as bacteria or viruses is so common, there is a certain temptation to regard inflammation as being **synonymous** with infection. This is certainly not true. Important causes of the acute inflammatory reaction include the following:

1. Mechanical trauma, such as cutting or crushing
2. Chemical injuries, such as those produced by acids, alkalis and phenols. An important cause of chemical injury of tissues in clinical medicine is the presence of physiological substances in inappropriate locations. For example, gastric juice is harmless in the stomach, its

31

natural milieu, but causes a striking inflammatory response in the peritoneal cavity after perforation of a peptic ulcer

3. Ultraviolet or x-irradiation

4. Injury due to extremes of cold or heat (burns and frostbite)

5. Injury due to a degree of reduction in the arterial blood supply sufficient to cause death of the underperfused tissue

6. Injury caused by living organisms such as bacteria, viruses, parasites, worms and fungi

7. Injury produced by the inappropriate or excessive operation of immune mechanisms

The Characteristics of Acute Inflammation

Any one who has suffered from a common 'boil' can give an excellent account of the clinical features of an acute inflammatory reaction. The affected area is **hot, red, swollen** and **painful**. These are the so-called **cardinal** signs of inflammation and were described by the Roman physician Celsus in the second century of the Christian era as **calor, rubor, tumor** and **dolor.**

The translation of these clinical observations into pathophysiological terms had to wait for the microscopic studies of Julius Cohnheim, who wrote a key paper on acute inflammation in 1867. Cohnheim studied the changes produced by mild injury in living tissues rather than in fixed and embedded material. Naturally he needed the most translucent possible preparations so chose thin membranes such as the frog mesentery. Simply exposing the living mesentery on the stage of a microscope was sufficient to cause some irritation and Cohnheim was able to see the rapid development of a series of changes in the small blood vessels. First the arterioles dilated and there was an obvious increase in and acceleration of blood flow in the whole vascular bed. Within a few minutes this accelerated blood flow slowed and large white blood cells began to line up along the walls of the venules, while the red cells flowed past. Then some of the white cells which seemed to have become adherent to the venule wall crawled through the blood vessel wall and thus reached the extravascular compartment. In some of the little blood vessels, the blood flow slowed so much that columns of red cells appeared not to move at all; in these vessels the red cells were tightly packed together as if the plasma had been lost. Fifteen years later Cohnheim took up this last observation again, and suggested that the plasma had escaped from the affected vessels because of **an increase in the permeability of the vessel walls.** Cohnheim's powers of observation were so acute and his descriptions of the rapidly changing pattern of events were so beautiful that, despite the simplicity of the

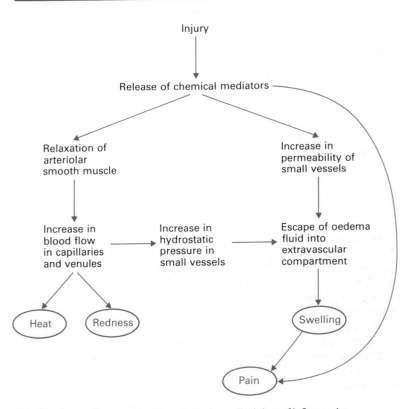

Fig. 4.1 The vascular events which underlie the cardinal signs of inflammation.

methods employed, they still stand as a model of scientific clarity and accuracy.

With the knowledge gained from these pioneering studies it is possible now to look at the cardinal signs of acute inflammation in the light of the series of events taking place in the microcirculation (Fig. 4.1).

Redness and heat

The only logical explanation for these features is persistent dilatation of small vessels and an increased blood flow in the affected area. This presupposes an increased filling of capillaries and venules, which is easy to imagine since only part of the capillary network in any tissue is filled with circulating blood at any one time. Since capillaries have no smooth muscle cells in their wall, their powers of constriction and dilatation are very limited (the constriction being mediated by the pericytes). They are, therefore, a rather passive set of channels whose blood content depends very largely on the flow in the feeding arterioles. Thus the redness and heat which are so striking a feature of acute inflammation must depend on an increase in the calibre of the arterioles feeding the injured area and this, in its turn, must represent the result of arteriolar smooth muscle relaxation.

The tone of these arterioles, which act as pre-capillary sphincters, is controlled in two ways. Under normal circumstances the circular smooth muscle coat of the arteriole is under the control of the autonomic nervous system, in particular the sympathetic vasoconstrictor nerves. These nerves are largely responsible for controlling the blood pressure, the cardiac output and the distribution of blood flow among the different organs and tissues. Blushing in response to some embarrassing circumstance constitutes an easily observed example of this control system in operation. However, the arteriolar smooth muscle cells also react to local chemical mediators, and it is believed that accumulation of such compounds at and around the site of injury plays a dominant role in the arteriolar dilatation of acute inflammation. Support for this view comes from the fact that acute inflammation in tissue which has long been denervated shows no essential differences from the process in areas with normal innervation. The reasons for the slowing of the blood flow within the microcirculation which occurs at a slightly later stage are better understood once the mechanisms underlying local swelling at sites of injury have been appreciated.

Swelling

In simple terms the presence of local tissue swelling must mean that something has been added to the bulk of the formed tissue elements or to the gel-like ground substance in that area. Chemical analysis of such a swollen area shows that this increase in bulk is due to the local accumulation of excess interstitial fluid which contains solutes and proteins derived from the plasma; such an accumulation of fluid in the extravascular compartment is called **oedema**. In inflammatory oedema the fact that there has been a net transfer from the intravascular to the extravascular compartment can be shown by injecting a small amount of the dye Evans' blue intravenously into a small animal. If, for example, a mild thermal injury is produced at some site, the skin at the site of injury shows blue staining. Since Evans' blue circulates in the plasma bound to albumin this result indicates that albumin has passed from the small vessels into the extravascular compartment.

The exudation of protein-rich fluid in inflammation

To understand the formation of the local inflammatory oedema, or of the **exudate** as it is often termed, we need to have some knowledge of the normal routes of transport across endothelial barriers and the forces which determine the rates of such transport. Endothelium of all types is permeable to a wide range of molecules. Most of the available data suggest the existence, in a functional sense, of a 'two pore' system. The large pore component appears to have a diameter of about 50 nm and the small pore one a diameter of about 9 nm. The structural equivalent of the large pore system has been shown by the use of appropriate ultrastructural tracers to be the plasmalemmal vesicles which are present in large numbers in endothelial cells and are concentrated along the luminal and abluminal membranes. Once these vesicles, which have a diameter of about 70 nm, have incorporated a large molecule by pinocytosis, they bud off from the luminal plasma membrane and travel across the endothelial cytoplasm towards the abluminal aspect of the cell. Here they fuse with the abluminal plasma membrane and discharge their contents. The structural equivalent of the 'small pore' system is more equivocal, but the available evidence suggests that it may correspond to the junctions between adjacent endothelial cells.

The mechanisms underlying the escape from the microcirculation of water and solutes on the one hand and plasma proteins on the other may well be different and merit separate consideration.

Ultrafiltration. Transport of water and solute across the endothelial cell barrier shows many of the features of ultrafiltration, in which the movement of fluid and electrolytes is controlled largely by physical forces. There are two sets of such forces which act in opposition to each other. Hydrostatic forces within the microcirculation tend to push fluid out into the extravascular compartment, and this process is aided by the osmotic pressure of extravascular tissue proteins and mucopolysaccharides. The intravascular osmotic pressure exerted by the plasma proteins and the hydrostatic pressure of the extravascular tissues combine to push fluid back into the vessels. Normally the resultant of these opposing sets of forces is a small net outflow of fluid from the microcirculation, which then drains from the extravascular compartment via the lymphatic channels. An increase in the intravascular hydrostatic pressure in the vessels of the microcirculation, such as occurs in acute inflammation, increases the amount of water and solute driven out of the vessels, though the oedema fluid produced in this way still has a relatively low protein content. Obviously loss of **protein** from the intravascular compartment potentiates this process, since the intravascular osmotic pressure falls and there is a corresponding rise in the osmotic pressure of the extravascular tissue fluid (Fig. 4.2).

Protein leakage. Chemical analysis of the extravascular fluid accumulations occurring in acute inflammation invariably shows a protein concentration which is simply not attainable by the process of

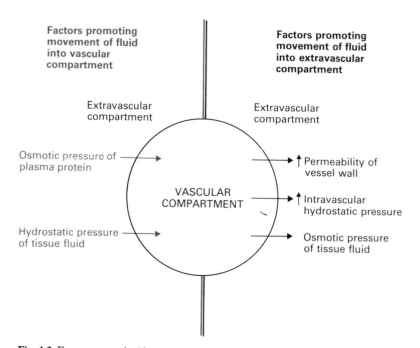

Fig. 4.2 Factors promoting the movement of fluid into and out of the microvascular compartment.

ultrafiltration or **transudation** discussed above. Some other mechanism for the appearance of relatively large amounts of plasma-derived protein must therefore exist. That very large molecules escape from the microcirculation in the course of the formation of inflammatory oedema can be shown very elegantly in small animals by the technique of vascular labelling, which serves the additional purpose of identifying those vessels in the injured area from which leakage has occurred. A few drops of indian ink are injected intravenously into a small animal such as a rat. Except in the liver and spleen where the endothelium is normally 'leaky', the tissues do not blacken and the vessels of the microcirculation are not outlined by the ink particles, which instead are taken up by phagocytic cells in the sinusoids of the liver and spleen. However, if a mild thermal injury is produced **after** the injection of the ink, some of the vessels in the injured area become outlined by the ink particles. On microscopic examination, these particles can be seen to have crossed the endothelial cells and to be lying piled up against the basement membrane, which they do not cross. Careful examination shows that the vessels which are labelled in this way are small venules measuring up to about 80 or 100 µm in diameter; capillaries, larger venules and arterioles are not labelled so long as the injury has been mild. Identical appearances can be produced by an intradermal injection of small doses of histamine, 5-hydroxytryptamine or bradykinin. Therefore, it is not without interest that a sting from a nettle (which contains histamine) invariably produces local swelling.

It is not clear on light microscopy what cellular events underly the passage of such large molecules as indian ink or ferritin across the normal endothelium. This question was answered by the electron microscopic studies of Guido Majno, who showed that when small doses of histamine or other vasoactive substances were injected into the cremaster muscle of rats, the endothelial cells in venules contracted, thus creating gaps through which the particles of indian ink could pass. In due time the endothelial cells presumably relax and the gaps disappear, since carbon particles can be found lying deep to apparently intact inter-endothelial junctions. It is not too surprising that such contractile shortening of the endothelial cells should take place, since a combination of ultrastructural and immunocytochemical studies has shown that these versatile cells contain contractile filaments.

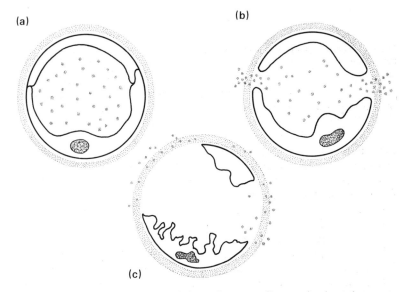

(a)   (b)   (c)

Fig. 4.3 Endothelial cell damage in relation to the escape of large molecules such as indian ink particles from the microvasculature. (a) Normal vessel. (b) If injury is mild, the endothelial cells contract and create gaps through which particles can pass. (c) In severe injury, the endothelial cells may be damaged or even killed, and the amount and duration of the escape of large molecules from the vascular compartment is greatly increased.

It should be stressed that the change in microvascular permeability described above is what is seen when the injury is mild in degree. In reality the alterations in vascular permeability following injury are more complex, both in nature and timing. The major factor affecting these changes appears to be the degree of severity of the injury, which is reflected in the magnitude of the functional and structural change in the endothelial cells (Fig. 4.3).

Most of the data relating to this come from studies carried out in small animals, where the experimental conditions, in particular the type and severity of injury, are clearly defined. It is likely that in human inflammatory disease the processes are much more complex. The patterns of increased vascular permeability following injury are

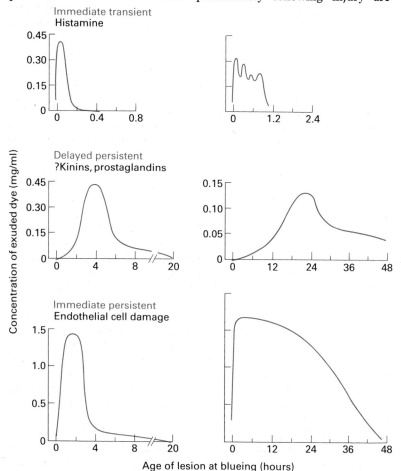

Fig. 4.4 Types of vascular permeability.

characterized in terms of two variables:

1. The time between infliction of the injury and recordable changes in microvascular permeability
2. The duration of the change in vascular permeability

On this basis then we can observe three patterns (Fig. 4.4):

1. The **immediate transient response**
2. The **delayed persistent response**
3. The **immediate persistent response**

The **immediate transient response**, as its name implies, follows almost immediately on mild injury. The alteration in vascular permeability reaches a peak within five minutes or so and returns to normal within 15 minutes. Carbon labelling shows that the escape of fluid is confined to small venules. The development of leaky venules extends more widely than the immediate area of injury, which suggests that a chemical mediator is involved. Since the increase in vascular permeability can be blocked by pre-dosing the animal with an antihistamine compound, it seems reasonable to suppose that this chemical mediator is histamine. The short duration of the change strongly suggests that the increase in venule permeability is brought about by endothelial cell contraction and that the endothelial cells are not seriously damaged.

The **delayed persistent response** takes longer to develop. In some instances the peak effect occurs about four hours after injury, while in others there may be an interval lasting up to 24 hours before the increase in vascular permeability becomes maximal. Increased permeability of this type is not blocked by the prior administration of antihistamines. In those cases in which the peak effect is noted after four hours, labelling with carbon shows that fluid and macromolecules escape from the capillaries. When the reaction peaks later (e.g. 24 hours after injury), both venules and capillaries are labelled. Some of the affected capillaries contain small aggregates of platelets, and damaged and broken up endothelial cells are also seen. While inter-endothelial cell gaps are found in affected venules, it is believed that these result from direct endothelial injury rather than from the operation of a chemical mediator such as histamine. A good example of the delayed type of response is to be found in **sunburn**. Exposure to sunlight on the first day of the holidays, while enjoyable, may be followed some hours after exposure has ceased by the onset of a very uncomfortable inflammatory reaction.

The **immediate persistent response** is associated, in experimental situations, with the application of relatively powerful agents. The affected vessels begin to leak within a few minutes and permeability becomes maximal 15 to 60 minutes after injury. Labelling studies show that small vessels of all types leak, and electron microscopy reveals severe damage to endothelial cells and pericytes, with sloughing away of the former from their basement membranes. Until the endothelial cells have been replaced by ingrowth of new cells, derived from the uninjured part of the vessel lining, along the basement membrane, exudation will continue. It may therefore last for many days and be of impressive proportions.

Understanding how the fluid exudate forms in acute inflammation leads naturally to an understanding of why the flow of blood slows in some parts of the microcirculation in injured areas. This change in flow is associated with packing or sludging of red cells. Loss of water from the leaking venules and capillaries leads to an increase in the concentration of blood cells in these vessels. Although plasma proteins also escape from the vessels, the loss of fluid may be so great as to increase the concentration of plasma protein within these vessels and this will add further to the tendency for there to be an increase in blood viscosity. Rouleaux formation by the red cells is enhanced by both these processes, and the tendency of white cells to adhere to the endothelial surface of the post-capillary venules and to each other may also impair flow through the injured vessels.

Pain

This is less well understood than the other cardinal clinical features of the acute inflammatory reaction and, indeed, may not always be present. Clearly the local increase in tissue turgor is one of the factors involved, and the denser the tissue in which the inflammation is occurring the greater the degree of pain. Palpating or squeezing an acutely inflamed area will either increase existing pain or produce pain where none existed; it seems reasonable to also ascribe this to the increase in local tissue pressure. However, it is known that some of the endogenous chemical compounds believed to be released in the course of the genesis of the acute inflammatory reaction are capable of causing pain in their own right when injected subcutaneously or intradermally. Therefore, these may also contribute to the pain experienced in many inflammatory reactions.

Chapter 5

Acute Inflammation II: Cellular Events

In phylogenetic terms, one of the first defences to develop against the presence of 'foreign' material, whether living or dead, was phagocytosis by specialized cells. The migration of phagocytic cells to a site of injury remains one of the most fundamental components of the host's response and, especially when the injurious agent is a living microorganism, is vital for a successful defence against such invaders. The central role of the phagocytic cell is demonstrated by the increased susceptibility to infections shown by persons who have insufficient phagocytic cells or whose cells cannot seek out, engulf or destroy pathogenic microorganisms.

Cell population of the inflammatory exudate

In the early stages of the inflammatory process most of the cells migrating to the injured area are **neutrophils**, though a small number of eosinophil and basophil polymorphs may also be present. Neutrophils are present in relatively large numbers in the blood, can be replaced rapidly from precursors in the bone marrow, and move more quickly than other leucocytes. The degree to which they accumulate in sites of tissue damage depends on the severity of such damage and on the nature of the injury. Physical injury rarely evokes a very significant neutrophil response, whereas infection by certain organisms such as *E. coli* or staphylococci elicits a very striking response.

Neutrophils make up 40 to 75% of circulating white cells. They have a diameter of about 15 μm, characteristically segmented nuclei and granular cytoplasm. Two types of granule are present in the cytoplasm. The first, which is larger and stains more densely with Romanowsky type dyes than its companion, contains lysozyme (which accounts for about one-third of its content), lysosomal enzymes, peroxidase and certain cationic proteins, the last of which may be important signals for the recruitment of further neutrophils. The smaller granules, which are also essentially lysosomal in nature, also contain lysozyme (about two-thirds of their content), together with alkaline phosphatase and lactoferrin, an iron-binding protein. The energy source of the neutrophil is glucose, which is normally stored as glycogen, and the cell can produce energy by glycolysis under anaerobic conditions, which is useful because oxygen tensions may fall to very low levels in areas of tissue damage.

In general, the early peak in the migration of neutrophils to an inflammatory focus is followed some hours later by another wave of cell migration, this time by mononuclear phagocytes (**macrophages**). This biphasic pattern of cell accumulation is found in most inflammatory reactions, but the precise timing may vary with the nature of the injury.

Neutrophil emigration

The mechanisms of emigration of the neutrophils from the microcirculation are not completely understood. With the change in the dynamics of blood flow the white cells, which are heavier than red cells,

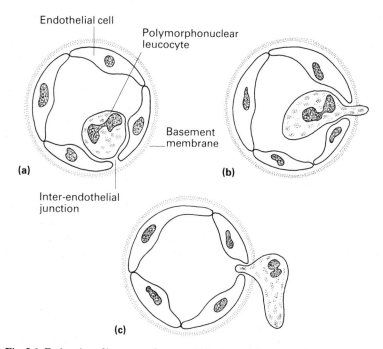

Fig. 5.1 Emigration of leucocytes from small blood vessels in acute inflammation. (a) Margination of white cells within the flowing blood occurs and granulocytes adhere to the endothelial cells. (b) The granulocyte inserts a cytoplasmic pseudopodium between adjacent endothelial cells. (c) The granulocyte has almost completely passed through the inter-endothelial gap and the underlying basement membrane and will soon be seen free in the perivascular space.

come to lie at the periphery of the column of flowing blood cells and some adhere to the endothelium. This is known as 'margination'. Adhesion of the leucocyte to the endothelium is clearly a fundamental step in the emigration of the neutrophil from the microcirculation and one which is difficult to understand, since the negative charges on the plasma membranes of the endothelial cells and the neutrophil might be expected to repel each other. However, divalent cations, especially calcium and magnesium, appear to play an important part in adhesion; the pretreatment of experimental animals with chelating agents which remove these cations inhibits the margination and adhesion of white cells. It is also known that exposure of neutrophils to chemotactic factors decreases their negative net surface charge and increases their adherence to endothelial cells. It has recently been suggested that exocytosis of lactoferrin from the specific granules of the neutrophil may be an important factor in making normal neutrophils stick to endothelium, and there has been a case report in which neutrophils deficient in lactoferrin would not stick to endothelium when stimulated by chemotactic factors. Once the neutrophils have come to lie in close contact with the plasma membranes of the endothelial cells, they put out pseudopodia which enter the gap between two adjacent endothelial cells and force it open. The neutrophils then move into the basement membrane substance, through which they soon pass (Fig. 5.1). This whole process takes from two to nine minutes. For reasons that are not clear, leucocytes from newborn infants and myeloblasts from leukaemic patients are not able to attenuate their cytoplasm sufficiently to squeeze through the inter-endothelial cell gaps.

Neutrophil function as a means of host defence

As part of the host's system of defence against infection by pathogenic microorganisms, the role of the neutrophil is to seek out, ingest and kill a wide range of these organisms. These processes can be looked at most easily as a set of operations, any of which can go wrong and thus render the neutrophil ineffective as a bacterial 'hunter-killer'.

The instruction to the neutrophil to emigrate from the local microvasculature and to proceed towards the invading microorganisms or the injured or dead tissue elements must involve, as does any instruction, the **giving** and **receiving** of an appropriate **signal**. **Transduction** of this signal must then take place, so that **migration** of the phagocytic cell **towards the point from which the signal emanated** can occur. This generation and reception of the signal and the vectorial movement which follows is known as **chemotaxis**.

Once the neutrophil has reached the invading microorganism or the dead or effete cells from which the chemotactic signal has been generated, a process of **attachment** between the neutrophil and the object to be phagocytosed occurs. This is facilitated by the latter being coated by either immunoglobulin or one of the components of complement. These substances are called **opsonins** and the coating process is termed **opsonization**. The foreign material is then engulfed by the plasma membrane of the phagocyte and comes to lie within a membrane-bounded vesicle called the **phagosome**. These two steps together constitute the process of **phagocytosis**.

Fusion then takes place between the membranes of the phagosome and a lysosome, resulting in the formation of a secondary lysosome or phagolysosome. In this way the contents of the lysosome are released into the lumen of the phagosome. The morphological correlate of this operation is loss of the granules in the cytoplasm of the neutrophil. If the occupant of the phagolysosome is a living organism, killing and digestion of that organism occurs. This is accomplished largely by oxygen-dependent mechanisms which will be discussed in more detail later.

Chemotaxis

Chemotaxis is the directional, purposive movement of phagocytic cells towards areas of tissue injury or death or the sites of bacterial invasion. As its name implies, it is mediated by a series of chemical messengers. **Chemotaxis** must be distinguished from **chemokinesis**, which is a chemically induced increase in activity of phagocytic cells which has no vectorial component. Clearly a process of this sort must, as indicated above, have two aspects: first, the signals which attract the phagocyte towards the appropriate area and, second, the ability of the phagocyte to respond to the signal by moving towards the point from which the signal has been generated.

That phagocytic cells are capable of responding in a directed way to a variety of stimuli has been shown in a number of ways. In my view the most elegant of these is the system devised in Oxford by Professor Henry Harris in which neutrophils are incorporated into clotted plasma between a coverslip and a slide. When such preparations are examined by dark-field microscopy, the cells show up as white spots against a black background, and movement in any direction can be recorded as white tracks by long exposure of a single photographic frame. Harris found that various bacteria were chemotactic under these experimental circumstances and some years later Ryan and Hurley showed that minced tissue fragments incubated with fresh serum also acted in this way. Another popular assay system for chemotaxis is the Boyden chamber. This consists of a small vessel separated horizontally into an upper and lower compartment by means of a millipore filter membrane, the pores of which are slightly smaller than the diameter of a neutrophil. A suspension of neutrophils is placed in the upper compartment and a solution of the substance to be evaluated for its chemotactic potential in the lower. If chemotaxis takes place the neutrophils crawl through the pores and come to lie either on the under surface of the membrane or in the solution in the lower compartment. In either case they can be counted and the attractant powers of one compound compared with another can be assessed. The possible drawback of this system is that it may simply be measuring chemokinesis rather than chemotaxis.

Generation and reception of signals

Using in vitro systems, many substances are now known to be chemotactic for neutrophils, though, of course, their significance in vivo is less clear. They include:

1. *Low molecular weight compounds*
   Formylated peptides with methionine as the N-terminal residue
   Arachidonic acid derivatives such as prostaglandin E_1

2. *Intermediate molecular weight compounds*
   The 5a fragment of **complement** and C5 derived peptides

3. *High molecular weight compounds*
   Caseins
   Partly denatured proteins (e.g. serum albumin, haemoglobin and immunoglobulin G)
   Lectins
   Lymphokines

Other substances which have been shown to have chemotactic properties are some members of the plasma cascade systems, which are believed to play an important part in bringing about changes in blood flow and vascular permeability. This aspect of their activity will be discussed later, when the question of chemical mediators in the inflammatory reaction as a whole will be considered.

Components of complement

One of the most important chemotactic factors for neutrophils is the 5a component of the **complement** cascade, though a trimolecular complex of C567 also operates as an attractant for phagocytes and some workers maintain that C3a also does. The complement cascade can be activated in at least two ways. The first of these, which is known as the **classical** pathway, is through the formation of antigen–antibody complexes. The second, which is known as the **alternate** pathway, operates via the direct cleavage of C3 with consequent activation of the rest of the sequence. The alternate pathway can be activated by certain lipopolysaccharides derived from gram-negative bacteria (endotoxins), by cobra venom and by polysaccharides derived from the cell walls of certain yeasts (zymosan). A number of aggregated immunoglobulins, notably IgA and IgE, will also act in this way, as will plasmin, a product of the fibrinolytic cascade, via both the classical and alternate pathways. In a later section we shall look at the interrelationship of these and other substances believed to operate as chemical mediators of the inflammatory reaction.

Formylated peptides

The formylated peptides (mentioned in the list above) have excited a considerable degree of interest. It is not certain whether such compounds as f-met-Leu-Phe (formylated methionine-leucine-phenylalanine) have any role to play in inflammation as we know it, but it is not without interest that in prokaryotes ribosomal synthesis of new proteins starts with formyl-methionine, which may later be cleaved. Since eukaryotic protein synthesis does not proceed in this way (except, interestingly enough, in mitochondria), this might provide a recognition system by which prokaryotic bacterial invaders could be distinguished from eukaryotic cells. A variety of chemical mechanisms for attracting neutrophils to sites of injury or infection is presumably of some advantage to the host, and the small molecular size of some of the 'signals' may enhance their access to phagocytes at distant sites through their ability to diffuse more readily through the ground substance gel.

Reception and transduction of the chemotactic signal

In the sense that chemotactic substances thus far identified are soluble molecules which act on cells at a distance from the point at which the chemical signal is generated, they can be likened to hormones. As with hormones, it is likely that the first site of interaction between the chemotactic molecule and the phagocyte is a specific receptor or series of receptors on the plasma membrane of the phagocyte. This view has been shown to be correct for at least two of the chemotactic signals mentioned above: the formylated peptides and the 5a component of the complement system. The peptides bind saturably and with high affinity to the surfaces of both human and rabbit neutrophils, and there appear to be definable populations of these peptide receptors on the neutrophil

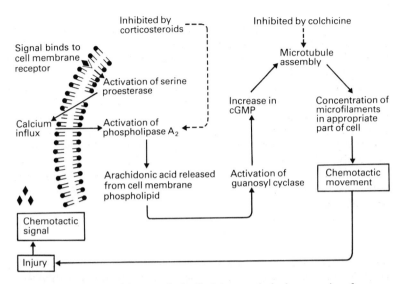

Fig. 5.2 Transduction of chemotactic signals. Injury results in the generation of chemotactic signals (for example, C5a) which bind to receptors on the cell membranes of granulocytes and macrophages. This triggers a series of intramembrane events which result in an influx of calcium and activation of phospholipase A_2 with release of arachidonic acid. This phospholipase A_2 activity is inhibited by corticosteroids. Arachidonic acid release is followed by guanosyl cyclase activation and release of cGMP. cGMP levels control microtubule assembly and hence microfilament orientation.

surface. It is unlikely that a single receptor on the plasma membrane of the phagocyte binds all the chemotactic substances mentioned, since exposing cells to excess amounts of the chemotactic peptides does not appear to block their ability to respond to C5a; the reverse is also true.

Signal transduction (Fig. 5.2) has been studied by exposing neutrophils to chemotactic peptides. This is followed by release of arachidonic acid from the cells, which suggests that a membrane phospholipase has been activated. This increase in arachidonic acid may directly or indirectly induce changes in membrane ion permeability (especially for calcium). Ion fluxes are now believed to play an important role in chemotactic signal transduction, changes in both sodium and calcium flux being involved.

The cyclic nucleotides appear to play an important part in the initiation of movement of the phagocytic cells. The balance between release of cAMP and cGMP may well constitute a control system for the activation and blocking not only of chemotaxis but also of certain other events (such as the release of active compounds from the granules of mast cells) in the acute inflammatory reaction. **cGMP** enhances chemotactic movement, the release of pharmacologically active substances such as histamine and leukotrienes from mast cells, and the release of lysosomal enzymes and lymphokines from neutrophils and T lymphocytes respectively. **cAMP** produces the **opposite** effect in each of these instances. The main effect of the cyclic nucleotides within the neutrophil is probably exerted on the cytoskeleton, the principal target being the microtubule system. The microtubules are hollow fibres with a diameter of 24 nm and they appear to be inserted at the periphery of the cell in the region where the contractile microfilaments are concentrated. The structural element of the microtubules is in equilibrium with the protein from which it is formed which is known as **tubulin.** This is a dimeric protein which, when assembled into tubules, plays an important role not only in chemotaxis and cell secretion but also, in other cells, in mitosis. A rise in intracellular cGMP promotes assembly of the microtubules, and a rise in cAMP inhibits tubule assembly. Anything which inhibits the assembly of the microtubules will inhibit the migration of neutrophils in response to chemotactic signals. This is the basis of an old, now discarded, treatment for acute gouty arthritis — colchicine. The acute local inflammation found in gout results from what might be regarded as a failure of normal neutrophil function. Sodium biurate crystals are deposited in the synovium as a result of an abnormality in uric acid metabolism. These 'foreign' bodies attract neutrophils which engulf them in the normal way. However, abnormal hydrogen bonds form between the surface of the urate crystals and the phagolysosomal membrane, with resulting rupture of the membrane and spillage of the lysosomal enzymes into the extracellular space. It is this that causes the intense pain. Colchicine, through its interference with microtubule assembly, prevents phago-cyte migration and interrupts this cycle of events. In contrast to this, drugs which **raise** the intracellular content of cGMP enhance the movement of phagocytes towards attractants. Among these is levamisole, which can be shown to reverse chemotactic deactivation in vitro and, more interestingly, has been shown to reverse the depression in movement of human neutrophils and monocytes induced by a number of viruses including herpes simplex.

The actual movement of phagocytic cells is accomplished by the shortening of microfilaments which are concentrated along the cell margins. These are about 6 nm in diameter and are composed of the contractile proteins actin and myosin. In a very real sense they constitute the homologue within the phagocytes of the muscle cells in more complex organisms.

Phagocytosis

Once the phagocytes have arrived at the site of tissue damage and/or bacterial invasion they must recognize which structures they should attack and must become attached to them. In vivo, phagocytes demonstrate remarkable selectivity as to what they will ingest, presumably by recognizing certain specific features on the surfaces of cells. For example, mononuclear phagocytes (macrophages) will ingest old or damaged red cells but will disregard normal ones.

Opsonization

It has been known for a long time that bacterial cells which are coated with immunoglobulin or damaged cells which have interacted with fresh serum are phagocytosed more readily than those which have not. This coating of particles with proteins is called **opsonization** (preparation for eating, the Greek word 'opson' meaning a 'relish') (Fig. 5.3).

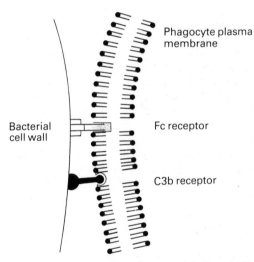

Phagocyte plasma membrane

Bacterial cell wall

Fc receptor

C3b receptor

Fig. 5.3 Opsonization through the medium of immunoglobulin and C3b.

The opsonins are either:

1. Specific antibodies of the IgG class. For opsonization to occur the Fc fragment of the Ig must be intact.
2. The C3b component of complement. This is a non-specific activity which is obviously of great biological value to the host, since invading microorganisms can be opsonized even if it is the first time that the host has been infected with these particular organisms.

The apparent restriction of opsonization to these two protein classes strongly suggests that the plasma membrane of the phagocytic cell

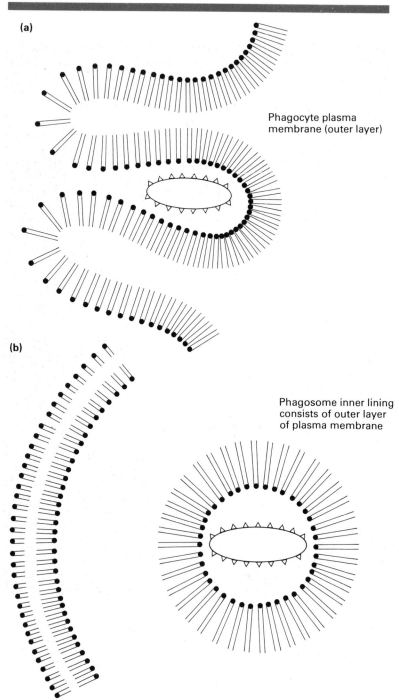

(a)

Phagocyte plasma
membrane (outer layer)

(b)

Phagosome inner lining
consists of outer layer
of plasma membrane

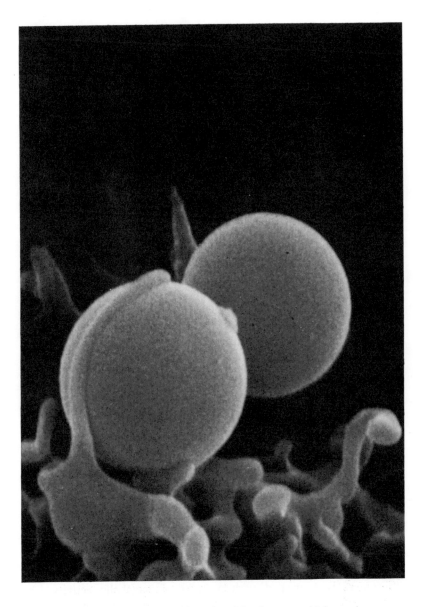

Fig. 5.4 (a) and (b) Phagocytosis and formation of the phagosome. (c) A scanning electron micrograph showing the attachment phase of phagocytosis of small latex particles by a macrophage. The surface membrane of the cell has an irregular 'ruffled' appearance and there are long processes thrown up from the cell surface which are closely attached to the surface of the latex spheres.

possesses specific receptor sites for the C3b subunit and for the Fc fragment of IgG.

Engulfment (Fig. 5.4)

Engulfment of the bacterium or foreign object takes place as a result of fusion of pseudopodia which project from the plasma membrane of the phagocyte in the form of long finger-like projections. The pseudopodia fuse on the far side of the object to be phagocytosed, thus locking it within a vesicle or **phagosome**, which then buds off from the plasma membrane of the phagocyte and lies within the cytoplasm of the neutrophil or macrophage. The membrane of this phagosome is obviously composed of part of the plasma membrane of the phagocyte which has become inverted; therefore the inner layer of the phagosome membrane is identical with the outer layer of the plasma membrane. Engulfment is an active, energy-dependent process which is inhibited by substances which interfere with the production of ATP. This is consistent with the hypothesis that a mechanism such as actin–myosin contraction 'drives' engulfment as well as migration. Some support for this view comes from the fact that colchicine also inhibits engulfment.

Lysosomal fusion and degranulation

Once the phagosome has formed, the lysosomal granules move towards it and apposition of their membranes followed by membrane fusion occur. The lysosomal granules disappear as this happens (hence the term 'degranulation of polymorphonuclear cells'). These events take place with very great speed; fusion of lysosomes with phagosomes occurs more or less in concert with ingestion and ends when the process of ingestion is over. Compounds known to inhibit migration and phagocytosis also inhibit degranulation.

Metabolic Events Associated with Bacterial Killing

Recognition of an invading microorganism and attachment to it by the phagocyte, as well as triggering ingestion and fusion of phagosomes and lysosomes, is associated with a burst of metabolic activity (the **respiratory burst**) which results essentially in the step-wise **reduction of molecular oxygen to hydrogen peroxide**. This respiratory burst is associated with a 2- to 20-fold increase in oxygen consumption compared with a resting cell and a considerable increase in glucose metabolism via the hexose monophosphate shunt.

The reduction of molecular oxygen is probably accomplished by a non-haem protein oxidase which is believed to be localized on the external surface of the phagocyte plasma membrane (which forms the **inner layer** of the phagosome membrane). The hydrogen donor for the reduction process is either NADH or NADPH. The presence of one or other of these pyridine nucleotides is an essential link in the chain, since if regeneration from NAD or NADP cannot take place, hydrogen peroxide will not be formed. Hence adequate amounts of glucose-6-phosphate dehydrogenase are required within the cell if bacterial killing is to proceed in the normal way.

In the reduction process the oxygen gains only one electron and is converted into the **superoxide anion** (O_2^{-}) (Fig. 5.5). About 90% of the oxygen consumed in the respiratory burst is converted into the superoxide anion. When two molecules of this anion react with each other, one is oxidized and the other reduced, forming **hydrogen peroxide** and oxygen in a dismutation reaction. This reaction is catalysed by the enzyme **superoxide dismutase**. Other highly reactive oxygen-derived metabolites have been identified or have been predicted to exist as a result of activation of phagocytic cells. These include an active hydroxyl radical ($OH\cdot$), singlet oxygen and hypochlorous acid.

There is abundant evidence that phagocytes are unable to kill ingested organisms in the absence of the respiratory burst and without the production of the superoxide anion. Both superoxide dismutase and catalase are capable of inhibiting phagocyte-mediated bacterial killing. However, superoxide itself appears to have little bactericidal effect on its own, and it is now widely believed that the most important bactericidal activity within the phagocyte stems from the production of hydrogen peroxide. Hydrogen peroxide by itself has significant bactericidal activity, but this is potentiated 50-fold when the H_2O_2 reacts with myeloperoxidase (one of the phagocyte's lysosomal enzymes) and halide ions. The most likely product, in chemical terms, of the hydrogen peroxide–myeloperoxidase–halide complex is hypochlorous acid (HOCl).

The mechanism of bacterial injury appears to involve halogenation or oxidation of the bacterial surface, but it is also likely that decarboxylation of cell walls and/or cell membrane proteins occurs, with the local generation of toxic aldehydes (Fig. 5.5). In addition to the activity of the hydrogen peroxide–myeloperoxidase–halide complex, there is a considerable body of evidence suggesting that hydroxyl radicals formed by the interaction between hydrogen peroxide and the superoxide anion are also important in bacterial killing; mannitol, a scavenger of hydroxyl radicals inhibits the bactericidal activity of an acetaldehyde–xanthine oxidase system which can trap and reduce molecular oxygen, generating active oxygen free radicals.

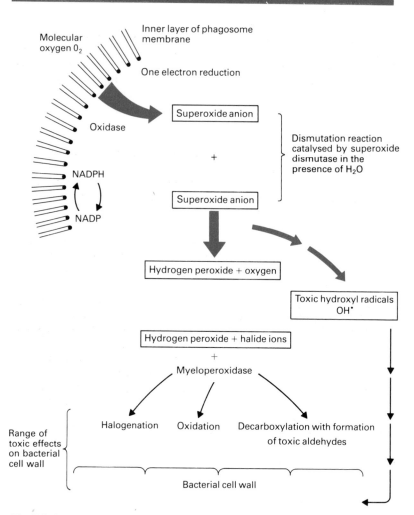

Fig. 5.5 Oxygen-dependent bacterial killing within phagocytes.

Detoxification of hydrogen peroxide

Since hydrogen peroxide can diffuse out of the phagosome, it is important that some control mechanisms should exist to prevent lipid peroxidation of the cell's own membranes. The scavenger systems involved are catalase and, perhaps even more important, glutathione peroxidase. The activity of the latter implies a need for a constantly replenished supply of reduced glutathione and this once again emphasizes the importance of glucose-6-phosphate dehydrogenase

(G-6-PD), since the reduced glutathione must be regenerated through coupling mechanisms linked to the hexose monophosphate shunt. Thus G-6-PD is involved both in the production of the bactericidal peroxides and in their detoxification.

Other mechanisms of bacterial killing

While the oxygen-dependent mechanisms described above are fundamental to the normal bactericidal activity of neutrophils and macrophages, there are other systems which may well be injurious to ingested microorganisms. These are related to various aspects of lysosomal function and include:

1. **Low pH within the phagolysosome.** The pH inside the vacuole is 3.5 to 4 — this in itself may be bactericidal or bacteriostatic. In addition, the low pH promotes the production of hydrogen peroxide from superoxide.
2. **Lysozyme.** This is a low molecular weight cationic enzyme which attacks the mucopeptide cell walls of some bacterial species.
3. **Lactoferrin.** This is an iron-binding protein which inhibits the growth of a number of microorganisms.
4. **Cationic proteins** with antibacterial activity also enter the phagosome in the course of fusion and degranulation.
5. **Lysosomal hydrolases** entering the phagosome in the course of phagosome–lysosome fusion may have some antibacterial activity, but are probably more important in digesting the remains of organisms which have been killed by other means.

Defects in Neutrophil Function

Neutropenia

Even if all the separate operations that have been discussed above can be carried out normally, this is of no avail in protecting the host if there are insufficient cells to cope with the number of invading microorganisms. This occurs in various forms of bone marrow failure:

1. Drug or poison-induced, e.g. chloramphenicol, benzene
2. Infiltration of the marrow by large numbers of tumour cells
3. Bone marrow fibrosis
4. Other forms of marrow aplasia

Disorders of migration and chemotaxis

These may occur as a result of an intrinsic defect in the cell, of inhibition of locomotion or of deficiencies in the generation of chemotactic signals.

Intrinsic cell defects

1. **'The lazy leucocyte syndrome.'** The precise point at which the defect occurs has not been identified.
2. **Job's syndrome.** This typically affects fair-skinned, red-haired girls and is characterized by recurrent 'cold' staphylococcal abscesses.
3. **Diabetes mellitus.** Leucocytes from diabetic patients whose diabetes is not well controlled show impairment of locomotion. This is at least partially reversed by adding insulin and glucose to the leucocytes.
4. **The Chédiak–Higashi syndrome.** This is a rare congenital autosomal recessive disorder that occurs in man, cattle, mink and certain strains of mouse. In all species it is characterized by partial albinism, the presence of giant lysosomal granules in neutrophils, and increased susceptibility to bacterial infection. In humans death usually occurs in childhood and is often preceded by the development of a malignant process involving lymphoid cells. Two major defects have been documented in the neutrophils of patients suffering from this syndrome. They fail to show directed movement in response to chemotactic stimuli both in vivo and in vitro, and they show a delay in intracellular bacterial killing which appears to result from a reduced rate of phagosome/lysosome fusion. It has been proposed that this combination of defects results from a failure in the assembly of microtubules from tubulin; the addition of cGMP or agents which increase intracellular cGMP generation to the neutrophils might reverse the situation.

Inhibition of locomotion

The sera of certain patients inhibit chemotaxis when added to neutrophils; certain drugs such as corticosteroids and phenylbutazone also do this.

Deficiencies in the generation of chemotactic signals

The most important of these are deficiencies in the complement system.

Disorders of phagocytosis

Opsonin deficiencies

These include deficiencies of complement or of IgG. Some patients with sickle cell disease have opsonic deficiencies, apparently associated with failure of alternate pathway activation of the complement system.

Defects of engulfment

These can be brought about by certain drugs, such as morphine analogues, and under hyperosmolar conditions, such as may be seen in patients with diabetic acidosis.

Disorders of lysosomal fusion

This may occur after administration of certain drugs, such as corticosteroids, colchicine and certain antimalarials. Failure of lysosomal fusion in the neutrophils of patients with the Chédiak–Higashi syndrome is mentioned above.

Disorders of bacterial killing

The most important of these is **chronic granulomatous disease of childhood**. This is a rare X-linked disease of childhood characterized by recurrent bacterial infections involving skin, lung, bones and lymph nodes. The affected children show increased susceptibility to infections by a rather curious mixed bag of organisms including *Staphylococcus aureus*, *Aerobacter aerogenes* and certain fungi such as *Aspergillus* species. Draining lymph nodes are often enlarged and show proliferation of mononuclear phagocytes lining the sinuses or aggregations of mononuclear cells tightly packed together to form granulomatous foci. The neutrophils in this condition respond normally to chemotactic signals and show no apparent difficulty in phagocytosis. However, once engulfment of the foreign organisms has occurred the expected burst of respiratory activity does not take place and there is no superoxide or hydrogen peroxide production. The precise nature of the defect is not clear, but may be an absence of the oxidase system associated with either NADPH or NADH. Interestingly, these neutrophils can kill certain pathogenic microorganisms such as streptococci and pneumococci. These organisms, produce a certain amount of H_2O_2 themselves but do not produce catalase. Within the phagosome the concentration of microorganism-produced hydrogen peroxide gradually rises until, in a sense, the organisms 'commit suicide'. However, those bacteria that also produce catalase are safe from the effects of their own hydrogen peroxide.

The role of G-6-PD in the production and detoxification of hydrogen peroxide has already been mentioned earlier. If the degree of deficiency of this enzyme is very severe then a clinical picture which resembles that encountered in chronic granulomatous disease of childhood may be seen. Absence of myeloperoxidase brings about some reduction in the efficiency of intracellular, oxygen-dependent bactericidal mechanisms, but the functional defect is usually not very severe.

Mononuclear Phagocytes in Acute Inflammation

The cellular component of the inflammatory response includes another type of phagocytic cell apart from the neutrophil — the mononuclear phagocyte, which exists in two forms. An intermediate form known as the **monocyte** circulates in the blood, and when it migrates into tissues it either matures or differentiates into the tissue **macrophage.**

The monocyte has a half-life of about 22 hours, which is approximately three times as long as that of the neutrophil. Despite the fact that it can be regarded as an intermediate cell form, it nevertheless possesses a range of functional activities shared with the mature tissue macrophage. Monocytes and macrophages are derived from bone marrow. If the bone marrow is destroyed by exposing an animal to x-irradiation, injury fails to elicit any mononuclear cell response, whereas if the thymus is removed a normal response is produced. Within the tissue the transition from a monocyte to a macrophage brings with it a considerable structural and hence, by implication, functional increase in the phagocytic, lysosomal and secretory apparatus. The cell becomes larger, the plasma membrane becomes more convoluted, lysosomes increase in number, and both the Golgi apparatus and the endoplasmic reticulum become more prominent. There is a considerable degree of overlap in the phagocytic functions of the macrophage and the neutrophil, so it is not a surprise to find that the plasma membrane of the macrophage has surface receptors for the Fc fragment of immunoglobulin as well as for complement components. Like the neutrophil, the macrophage depends on glycolysis for its energy needs in the course of phagocytosis and also exhibits a respiratory burst following bacterial engulfment. However, since it has a well developed protein secretory apparatus, the macrophage can synthesize and replace depleted enzymes and this allows it to act for a much longer time than does the neutrophil.

Many pathogenic microorganisms are phagocytosed by the macrophage and a large number of these are destroyed within phagosomes with a facility no less than that of the neutrophil. However, some organisms parasitize macrophages and multiply within the phagosomes. Such organisms include *Listeria, Brucella, Salmonella, Mycobacterium, Chlamydia, Rickettsia, Leishmania, Toxoplasma, Trypanosoma* and *Legionella*. This symbiotic relationship is destroyed by **activation** of the macrophage, which then becomes highly dangerous to its previous symbiotes.

Chemical influences on macrophage function

Macrophage chemotactic factors include those which have already been described in relation to the neutrophil, such as complement cleavage products, microbial products, N-formyl methionyl peptides and fibrin degradation products. In addition, however, there is a very important group of chemical activators which trigger a wide range of macrophage functions apart from chemotaxis. These are called **lymphokines** and are secreted by activated T lymphocytes. The concept that sensitized T lymphocytes reacting with specific antigen can release products that activate macrophages, both in vivo and in vitro, is now well accepted. The lymphokines include a **macrophage chemotactic factor** which can recruit macrophages into sites of infection, contact type hypersensitivity or inflammation, a **migration-inhibition factor** which can immobilize macrophages in certain lesions, and factors which stimulate the secretion of hydrolytic enzymes by the macrophages, making them able to kill neoplastic cells and to limit the ability of intracellular organisms to reproduce themselves. Other types of macrophage activation, for example via the action of complement cleavage products, lead to other forms of activity which are listed in Table 5.1.

Table 5.1 Secretory functions of the macrophage.

Secretion of enzymes into the extracellular environment
Release of activated complement components
Increased capacity to kill tumour cells or prevent their multiplication
Increased capacity to kill intracellular organisms or limit their multiplication
Production of interferon, which can provide short-term protection against viruses and some microbial pathogens
Secretion of endogenous pyrogen, which explains the fever elicited by endotoxin, microbial cell walls and certain synthetic materials
Release of colony-stimulating activity, which increases the production and release of neutrophils
Formation of tissue thromboplastin
Secretion of plasminogen activator
Secretion of metabolites of arachidonic acid, including those derived via the lipoxygenase pathway
Release of factors which stimulate the proliferation of fibroblasts and the synthesis of collagen

Chapter 6

Acute Inflammation III: Chemical Mediators

Repeated reference has been made to the fact that most of the events, both vascular and cellular, which occur in the course of the inflammatory response are triggered by the generation and reception of chemical signals, and some of these signalling systems have already been mentioned, chiefly in relation to the functions of phagocytic cells. In this section we shall seek to identify other chemical mediators and to see how some of the systems interact with one another.

Sir Thomas Lewis, who described the vascular 'triple response' elicited by mechanical trauma, suggested in 1927 that some of the features of acute inflammation might be ascribable to histamine. Many other substances are probably also involved in the mediation of the acute inflammatory reaction.

In theory we should not label any substance a chemical mediator of acute inflammation unless, when given in the concentrations likely to be found in human disease, it can reproduce the features of inflammation, and unless it can always be identified at the sites of inflammatory reactions. However, it is not possible to operate with such a degree of certainty in many instances and some of the compounds discussed here retain for the present a putative rather than a proven role.

The main sources for **endogenous mediators** are the **plasma** and the **tissues**; these will be considered separately.

Mediators Derived from Plasma

These include:

1. The **kinin system,** of which the archetype is bradykinin
2. The **complement system,** of which C3a, C5a and the trimolecular complex C567 are the active components in this context
3. The **clotting system,** in which fibrinopeptides and fibrin degradation products are active
4. The **fibrinolytic system,** in which plasmin plays a key part in maintaining the inflammatory response

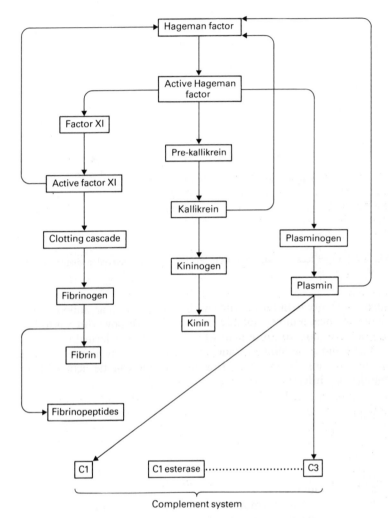

Fig. 6.1 The interrelationships between the plasma cascade systems and acute inflammation.

All these plasma systems are interconnected (see Fig. 6.1), the interconnections serving the purpose of **positive amplification loops** (Fig. 6.2).

The kinin system

The kinin system is a series of enzymatic steps which lead to the conversion of certain plasma precursors into active polypeptides which

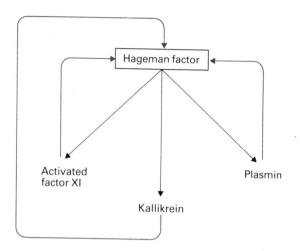

Fig. 6.2 Positive feedback mechanisms in relation to plasma-derived mediators of acute inflammation.

share an ability to induce change in the tone of vascular smooth muscle. Some of these kinins, notably bradykinin, are powerful vasodilators and are also able to cause pain when injected intradermally.

The kinin generating cascade starts with the activation of Hageman factor (clotting factor XII). Hageman factor can be activated by a number of different substances including:

glass
kaolin
collagen
basement membrane
cartilage
trypsin
sodium urate crystals
kallikrein (a later member of the kinin forming cascade)
plasmin (the fibrinolytic enzyme)
clotting factor XI
bacterial endotoxins

This wide range of activators signifies its central and important position. Once Hageman factor is activated, it acts on three plasma proenzymes to convert them to their active form. Clotting factor XI is activated to initiate the intrinsic clotting cascade. Plasminogen proactivator is activated to plasminogen activator with the ultimate formation of plasmin, the fibrinolytic enzyme, and prekallikrein is changed to kallikrein, thus leading to kinin generation. Plasma kallikrein (which, incidentally, is chemotactic for neutrophils) cleaves a plasma substrate kininogen to release the active nonapeptide bradykinin. Bradykinin is a very powerful hypotensive agent and produces both vascular dilatation and increases in vascular permeability in extremely small doses. Bradykinin is destroyed by two peptidases, and the other enzymes of the kinin-generating system can be interrupted at various points along the cascade. The precise role of the kinin system in inflammation has yet to be determined. Clearly it is not the only system involved since patients who suffer from a deficiency of Hageman factor can still mount a normal inflammatory response. It may be that the kinin system is important because of its interrelationships with other inflammation-mediating plasma cascades.

The complement system

Mention has already been made of the role of some of the components of the complement cascade in relation to the chemotactic attraction of neutrophils and macrophages, and of the chief ways in which complement activation can be achieved. However, the part played by the complement system extends beyond the bounds of chemotaxis to involve the vascular changes in the acute inflammatory reaction as well. The increased vascular permeability produced by activation of the complement cascade has been attributed to the formation of what have been called 'anaphylatoxins', which we now know are the cleavage products of C3 and C5 — C3a and C5a. If C3a and C5a are injected into human skin they cause local reddening and leakage from the microvasculature; C5a is 1000 times more active than C3a in this respect. Thus both C3a and C5a are deemed to be mediators of the vascular and cellular components of the inflammatory reaction, C5a being the more active, while the C567 complex exerts its effect solely in respect of chemotaxis. In addition C3 fragments can induce the release of neutrophils from bone marrow reserves, while C5a may induce the release of lysosomal enzymes.

The clotting system

The activation of Hageman factor also activates clotting factor XI. This active form of factor XI feeds back to activate more Hageman factor, thus providing the third positive amplification loop. Of the three enzymes which act in this way — factor XI, plasmin and kallikrein — the last is by far the most active on a molar basis. The fibrinopeptides released from fibrinogen by the action of thrombin may both induce vascular leakage and be chemotactic for neutrophils.

The fibrinolytic system

Activated Hageman factor, as mentioned above, also triggers the fibrinolytic system, leading to the production of **plasmin**. Apart from its fibrinolytic powers, plasmin is well fitted to play an important part in the generation and maintenance of the inflammatory reaction. It feeds back to activate more Hageman factor and also digests the Hageman factor into particles which tend to activate prekallikrein rather than clotting factor XI. Thus plasmin forms the second positive amplification loop in the kinin-generating system (kallikrein itself constituting the first). In some species, when fibrin is cleaved by plasmin, fibrin degradation products which are chemotactic for neutrophils are formed; these also have the ability to enhance vascular permeability. Plasmin also activates C1 to trigger the classical pathway of complement activation and can cleave C3 directly, thus also initiating the alternate pathway of complement activation.

Mediators Derived from the Tissues

Vasoactive amines

The first of these to be linked with the acute inflammatory reaction was **histamine**. Histamine, which is formed by the decarboxylation of histidine, is found in the granules of mast cells and in the parietal cells of the stomach mucosa. Mast cells are distributed throughout the body and can usually be found in relation to small vessels in the connective tissue. They are recognized by their metachromatic reaction with blue-violet dyes such as toluidine blue — their intracytoplasmic granules stain red. This reaction is due to the presence of sulphated mucopolysaccharides within these granules. In addition to histamine the granules contain heparin, 5-hydroxytryptamine (in rats and mice) and a variety of other enzymes. The name 'mast' cell seems rather curious; it stems from a failure to translate from the German description of these cells (*mästen*) meaning to stuff or fatten, presumably because of the large number of granules in the cytoplasm. They obviously have a very considerable pharmacological potential and play a significant part in the early phases of the acute inflammatory response and in type I hypersensitivity reactions (anaphylaxis).

There is a wide range of non-cell killing stimuli for the release of mediators from the mast cell granules. These include physical injury such as heat, mechanical trauma and irradiation; chemical agents such as immunoglobulins, snake venoms, bee venom, dextrans, chymotrypsin and trypsin, certain surfactants and cationic proteins released from the lysosomes of neutrophils, C3a and C5a; and, in connection with

Type I hypersensitivity reactions, an antigenic challenge to IgE-coated cells. The mechanism of release of granule contents depends on an increase in intracellular cGMP and a corresponding inhibition of cAMP. Any treatment which increases cAMP in the mast cell will inhibit release, not only of histamine but of certain other active substances which are not preformed within the cell but which are synthesized and released following on a rise in cGMP. Both histamine and, in appropriate species, 5-hydroxytryptamine cause vascular dilatation and increase vascular permeability. However, as pointed out previously, when antihistaminic compounds are given, only the immediate phase of vascular permeability change is inhibited, suggesting that these amines are of significance only during this early period of the inflammatory reaction.

Acidic lipids — the products of arachidonic acid peroxidation

In 1970 the discovery was made that certain 20-carbon-chain fatty acids were released in experimentally induced inflammatory states and in type I hypersensitivity reactions. These are known as prostaglandins (so named because they were first identified in seminal fluid). This was followed by a series of studies in which it was demonstrated that peroxidation of arachidonic acid, a major constituent of the lipid in cell membranes, took place in many inflammatory conditions in a wide variety of species (including man) and that the injection of prostaglandins produced the vascular changes of the acute inflammatory response. It is a matter of very considerable interest that some potent anti-inflammatory drugs, most notably aspirin and indomethacin, selectively inhibit prostaglandin synthesis. Corticosteroids, the other major group of anti-inflammatory agents, do not inhibit prostaglandin synthesis but stabilize membranes and in so-doing may block the release of fatty acids from membrane phospholipids and thus cut off the supply of starting material for the synthesis of prostaglandins.

Arachidonic acid can be metabolized in two ways. The stable prostaglandins, such as prostaglandin E_2, the potent vasoconstrictor and platelet aggregator thromboxane A2, and the dilator and anti-aggregatory compound prostaglandin I_2 are all produced via two unstable endoperoxides. These are produced from arachidonic acid via an enzyme pathway known as the **cyclo-oxygenase pathway.** This cyclo-oxygenase system is blocked by aspirin and indomethacin. Both prostaglandin E_2 and I_2 have a strong vasodilator effect and also produce some increase in vascular permeability. Prostaglandins of the E series are hyperalgesic and also act synergistically with other pain-producing mediators of inflammation such as bradykinin.

Another pathway of arachidonic acid peroxidation exists which is known as the **lipoxygenase pathway**. This can occur in platelets, neutrophils and mast cells, and the initial step is the formation from arachidonic acid of an intermediate, 5-hydroperoxy-eicoso-tetraenoic acid. From this intermediate a family of compounds can be produced which are known as the leukotrienes. Much less is known about the inflammatory activity of these compounds than of the prostaglandins, but some are certainly chemotactic and others chemokinetic. One of the leukotrienes (leukotriene C) is now known to be identical with a compound discovered over 40 years ago known as **slow reacting substance A**, which is remarkable for its ability to produce slow and sustained contraction of smooth muscle in contrast to the more rapid and short-lived effect of histamine. This substance can be found in the lungs of sensitized guinea pigs challenged with the appropriate antigen, and is believed to be the effector substance which causes contraction of bronchiolar smooth muscle leading to narrowing and obstruction of small airways in type I hypersensitivity reactions. Interestingly enough, in view of the tendency for eosinophils to accumulate in the tissues of patients with type I hypersensitivity reactions, it is now known that eosinophils contain large amounts of aryl sulphatase which can destroy slow reacting substance A. Thus the eosinophil reaction in tissues, for so long regarded just as a useful marker of allergic injury, can now be seen to be the expression of a protective function against excess leukotriene.

Compounds released from lysosomes

The cell population of an acutely inflamed area can contribute a number of potential mediators derived from lysosomes. This applies not only to the neutrophils, but also to other cell types, notably platelets. Some of these candidates for the role of mediators are:

1. **Cationic proteins.** Some of these can attract mononuclear phagocytes when tested in in vitro systems, while others induce the release of histamine from mast cells and so have some effect on vascular permeability.

2. **Acid proteases.** The lysosomes of neutrophils contain many proteases which are most active at approximately pH 3.0. In areas of acute inflammation, the pH tends to fall because of the increased production of lactic acid consequent on the glycolysis occurring in the neutrophils, but the pH does not usually fall so far as to provide the optimal condition for activity of these enzymes.

3. **Neutral proteases.** The objection raised above to a significant role for acid proteases does not apply to the lysosomal enzymes which are

active at neutral pH. It is believed that these are of considerable importance in causing tissue breakdown in a number of pathological situations. The range of targets which may be attacked in this way is wide, since neutrophil lysosomes contain collagenases, elastases, and enzymes which degrade cartilage and basement membranes. It may well be that tissue damage caused by the exocytosis of lysosomal contents and the generation of oxygen free radicals occurs much more frequently and is of much greater significance than has hitherto been appreciated. Apart from the direct tissue damage which may be caused by release of lysosomal enzymes, some of these can also generate chemotactic fragments from C5 and produce kinins from plasma precursors. In addition, damaged or activated neutrophils release substances which attract other neutrophils by a mechanism independent of complement.

Chapter 7

Factors which may Modify the Inflammatory Reaction

The processes that have been described occur to a greater or lesser degree in all acute inflammatory responses to injury, but it must be obvious from personal experience that there are considerable differences between one inflammatory reaction and another and that these differences involve a number of variables; for example, a 'boil' on the neck differs very much from an area of 'sun-burn'. The outcome of any injury is the resultant of interaction between the injurious agent and the host, and variations in either of these may exert a considerable effect. Factors related to the injurious agent include:

1. The amount or dose of the agent
2. Its strength (or, in the case of a pathogenic microorganism, its virulence)
3. The duration of exposure in the case of physical or chemical agents
4. The intrinsic nature of the agent

The degree of injury produced by any noxious agent, whether living or not, is a function of its inherent toxicity and the time during which it is allowed to exert its effect. Duration of exposure is of particular importance in injuries produced by physical and certain chemical agents such as heat, cold, actinic rays, acids and alkalis. In injury produced by pathogenic microorganisms, clearly the inherent power of the organisms to produce tissue damage is of great importance, but here too the **dose** of the agent may well determine the outcome of the infection.

Morphological features related to the injurious agent

The intrinsic nature of the agent may produce a morphological reaction in the tissues which is quite distinctive. In some cases the type of structural change may be of considerable help to the histopathologist in making an aetiological diagnosis. For example, certain organisms, such as **Staphylococcus aureus**, tend to elicit an inflammatory response which is characterized by a massive emigration of neutrophils to the site of infection. Many of these neutrophils die after phagocytosis of the invading microorganisms and release large amounts of lysosomal enzymes into the damaged area. Since the organisms also produce substances (exotoxins) which damage tissues directly, the end result is a central area of liquefaction necrosis which contains tissue debris and many dead and dying neutrophils. This forms a rather thick, opaque, yellowish-green fluid which is known as **pus**. Organisms which elicit this reaction are termed **pyogenic** (i.e. pus forming). The process by which such tissue necrosis associated with the formation of pus occurs is termed **suppuration** and the localized suppurative lesion is called an **abscess**.

Corynebacterium diphtheriae and *Clostridium difficile* produce exotoxins which kill surface epithelia. The fluid which exudes from the small, subepithelial blood vessels is very rich in fibrinogen. This becomes converted to fibrin and then becomes densely infiltrated by neutrophils. The end result is the presence on the affected surface of an opaque greyish-white membrane which consists of a mixture of dead epithelial cells, fibrin and neutrophils. This type of reaction is known as **membranous** or **pseudo-membranous**. In the case of the diphtheria organism, the target area is the pharynx and larynx; the clostridium causes pseudo-membranous enterocolitis, particularly in those whose bowel bacterial flora has been altered by previous antibiotic treatment.

Salmonella typhi, the organism responsible for typhoid fever, does not elicit a neutrophil response, though in vitro it is chemotactic for the neutrophil. The lesions of typhoid, which may occur in the gut, the lymph nodes, the liver and less often at other sites, are therefore characterized by a cellular infiltrate in which the macrophage is the predominant cell.

Some organisms appear to attack small blood vessels and thus produce lesions in which bleeding is a prominent feature. This is seen in certain rickettsial diseases such as typhus, in anthrax, and in some cases of pneumonia caused by the influenza virus.

Inflammatory reactions due to the impaction or formation of antigen/antibody complexes in small blood vessels or due to irradiation are characterized by a tissue reaction in which both blood vessels and intercellular collagen show a curious form of necrosis. In sections conventionally stained with haematoxylin and eosin, the affected vessels or collagen fibres show a smudgy appearance and are deeply eosinophilic. Appropriate special stains show fibrin to be present in these areas, and this type of tissue damage is accordingly known as 'fibrinoid necrosis'.

In cases in which the inflammatory reaction is due to infection by a pathogenic microorganism, whether or not the organisms can spread through the tissues is an important modifying factor. It is of prime importance whether the tissue reaction will keep the infection localized or whether spread to the surrounding tissues or to distant sites can occur. Factors which may influence this include:

1. The elaboration of **spreading factors** by the infective agents. A wide variety of such agents exist, including exotoxins which can hydrolyse the mucopolysaccharide ground substance in the extracellular space, such as the hyaluronidase which is produced both by **Streptococcus pyogenes** and **Clostridium welchii**, both of which characteristically cause spreading types of inflammation. Streptococci produce streptokinase, which lyses the polymerised fibrin laid down in the course of formation of the protein-rich inflammatory exudate; this too may inhibit attempts to localize the infection. The clostridia which produce **gas gangrene** (*C. welchii*, *oedematiens* and *septicum*), in addition to producing exotoxins such as hyaluronidase and collagenase which facilitate spreading of infection, also modify the local reaction by their release of powerful necrotizing toxins which break down muscle. The muscle carbohydrate is then fermented by appropriate enzymes also produced by these organisms, forming bubbles of gas which make the affected tissues feel crepitant (crackly).

2. The presence of **lymphatic blockage** may also assist in localization of infection. Such blockage is presumably mediated by the coagulation of lymph with the formation of fibrin, and appears to be inhibited if the invading pathogens (such as *Streptococcus pyogenes*) are able to elaborate lytic enzymes.

3. The susceptibility of the infecting microorganisms to the normal defensive process of phagocytosis is obviously an important variable in shaping the events which follow infection. Some organisms have surface material (capsules) which makes phagocytosis of them difficult. This material may be carbohydrate in nature, such as the capsular polysaccharide of the *Pneumococcus*, or a protein. **Staphylococcus aureus** has a protein (protein A) in its wall which combines with the Fc fragment of antibody attached to the organism and thus blocks attachment of this fragment to the Fc receptor on the phagocyte. **Streptococcus pyogenes** and **Staphylococcus aureus** elaborate exotoxins which can kill the threatening phagocytes. These few examples serve to indicate the range of defensive options evolved by prokaryotes against phagocytosis and killing.

Factors related to the host

Factors related to the **host** operate predominantly but not exclusively in relation to the injuries produced by microorganisms. Some of these may be inferred from material presented in earlier sections, especially in relation to chemotaxis, phagocytosis and bacterial killing. The general physiological state of the host is clearly important; if the host is debilitated, undernourished or severely anaemic, infections which under normal circumstances might be regarded as fairly trivial may become life-threatening. For example, measles, which occurs principally in childhood, is a disorder which we regard as mildly unpleasant and inconvenient. In those populations where malnutrition is rife, measles is one of the major causes of death in infants and children.

Just as defects in the phagocyte system render the host much more susceptible to infection, so do defects in the B and T cell elements of the immune system. Such defects may occur as part of a congenital syndrome or may be acquired either through some disease process which is associated with immunosuppression (such as Hodgkin's disease) or as a result of some treatment in which immunosuppression is induced either deliberately (as in patients receiving allogeneic transplants) or as a side-effect (as in patients receiving cytotoxic therapy for malignant neoplastic processes, particularly those involving the lymphoreticular system).

The Classification of any Individual Inflammatory Reaction

The classification of any inflammatory lesion can be regarded essentially as an exercise in simple **set theory**. The **sets** which we can usefully consider are:

1. The **duration** of the inflammatory reaction
2. The **type of exudate** associated with the particular type of injury. This may be:

> serous
> fibrinous
> haemorrhagic
> catarrhal
> purulent (suppurative)
> membranous or pseudo-membranous
> combinations of the above

3. The influence on lesion morphology and natural history of the **anatomical location** of the injury. This can be considered under the following simple headings:

> **solid tissue**
> **epithelial lined surfaces**
> **serosal surfaces**

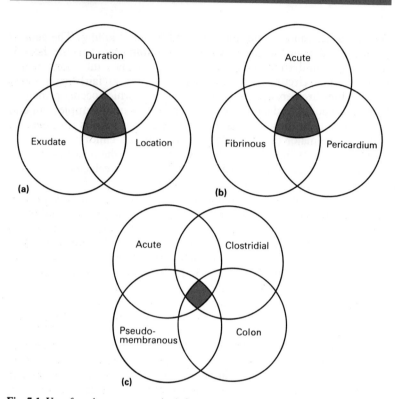

Fig. 7.1 Use of set theory to categorize inflammatory reactions. (a) Chosen sets. (b) Fibrinous pericarditis. (c) Pseudomembranous colitis.

Examples of the use of a **common set** as an expression of a particular inflammatory reaction are shown in Fig. 7.1.

Duration

If the duration of the inflammatory reaction is fairly short (e.g. days) it is termed **acute.** A reaction lasting for some weeks is termed **subacute,** and long lasting inflammatory reactions (months or even years) are called **chronic.**

Types of exudate

Serous exudate

This is characterized by the outpouring of fluid which has a rather low protein content, in particular of fibrinogen so that there can be little formation of polymerized fibrin strands. This type of reaction is frequently seen in relation to surfaces which are lined by mesothelial cells, such as the joint spaces or the pleural cavities. The fluid which accumulates in a common blister, such as that seen after mild repetitive trauma (e.g. chopping wood or rowing by those not used to the exercise), is a typical example of serous exudation. Similar serous effusions are seen not uncommonly as an expression of tuberculous pleurisy particularly in young adults.

Fibrinous exudate

This type of exudate is rather less in volume and has a high protein content, with large amounts of fibrinogen being present and being converted to fibrin. It tends particularly to occur in relation to serosa-lined cavities such as pleura, pericardium and peritoneum. The mesothelial linings involved characteristically lose their moist, shiny-looking surface, which becomes dull, granular and opaque as they become covered by polymerized fibrin. Some forms of pneumonia, notably **lobar pneumonia** caused by the *Streptococcus pneumoniae*, are dominated by the outpouring of a fibrin-rich exudate into the alveolar spaces with obvious, serious consequences for gas diffusion within the lungs. Two contiguous surfaces covered in fibrin tend to stick together, and, if the fibrin is not lysed later in the inflammatory process, scar tissue is formed, with permanent loss of function. One important example among many is post-inflammatory stenosis of the aortic or mitral valves.

Haemorrhagic exudate

This is usually an example of fibrinous exudation where damage to small blood vessels has been sufficiently severe to allow the escape of red cells from the lumena into the extravascular space. This may be seen in certain bacterial infections such as anthrax, in rickettsial infections such as typhus and rocky mountain spotted fever, and in some viral conditions such as influenzal pneumonia.

Purulent exudate

As indicated earlier, certain pathogenic microorganisms elicit an inflammatory reaction in which the neutrophil is the dominant element. Largely because of the large number of cells present, the exudate is opaque. The organisms concerned often also liberate toxins which produce tissue necrosis, and the lysosomal enzymes liberated from the dying neutrophils cause liquefaction of the dead tissue, so that the centre of the lesion consists of the fluid material called pus. Not infrequently we see a combination of fibrinous and purulent exudation, often in relation to serous surfaces such as the peritoneum. This is called a fibrino-purulent exudate.

Catarrhal exudate

This variety of exudate is usually seen where mucous membranes are involved in inflammatory reactions. The exudate is initially serous in character, but this phase is followed by a profuse discharge of mucus from the glands in the mucosa which converts the exudate into sticky, viscous material. An upper respiratory tract viral infection, such as a common 'cold', is a good example of such a reaction.

Membranous and pseudo-membranous exudates have been considered in an earlier section (p. 69).

Anatomical location and the inflammatory reaction

The type of tissue in which injury and the consequent inflammatory reaction take place affects the course of events and hence the structural changes which occur.

Abscess formation

If the injury takes place in the substance of what one might regard as a **solid block** of tissue such as the dermis, the liver, the kidney or the brain and the causal agent is a pyogenic organism, suppuration is likely to occur. If the process is localized the lesion with its necrotic pus-filled centre is termed an **abscess**. If the inflammatory reaction is a spreading one, it is termed **cellulitis.**

Within an abscess, the inflammatory reaction at a number of different points in its development can be seen, especially if thought of in three dimensions. The centre of the roughly spherical mass which constitutes the abscess is made up of partly or completely liquefied dead tissue admixed with the remains of dead or dying neutrophils. This is surrounded by a layer in which fibrin and living neutrophils are present. At the periphery of this is a membrane made up largely of proliferating fibroblasts, new capillaries and young collagen fibres. This last layer represents the **repair process**, which is one of the possible lines of development in the natural history of acute inflammation. This zone of fibroblastic proliferation serves as a barrier to the further spread of the inflammatory process, but also prevents the discharge of the abscess contents without which healing cannot occur.

It is often necessary, therefore, to lay the abscess open so that it may discharge adequately, or, in some cases such as the lung or the brain, to remove the lesion completely with a rim of surrounding tissue.

Ulcers

In epithelial-lined tissue such as the skin, gut, pharynx, larynx or trachea, a number of different reactions may occur. One, which has been discussed earlier, is the pseudo-membranous reaction, in which the surface epithelium becomes necrotic and, together with fibrin and inflammatory cells, forms part of a membrane which can be detached showing the raw, subepithelial tissue beneath. A more common type of inflammatory lesion in epithelial surfaces is the **ulcer**. An ulcer can be defined as a local defect in an epithelial surface, the defect being produced by the shedding of dead epithelial cells.

Inflammation on serosal surfaces

On serosal surfaces such as the pleura or peritoneum the reaction is most often serous, fibrinous or fibrino-purulent. Because of the arrangement of the tissues in what are basically flat mesothelial-lined sheets, there is little or no tendency for the process to become localized other than by the 'glueing' together of contiguous affected membranes.

Biological Effects of the Inflammatory Reaction

Earlier the question was raised as to whether inflammation should be regarded as helpful or harmful, and it was stated that the processes subsumed in the acute inflammatory reaction are basically defensive in nature; it is now appropriate to consider how this defensive function is mediated.

Inflammation as a defence mechanism

Role of the exudate

The outpouring of fluid exudate might serve in a number of possible ways. If the injurious agent is a chemical poison or if, in the course of infection, tissue-damaging exotoxins are released by the pathogen, the fluid exudate might dilute the toxin. Since exudation implies the escape from the microcirculation of proteins as well as fluid and solute, antibodies and complement are likely to form part of the exudate and will contribute to the killing of microorganisms and/or the neutralization of their toxins. The transformation of fibrinogen to fibrin and the polymerization of the latter into tough strands may serve some localizing function, and the presence of fibrin assists the phagocytosis of non-opsonized organisms, this process being known as **surface phagocytosis.**

Role of phagocytic cells

The benefit which accrues to the host through the action of phagocytic cells must be obvious from what has been said earlier. The protective role of these cells as a primary means of defence against the consequences of infection is made clear by the greatly enhanced risk of serious infections in patients in whom either the number of circulating neutrophils is significantly reduced or one of the functions of these cells is seriously compromised.

Possible harmful effects of inflammation

Inflammation, in the broadest sense, also forms the basis of a series of potentially life-threatening or functionally crippling diseases, and it is worthwhile to examine some of the ways in which the basic processes we have considered can operate to the disadvantage of the patient. At a fairly simple level the presence of inflammatory oedema may have serious consequences. For example, if the larynx is involved in a patient with a parainfluenza virus infection of the upper respiratory tract laryngeal oedema may develop and obstruct normal airflow through the quite narrow lumen of the larynx. The patient will experience great difficulty in breathing, the inspiratory and expiratory efforts will be accompanied by a loud noise (stridor) and the patient may become cyanotic through lack of oxygen. This event, which is comparable to being strangled, is a medical emergency. The patient may well require tracheostomy to restore normal airflow until such time as the laryngeal oedema has subsided. Cerebral oedema, which can occur as a consequence of inflammation as well as in certain other situations, may also have disastrous consequences. Swelling of the brain within its rigid box, the cranium, means that any increase in pressure must be transmitted downwards and backwards through the only available potential avenue of escape, the foramen magnum. This displacement puts severe shearing stresses on the small perforating blood vessels at the base of the midbrain and may cut off the blood supply to important areas. At post-mortem examination the presence of such displacement due to cerebral oedema may be expressed by the presence of deep grooves (formed by the pressure of the tentorium) on the midbrain or by grooves produced in relation to the cerebellar tonsils if they have herniated through the foramen magnum.

Very rarely, unpleasant consequences may arise from failure to control the generation of one or other of the chemical mediators of inflammation. One such example is a condition known as hereditary angio-neurotic oedema, in which patients develop localized areas of oedema in a wide range of anatomical locations, the oedematous areas often being painful. This is believed to be due to the unrestrained activity of a kinin-like particle liberated in the course of activation of the C2 component of complement. Normally this is inactivated by an esterase, but in sufferers from this disease the inactivator substance is not synthesized.

In addition to the purely mechanical problems which may arise from inflammatory oedema, the presence of certain types of exudate in particular locations may produce profound and dangerous functional changes. In lobar pneumonia caused by *Streptococcus pneumoniae*, an exudate rich in fibrin is formed and this sweeps through the pores of Kohn to involve large areas of the lung tissue. The presence of the exudate causes some difficulty in oxygen diffusion and in gas exchange across the alveolar septa. Fortunately in most cases blood oxygen levels are not significantly reduced, but if the process involves enough lung tissue a considerable disturbance in blood gases may occur. In under-privileged communities this condition is still an important cause of death, even though it has become much rarer in Western countries.

So far as the phagocytic cells are concerned, tissue damage may result either through some interruption of phagosome–lysosome fusion or, on a wider scale, through inappropriate triggering of some of their secretory or metabolic functions.

Examples of abnormalities in lysosomal fusion which might lead to tissue damage are found, in the case of the neutrophil, in acute gouty arthritis, and, in the case of the macrophage, in silicosis. The former has already been discussed on p. 15. In silicosis the silica particles are inhaled and deposited in the respiratory bronchioles. They are then phagocytosed in the normal way by macrophages and come to lie within phagosomes. Silicic acid forms on the surface of the silica particles and when the primary lysosome fuses with the silica-containing phagosome, hydrogen bonds form between the silicic acid and the lysosomal membrane. This leads to rupture of the lysosomal membrane with spillage of its enzymes into the cytoplasm. The macrophage then dies and the lysosomal enzymes and the offending silica particle are released into the interstitial tissue. The lysosomal enzymes (which include collagenase and elastase) cause tissue damage, and the silica particle is once again available for phagocytosis, so the cycle starts again.

It is not unlikely that phagocytic cells may secrete lysosomal enzymes in response to a variety of stimuli. The potential ill effects of such secretion are avoided by the presence within both plasma and extracellular fluid of glycoproteins which inhibit the proteolytic effects of lysosomal enzymes. As in so many fields in pathobiology, the importance of such inhibitory mechanisms is only discovered when they fail. An example of this can be seen in the inherited condition known as **alpha-l-antitrypsin deficiency.** The ability to synthesize this protease inhibitor (in the liver) is governed by the possession of a normal allelic pair of genes. Absence of both members of this pair renders the affected person homozygous for the deficiency and such people may develop destruction of the alveolar and bronchiolar walls in the lung leading to **panacinar emphysema** and also show an enhanced risk for liver damage leading to **cirrhosis.** Absence of one member of the pair of genes (the heterozygous state) leads to an increased risk of lung damage if the subject is a smoker, though he or she will not as a rule develop signs of tissue damage if other potential noxious substances, such as smoke, are avoided.

Another way in which tissue damage may be brought about by the action of phagocytic cells is by the release of oxygen-derived free radicals. Many experimental studies have shown that oxygen metabolites released from activated neutrophils and macrophages may be toxic to a wide variety of eukaryotic cells, including red cells, endothelial cells, fibroblasts, tumour cells, platelets and spermatozoa. Damage to endothelial cells, especially in the pulmonary capillary bed, can certainly be produced by oxygen-derived free radicals and this may well be the most important pathogenetic mechanism underlying the respiratory distress syndrome seen in association with a number of clinical states. Another area in which such a mechanism may be operative is the tissue damage which follows lodgement of antigen/ antibody complexes in various locations. Such lodgement is often associated with the presence of phagocytic cells and in experimental systems tissue damage may be avoided by the administration of superoxide dismutase, even though the normal inflammatory cell response takes place. Similarly in experimentally produced antigen/ antibody complex mediated injury in the lung, tissue damage can be reduced by administering catalase whereas antiproteases have no such protective effect. A great deal of work still remains to be done in humans to establish the role of oxygen metabolites in tissue injury, but the following situations have been suggested, at least in part, to result from cellular injury produced by an increased flux of free radicals:

ischaemic damage in the brain or heart
paraquat poisoning
some drug-induced haemolytic anaemias
ageing
rheumatoid arthritis

ulcerative colitis
some immune complex mediated disorders
radiation damage
damage due to smoking

Chapter 8

The Natural History of Acute Inflammation I: Healing

The end results of tissue injury and the acute inflammatory reaction which it elicits encompass a wide spectrum of biological events. These range from a complete return to both structural and functional normality to scar formation or the persistence of the inflammatory process for weeks, months or years (Fig. 8.1). The factors which determine which of these will follow a given inflammatory reaction relate to the nature of the injurious agent, the target of the attack and

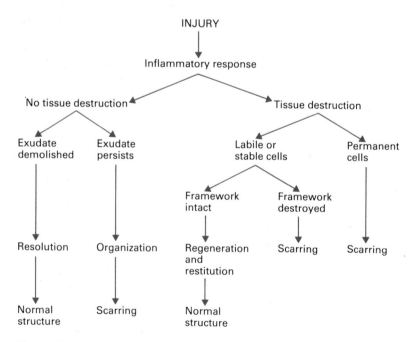

Fig. 8.1 The natural history of acute inflammation.

the host response. The basic processes which are involved are, in phylogenetic terms, some of the oldest known. They include:

1. Removal of foreign material whether living or dead
2. Clearance from the tissues of the elements of the inflammatory response
3. Regeneration of lost tissue components where possible
4. Replacement of lost tissue elements by well vascularized connective tissue

Resolution

This is the term used to imply a more or less complete return of an inflamed part of an organ or tissue to the state existing before the onset of the inflammatory reaction. Also implied is the fact that for resolution to occur, **no** loss of tissue should have taken place, the injury being severe enough to elicit the formation of an inflammatory exudate but not so severe as to cause tissue destruction. Removal of the inflammatory exudate is accomplished largely by the fibrinolytic system, though phagocytosis by macrophages also plays a part.

A striking example of resolution is to be seen in the natural history of lobar pneumonia, an acute inflammatory disorder affecting the lung parenchyma and involving large areas of lung tissue in continuity (Fig. 8.2). Invasion of the air spaces by *Streptococcus pneumoniae* evokes a

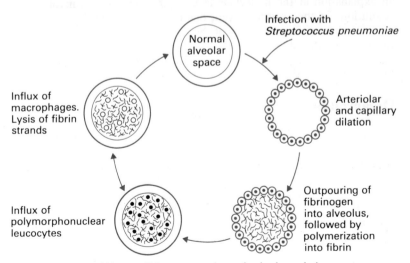

Fig. 8.2 The natural history of lobar pneumonia terminating in resolution.

severe acute inflammatory reaction characterized by a massive outpouring of a fibrin-rich exudate into the air spaces. This exudate spreads rapidly through the adjacent airspaces, probably via the pores of Kohn. The appearance of the exudate is followed by a cellular reaction, the majority of the cells at the height of the inflammatory process, while organisms are still present, being neutrophils. At this stage, microscopic examination of affected areas of lung shows the air spaces to be filled with exudate; as a result, the affected portion of lung is airless. However, the walls of the air spaces are intact and show only the vasodilatation expected with any acute inflammatory reaction. The infecting organisms are cleared, largely through phagocytosis by neutrophils, many of which die in the process. Once this has occurred, the cell infiltrate changes, macrophages being recruited to the inflamed areas. At this point the fibrin meshwork becomes broken down by the action of plasmin. It is possible that the macrophages act as the trigger for this process since **plasminogen activator** is one of the substances they can release. The macrophages themselves phagocytose much of the cellular and bacterial debris and their release of lysosomal enzymes by reverse endocytosis accounts for the breakdown of non-phagocytosed debris. All this material leaves the inflamed area via the lymphatics, the protein content of the draining lymph becoming considerably elevated. At the end of the resolution process all the exudate should have been removed from the affected alveoli and these can once again become aerated.

This more or less empirical account makes no pretence of providing an explanation at the molecular level of the mechanisms involved in resolution. In the example given, one of the most puzzling aspects is why at a time when proteolysis of the fibrinous exudate is taking place, the walls of the alveoli seem to be immune from enzyme-mediated damage.

Organization

If exudate demolition does not take place and the exudate persists, another process which is known as **organization** is triggered. The persisting exudate is invaded by many macrophages, fibroblasts and new capillaries. It is either totally or partially removed, largely as a result of the activity of the macrophages, and is replaced by collagenous tissue in which, in the early stages, many thin-walled blood vessels are present. Eventually these blood vessels regress and some shortening of the collagen fibres occurs. The end result is a **scar**. This process of organization, the details of which are discussed later in relation to wound healing, is not only evoked by the persistence of inflammatory reactions but also by thrombus or blood clot and by the presence of dead tissue which cannot regenerate such as infarcted heart muscle.

Organization taking place in relation to persistent inflammatory reactions can produce serious functional disturbances in the affected areas. For example, the inflammation in the heart valves which occurs in acute rheumatic carditis often leads to organization, the commissures of the valves becoming fused by scar tissue with resulting narrowing of the valve orifice. This stenosis imposes a high pressure overload on whatever chamber of the heart is immediately proximal to the affected valve, and in due time this can lead to significant haemodynamic disturbances ending in cardiac failure. In the lung affected by pneumonia, persistence of exudate leads to the affected alveoli becoming filled with connective tissue and being solid rather than spongy and aerated. Serosal cavities such as the pericardial or pleural cavities can be partly or completely obliterated by scar tissue formed in relation to persistent exudate. In some instances the heart may be ensheathed in a thick layer of scar tissue (**constrictive pericarditis**) which interferes both with the relaxation of heart muscle (diastolic compliance) and with systolic contraction, leading to severe, predominantly right-sided cardiac failure.

Regeneration

If tissue has been destroyed as a result of injury the resulting defect, whether large or small, must be replaced by new, living tissue. This may be accomplished by the normal constituents of the damaged tissue proliferating and replacing the lost cells. If this takes place in an orderly fashion the lost tissue elements are replicated and the end result is a tissue which is 'as good as new'. This process is known as **regeneration** and can be seen to operate most effectively in non-mammalian species such as the salamander which can readily replace an amputated limb.

Successful regeneration depends on two factors. First, the lost cells must be capable of being replaced by identical cells; second, the connective tissue and vascular framework along which the parenchymal cells of any particular organ or tissue are arranged must be preserved.

Cell type

From the point of view of their potential regenerative ability, mammalian cells can be divided into three classes:

labile cells
stable cells
permanent cells

Labile cells are those which divide and proliferate throughout postnatal life. They have a predetermined lifespan and hence are 'turned over' with a considerable degree of regularity. They fall into two main groups:

1. The covering epithelia. These include the stratified squamous epithelium of the skin, mouth, pharynx, oesophagus, vagina and cervix; the transitional epithelium of the urinary tract, the linings of the ducts of exocrine glands, the gut and the uterus, Fallopian tubes, etc.
2. Cells of the blood and lymphoid tissue. In both these, loss of cells can be made good with relative ease.

Stable cells are normally quiescent insofar as division is concerned and under normal circumstances mitoses are rare. However, a variety of stimuli, including a sudden decrease in the cell number, can stimulate cell division and when such cells are lost they can be replaced quite rapidly. This group includes the parenchymal cells of the liver, renal tubular epithelium, the parenchymal cells of endocrine glands, bone, and fibrous tissue.

Permanent cells are those which normally only proliferate during fetal life and which, therefore, cannot be replaced. Neurones, cardiac muscle cells and the cells of voluntary muscle fall into this category, though voluntary muscle cells do have some rather limited powers of regeneration.

The preservation of a normal stromal framework is essential for a return to full normality

The replacement of lost cells is only one part of the process leading to a return to normal tissue structure, albeit the most important. If the architectural arrangement of the connective tissue framework of an organ or tissue is destroyed, the arrangement of the regenerating cells will be abnormal and this can have serious functional consequences.

Such a situation is well exemplified in the liver. The stable parenchymal cells show a marked ability to divide and proliferate after damage sufficient to lead to a decrease in the normal cell population. In experimental situations it is possible to excise 80% of the liver and, a few weeks later, to find a liver of normal weight and normal appearance. However, in certain cases of either continuing or acute liver cell necrosis, there may be either collapse or destruction of the reticulin framework. Regenerating hepatocytes, instead of being orientated along vascular sinusoids or along bile canaliculi, grow in the form of disorganized nodules. Thus normal hepatic **mass** will be restored but not normal hepatic **architecture.** Such a process can lead to a marked disturbance of normal blood flow patterns in the liver, leading to abnormally high blood pressure in the portal venous system and shunting of portal blood into the systemic venous circulation. This abnormal regeneration pattern and its functional consequences are important components of the clinical and pathological picture seen in **cirrhosis** of the liver.

If, as already pointed out, the processes of resolution or regeneration cannot take place then either persistent exudate or lost tissue must be replaced by **organization**. In internal organs, replacement of lost tissue is most frequently encountered in the replacement of dead cardiac muscle by scar tissue. Formation of scar tissue is allied with regeneration in **wound healing** which, apart from its fundamental biological significance, provides a useful model in which these phenomena can be studied.

Wound Healing

The mechanisms involved in the healing of wounds are basically the same whatever the type of wound; such differences as are described are of degree rather than of kind. However, almost by convention, the healing of cleanly incised wounds where the edges are in close apposition tends to be considered separately from those where there is a large tissue defect which has to be filled in by scar tissue and where the edges cannot be stitched together. Indeed, this is an area where terminology of the most archaic kind persists, healing of the first type of wound being described as being by 'first intention' and that of the more open type as being by 'second intention'. These terms first appear in a surgical treatise published in 1543, though Thomson in *Lectures on Inflammation* (1813) gives the credit for the introduction of the terms to Galen.

Healing of incised wounds

The minimal loss of tissue in this situation makes the close apposition of the wound edges using stitches or clips a matter of ease. The incision obviously severs many small blood vessels so that the first tissue reaction is haemorrhage. Such free blood as remains within the narrow wound cleft clots; this fibrin-rich clot tends to glue the sides of the wound together. This process is aided by the normal inflammatory exudation which follows the injury.

Epidermal events

Within a few hours of wounding a single layer of epidermal cells starts to **migrate** from the skin edges to form a delicate covering over the raw area of dermis. This migratory process can be studied in isolation by observing the behaviour of epidermal cells when fragments of skin are placed in nutrient media and cultured at 37°C. Under these circumstances the epidermal cells begin to migrate in much the same way as in wound healing and eventually spread round the cut edges of the dermis so that the whole block of tissue becomes covered by epidermis (this process being known as **epiboly**). Substances which are known to inhibit cell movement, such as cytochalasin B, also prevent epiboly. This suggests that the significant process involved in this phenomenon is epidermal cell movement. The controlling mechanisms for this epidermal cell migration are not known. In vitro it cannot take place unless serum is present, but the serum factor(s) have not been identified.

While epidermal cell movement, by itself, may be able to provide an epithelial covering in some very small wounds, in most instances this cannot be accomplished without proliferation of epidermal cells in the basal layers of the epidermis near the wound edges. From about 12 hours after wounding, there is a marked increase in mitotic activity in the region of the epidermis approximately three to five cells from the cut edge. This is preceded by an increase in DNA production of about 30%. Similar cycles of increased DNA synthesis and mitosis follow. The new epidermal cells grow under the surface fibrin clot and for a little distance down the gap between the cut edges so as to form a little 'spur' of epithelium which afterwards regresses. If the wound has been sutured a similar type of epidermal growth occurs in relation to the suture tracks.

Dermal events

Some 38 to 72 hours after the wound has been produced, the predominant cell in the inflammatory infiltrate is seen to be the macrophage. Experimental manoeuvres which inhibit the local macrophage response have been reported as causing inadequate healing and it seems likely that the macrophage exercises functions in wound healing which transcend its role as a phagocyte. Macrophage infiltration is followed a day or two later by the proliferation of fibroblasts, cells which produce collagen and other tissue proteins. By the sixth day, thick fibres which show the staining reactions of collagen appear and these tend to be orientated in the normal direction, i.e. parallel to the skin surface and across the wound axis.

Both macrophage infiltration and fibroblast proliferation are accompanied by ingrowth into the wound of small capillary buds which are derived from intact dermal vessels near the wound edges. Initially these buds consist of solid ingrowths of endothelial cells, but they soon acquire a lumen. At this stage these rudimentary new vessels have little basement membrane substance and, compared with a normal capillary, are extremely leaky. This newly vascularized, collagen-producing tissue is called **'granulation tissue'**. This relatively meaningless term is derived from the fact that when the raw area of a wound in which there is a large tissue defect is examined the surface appears granular and each of the little granules contains a loop of new capillaries and thus bleeds easily.

Healing of wounds associated with a large tissue defect

A large area of tissue loss can occur in cases of severe trauma or extensive burns, or much less frequently in relation to surgical procedures. There are few significant differences between the process of healing of an incised wound and those of a large tissue defect in which the skin edges cannot be apposed, other than those of degree. The formation of well vascularized granulation tissue must necessarily occur on a much larger scale than in the case of the incised wound where loss of tissue is minimal. One feature of the healing process not seen in relation to incised wounds is **wound contraction.**

Wound contraction

In the case of large open wounds, after two or three days the wound area starts to decrease. This is a real movement of the wound margins and is quite independent of the rate at which covering by new epithelium takes place. In some fur-bearing animals the wound area can decrease by 80% in two weeks and sometimes the degree of contraction may be sufficient to close the wound completely.

Since wound contraction occurs at a time when there is relatively little collagen being formed, it seems improbable that shortening of collagen fibres at the wound margins can play any significant part in the process. Indeed, inhibition of collagen synthesis does not interfere with the process of contraction. The currently favoured hypothesis is that the contraction is brought about by the action of cells which appear at the wound margins in the first week and which, on examination with the electron microscope, show features of both fibroblasts and smooth muscle cells (hence the name **myofibroblast**). Use of the appropriate labelled antibody shows that these cells contain actin. The view that wound contraction is mediated through the action of contractile protein is strengthened by the observation that strips of granulation tissue can be made to shorten in vitro by the same pharmacological agents which cause smooth muscle cells to contract. It is not without interest that such myofibroblasts have been identified in some disorders in which spontaneous contracture of dermal connective tissue occurs, such as Dupuytren's contracture.

Mechanisms involved in the various phases of healing

Epithelialization

The three processes involved in the covering of a denuded surface by new epithelium are:

migration of cells
proliferation
differentiation

While these follow each other in sequence, there is a considerable degree of overlap.

Migration.   In considering the question of how and why epithelial cells can move over a raw surface and, in this way, contribute to its covering, it might be profitable instead to ask why it is that normal epithelial cells do not behave in this fashion. Data derived from cell culture studies suggest that a factor which might be important is '**contact inhibition**'. When a monolayer of cells is grown on a surface, the initial cell colony proliferates and the cells spread over the surface. Once the growing cells come into contact with other cells which have been seeded onto the surface, both cell movement and cell proliferation cease. In any wound the epithelial cells at its edge have no neighbours on one side and thus loss of normal contact inhibition occurs, with the result that the cells spread across the raw surface until cell-to-cell contact is restored. In addition to this loss of normal restraints on migration, it is possible that some positive stimulus to cell movement may also play a part. Within a few hours of wounding, a glycoprotein known as **fibronectin** appears on the raw surface. In cell culture systems this molecule is known to have significant effects on adhesion between cells and various substrates and in addition can be shown to promote migration.

Epithelial cell proliferation. There are two theoretical models, each with some evidence to support them, that can be considered in relation to the genesis and control of epithelial proliferation in wound healing. First, it can be postulated that the increase in cell division occurs as the result of a **loss of some normal restraining function** that controls the rate of cell turnover and mitosis in labile cells and for the most part represses cell division in postnatal life in stable cells.

It has been suggested that such a suppression of normal mitotic activity is mediated by a group of substances which have been extracted, but not purified, from a number of cell types of which the epidermis is one. These substances, which appear to be glycoproteins, have been called **chalones** — a term derived from the Greek *chalinoeion* which means to 'bridle' or 'restrain'. In this model it is postulated that normal cell numbers are maintained as a result of the secretion of chalones from differentiated cells, the result being a damping down of division in the stem cell population. When, for example, epidermal cells become effete and keratinized and are shed, the chalone level would fall slightly and new cells would be recruited as a result of the restraint on stem cell division being decreased. If cell loss on a large scale occurs, as in an open wound, there would be a sudden marked drop in local chalone concentrations and a corresponding wave of mitotic activity (Fig. 8.3) until the cell mass had been restored. The

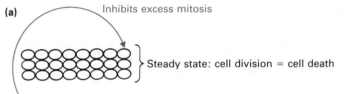

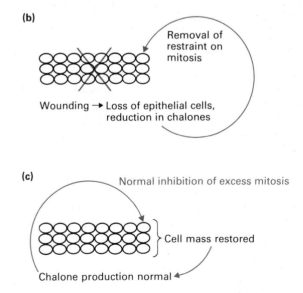

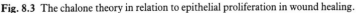

Fig. 8.3 The chalone theory in relation to epithelial proliferation in wound healing.

chalone theory is an attractive one and there is a certain amount of experimental evidence which can be interpreted as being in support of it. However, much work remains to be done before complete acceptance has been earned and, for the present, it seems safer to apply the Scottish verdict of 'not proven'.

The mirror image of the chalone theory is that cell turnover is controlled by factors which directly **stimulate** cell division. A number of such factors have now been described, though, since most of our knowledge of these is derived from cell culture systems, their role in vivo is still undefined. An **epidermal growth factor** has been identified and characterized. This substance, which was first identified in the salivary glands of mice, bears a strong resemblance to human urogastrone. It accelerates the eruption of incisor teeth and eye opening in newborn mice and has been shown to stimulate cell division in human epidermis kept in cell culture and in vivo. It has also been shown to promote keratinization and to aid in the migration of epidermal cells. It exists as a precursor, complexed with protein, from which it is released through the action of arginine esterase, which also releases other active peptides that have a role in the reaction to tissue injury.

Other substances which are released in the course of the inflammatory reaction following injury may also have a role to play in repair. This certainly appears to be the case with prostaglandins of the E series, which can be shown to increase DNA synthesis in the epidermis in a number of model systems.

The formation of new vessels and fibrous tissue

The invasion of fibrin clot, dead tissue or inflammatory exudate by macrophages and granulation tissue capillaries takes place quite rapidly. The new vessels appear within the first week and can grow into the area which is to be repaired at rates of between 0.1 and 0.6 mm/day. They first appear as solid buds of endothelial cells which grow out from the intact capillaries at the wound edges as a result of mitotic division of endothelium in these parent vessels. As the solid buds push in towards the centre of the wound, the cells about 0.5 mm proximal to the tip of the bud also undergo mitosis and join with each other to form loops. Within a few hours of the formation of such loops, the cords of cells acquire a lumen and blood begins to flow through the new capillaries, though they are very leaky and thus tend to be surrounded by blood cells which have escaped. The mechanisms controlling the ingrowth of these new capillaries and their dying back later once well formed scar tissue is present are not understood. Many substances have been suggested as possibly playing the role of stimulator of endothelial growth and attractant for the buds of endothelium thus formed. These include compounds released by macrophages, heparin derived from the mast cell, and metabolic products resulting from the low oxygen tension within the wound centre. It seems likely that the process is a multifactorial one.

The formation first of granulation tissue and then of scar tissue is preceded by changes in the extracellular matrix of the wounded area. Within a short time of wounding, the content of fibronectin within the damaged area increases sharply. The fibronectins are a group of structurally related large glycoprotein molecules. One type exists in the plasma and other body fluids in soluble form, while another insoluble variety exists on the surface of cells. Numerous biological functions have been attributed to the fibronectins, though it is fair to say that most of our knowledge is derived from studies carried out using ex vivo systems. They appear able to promote cell–cell aggregation, they promote cell spreading on surfaces and mediate adhesion of many cell types to various underlying substrata, they promote microfilament organization within cells, stimulate particle clearance by phagocytic cells, and bind to a large number of macromolecules including fibrin.

Since the accumulation of fibronectin within wounds precedes the proliferation of fibroblasts, it has been suggested that, in addition to contributing to the bulk of the fibrin clot, fibronectin may stimulate the migration into the wound of macrophages, fibroblasts and, as stated earlier, epithelial cells. This could be brought about by the provision of areas of preferential cell adhesion compared with the surrounding matrix. Since it can also act as an opsonin, fibronectin might help to promote the phagocytosis of denatured collagen and other matrix proteins within the wound.

The origin of the **fibroblasts** which play such a dominant role in the formation of scar tissue is still somewhat controversial. At various times it has been suggested that they are derived from resting cells which have been stimulated to proliferate and to secrete procollagen, from undifferentiated mesenchymal stem cells, or from mononuclear cells which have arrived at the site of tissue damage via the bloodstream. The last of these seems unlikely to be correct since irradiation of the bone marrow does not suppress the formation of local scar tissue, while local irradiation of a wound does. The chief function of the fibroblast in respect of wound healing is a secretory one; it produces both collagen and the other major constituent of the extracellular connective tissue matrix, the glycosaminoglycans.

The development of **tensile strength** in a wound depends on the **production of collagen.** This is the only protein to contain large amounts of the amino acids hydroxyproline and hydroxylysine. Within 24 hours of wounding, protein-bound hydroxyproline appears within the damaged area and within two or three days a few fine fibrils are also seen to be present, though these lack the dimensions and the 64 nm banding of polymerized collagen. Within three weeks of the production of a surgical wound the tensile strength of the newly formed collagen reaches normal levels, though a considerable amount of remodelling takes place over the ensuing months.

Each type of collagen (there are five) consists of three peptide chains. These are synthesized in the rough endoplasmic reticulum of the fibroblast following translation of the messenger RNA for each chain. They then undergo post-translational hydroxylation of their proline and lysine components and glycosylation of hydroxylysine. Linkage of the chains occurs through the formation of disulphide bonds. The three chains become twisted into a helix and the molecule passes to the Golgi zone within vesicles. Assisted by the microtubules, the soluble procollagen molecules are secreted into the extracellular environment. Solubility is conferred by the presence of an extra peptide. This is removed by a peptidase and the cleaved molecules then spontaneously assemble into fibres which gain tensile strength by cross-linking. The typical 64 nm periodicity of the collagen fibres is due to the assembled molecules having a staggered arrangement. On some occasions the control mechanisms which determine that the amount of collagen formed in the course of wound healing is appropriate appear to be faulty and excess collagen may be formed, leading to the formation of a bulky scar which stands proud of the surrounding surface. Such a scar is known as a **keloid**.

Factors which interfere with the healing process

Foreign bodies or infection

The presence of a foreign body or infection in the wound will increase the intensity and prolong the duration of the inflammatory response to the injury and will inhibit a satisfactory conclusion to the healing process. It is worth remembering that a patient's own dead tissue, such as fragments of necrotic bone (sequestra) in patients with osteitis, can act as a foreign body and keep an inflammatory reaction smouldering on.

Mobility

Excess mobility will, inevitably, lengthen the healing process. This is of particular importance in relation to fracture healing, but operates to some extent in other situations as well.

Nutrition

The state of nutrition of the patient is undoubtedly a potent factor in the healing process. In generalized protein undernutrition the formation of collagen appears to be inhibited to a considerable extent. Sulphydryl-containing amino acids such as **methionine** seem to be particularly important; giving methionine alone can partially offset the effects of protein deficiency on the healing process.

Among the individual dietary factors which could affect healing, **vitamin C** holds a prominent place. It has been known since the seventeenth century that scurvy is associated with poor healing of wounds and fractures. Indeed there are many colourful descriptions of healed wounds, acquired honourably or otherwise years before, breaking down after the onset of scurvy. Once the vitamin had been discovered, it was soon shown that its lack had an inhibiting effect on the production of collagen fibres by fibroblasts and similarly, that local applications of vitamin C accelerated wound healing. Two processes appear to be modulated by the vitamin. The first of these is the hydroxylation of proline within the endoplasmic reticulum of the fibroblast. The second is the formation of chondroitin sulphate in granulation tissue. Lack of vitamin C is associated with a deficient production of galactosamine, an essential component of the chondroitin sulphate. Vitamin A also accelerates the process of wound healing in a variety of species.

The role of **zinc** in wound healing was discovered accidentally. In a study on the effects of certain amino acids on wound healing a phenylalanine analogue which should have impaired wound healing was found instead to accelerate it. Careful study of the analogue revealed that it was contaminated by zinc. Further studies were then carried out on the healing of experimental wounds and showed that zinc did indeed promote healing. Some surgical patients who are debilitated or who have been maintained on parenteral nutrition for a long time have been found to be lacking zinc and this has also been observed in patients suffering from severe burns. Even in a number of healthy young patients who had granulating wounds, the administration of zinc increased the rate of wound healing.

Steroid hormones

There have been many reports that glucocorticoids have an inhibitory effect on healing and the production of fibrous tissue. Indeed, corticosteroids are sometimes given in an attempt to inhibit the process of fibrosis where it is harmful rather than helpful. It is still not clear whether steroids have a direct effect on the healing process or whether they exert an indirect effect by inhibiting the inflammatory response.

The blood supply

Vascularization of damaged tissue is a key process both in inflammation and, more particularly, in repair. In situations where the blood supply is compromised, a quite trivial injury may give rise to tissue damage out of all proportion to the injury. This is often seen in older patients with a poor blood supply to the lower limbs. In such patients a minor injury may lead to the formation of large ulcers which heal only slowly and with great difficulty.

Repair in some Specialized Tissues

Bone

The processes involved in the healing of bone are best studied by observing the local events which follow the fracture of a long bone. The tissue defect in a fracture is first made good by new connective tissue in a manner analogous to that seen in the healing of large open wounds. However, important differences are then imposed on the basic model of healing. These differences are induced by the need for mechanical and weight-bearing efficiency of a high order and are brought about by specialized cells — the **osteoblasts** which lay down seams of uncalcified new bone (osteoid) and **osteoclasts**, a variety of multinucleated macrophage which resorb bone and thus are responsible for remodelling of new bone formed in the course of fracture healing.

Stages in fracture healing (Fig. 8.4)

1. When a bone is fractured, tearing of blood vessels takes place and haemorrhage ensues, the defect between the fractured ends being filled with clotted blood.
2. The injury elicits an acute inflammatory reaction. The combined presence of blood clot and inflammatory oedema causes some loosening of the periosteal attachment to the surface of the bone; this results in a fusiform swelling at the fracture site.
3. Macrophages invade the blood clot and begin the normal process of demolition. This is followed by the ingrowth of granulation tissue capillaries. After about four days the vascular granulation tissue has completely replaced the blood clot and extends upwards and downwards within the marrow cavity for a considerable distance from the fracture line. Within this mass of granulation tissue small groups of cartilage cells are forming.
4. Some islands of cartilage now appear, chiefly on the periosteal aspect. The fractured ends are now united by a sleeve of vascular

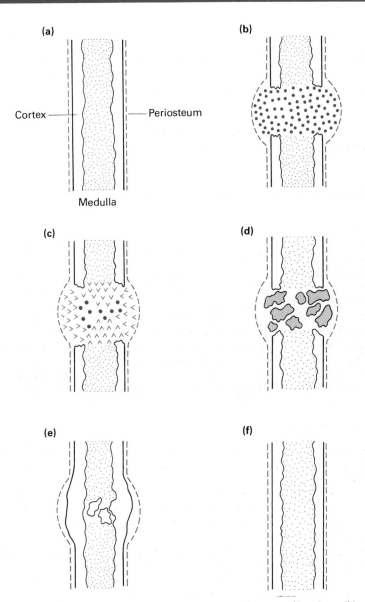

Fig. 8.4 Stages in the healing of fractures in long bones. (a) Anatomy of long bone. (b) Fracture leads to bleeding from severed vessels. Blood clot accumulates in the gap and elevation of the periosteum occurs. This is followed by a brisk inflammatory reaction. (c) Granulation tissue is formed. (d) Osteoid and cartilage appear. This is known as the 'provisional callus'. (e) The callus is replaced by new bone. The ends are now firmly united. (f) The new lamellar bone is remodelled.

granulation tissue and cartilage, the whole having a fusiform shape. This material is known as the '**provisional callus**'. It is fairly firm but still pliable and adequate immobilization of the fractured bone is of prime importance at this stage if the provisional callus is to be replaced by true bone.

5. At the end of the first week some calcium is deposited in the islands of cartilage and the new osteoblasts begin to produce seams of osteoid which traverse the callus. Most of this new bone formation up to this stage has been subperiosteal, but now endochondral ossification becomes established and this adds considerably to the bulk of new bone formed. The callus becomes calcified and eventually the fractured ends of bone are united by a rather irregularly shaped bony callus.

At this stage, however, there is excess bone both within the marrow cavity and subperiosteally. Because of the latter, the site of the union is irregular and there is a distinct swelling at the fracture site. Most of the new bone is **woven** rather than **lamellar** bone, i.e. the collagen fibres in the osteoid seams are arranged apparently haphazardly in short bundles and lack the 'onionskin' lamellar pattern of normal bone arranged in Haversian systems.

6. Remodelling of the bony callus now takes place as a result of the resorptive action of osteoclasts. The marrow cavity is restored to its normal dimensions and the excess cortical bone lying beneath the periosteum is gradually smoothed away, leaving a normal outline. By five weeks an almost new cortex,thicker and as dense as the old, has been formed, and by seven weeks the structure of the fractured bone has almost completely returned to normal. The direction of mechanical thrust in the bone is an important factor in controlling the remodelling process, and if the ends of the fractured bone are not in good alignment the remodelling may be less than perfect and a lumpy, rather irregular site of union may result.

Abnormalities of fracture healing

Any of the factors listed earlier which interfere with healing can cause delay in the union of a fracture. Those that have a special relevance are:

movement of the separated bone ends
a poor blood supply
infection

Occasionally where there has been excessive movement at the fracture site the union will consist of fibrous tissue only rather than bone; this can be replaced by bone only with extreme slowness.

Nervous tissue

With the possible exception of the granular layer of the cerebellum, mitotic activity ceases in the nervous system once neuronal differentiation has been achieved. As in the case of cardiac muscle, this places the mature nervous system at a striking disadvantage in respect of healing and regeneration as compared with most other tissues, and regeneration can be accomplished only by the regrowth and reorganization of neuronal processes.

Central nervous system

Most neurones cannot be replaced once lost, though there is some evidence to suggest that regeneration can take place in the hypothalamic–neurohypophyseal system. In contrast to the peripheral nervous system, where injury is not associated with any marked tendency towards scarring, necrosis within the central nervous system elicits the proliferation of glial cells and the formation of glial fibres which, together with the ingrowth of capillaries, may constitute a physical barrier to the regeneration of new neuronal fibres.

Peripheral nerves

When an axon is severed the nerve cell shows chromatolysis, i.e. it swells and the Nissl granules (which represent zones of the endoplasmic reticulum studded with many ribosomes) disappear. The axon swells and becomes irregular and its lipid-rich myelin sheath splits and later breaks up. The surrounding Schwann cells proliferate and accumulate some of the lipid released from the damaged myelin.

Soon new neurofibrils start to sprout from the proximal end of the severed axon and invaginate the Schwann cells, which act as a guide or template for the new fibrils. These neurofibrils push their way down through the Schwann cells at a rate of about 1 mm/day. Eventually they may reach the appropriate end organ and, with the reforming of their myelin sheaths as a result of the secretory activity of Schwann cells, some degree of functional recovery is possible. In some instances neurofibril sprouting takes place, but the fibres do not grow down pre-existing endoneurial channels, growing instead in an undirected fashion. The end result may be a tangle of new nerve fibres growing in a mass of fibrous tissue, the whole being called a **traumatic neuroma**.

Chapter 9

The Natural History of Acute Inflammation II: Chronicity

If an inflammatory process lasts for months or years, it must, ipso facto, be termed **chronic**. Many important and common diseases are expressions of chronic inflammation. They are diverse in their origins and in their manifestations, but all share certain histological characters which, in themselves, are markers of a long-lasting process.

The difficulties in classification due to the heterogeneity of chronic inflammatory processes may be slightly eased by considering them as members of three major groups. These are:

1. Conditions in which there has been a significant phase of acute inflammation, e.g. chronic osteomyelitis
2. Conditions where the tissue damage has been accomplished by the entry into the host tissues of **non-living** foreign material. Such irritants can persist within the tissue for a very long time. The inflammatory response elicited is dominated by the macrophage and by evidence of repair, e.g. silicosis.
3. Conditions in which the acute inflammatory phase is short-lived and mild, and the process is predestined by the nature of the injury to be chronic. The lesions in this group are also characterized by the focal accumulation of macrophages and lymphocytes. Necrosis of a greater or lesser degree may be associated with the macrophage aggregates and there may be extensive scarring. Cell-mediated immune reactions play a significant role in the pathogenesis of this group of diseases, which includes such important conditions as tuberculosis and leprosy.

The rather special type of reaction mentioned in the second and third groups is termed **granulomatous inflammation**. It is dealt with in some detail in Chapters 14 and 15 and will not be considered further here.

Chronic Inflammation Occurring as a Complication of an Acute Inflammatory Process (Non-specific Chronic Inflammation)

Complete healing of an acute inflammatory process occurs only when both the initial cause and any factors likely to prolong the inflammatory reaction are removed. The exudate formed in the course of the reaction must be demolished and, if suppuration has taken place deep within the tissue, the resulting pus must be drained adequately. A good blood supply to the affected area is also mandatory. If all these conditions are not met then a type of pathological process is likely to develop in which there is a mixed morphological picture characterized by:

1. Evidence of persisting acute inflammation, not infrequently associated with some tissue necrosis
2. Evidence of attempts at demolition of the inflammatory exudate and removal of dead tissue in the form of a cell infiltrate in which large numbers of macrophages are seen
3. Evidence of repair with the formation of granulation tissue and scar tissue. The neighbouring arteries frequently show severe narrowing of their lumina as a result of proliferation of connective tissue in their intimal layers. This is known as **endarteritis obliterans.**
4. Evidence of some degree of regeneration
5. The presence of numerous lymphocytes and plasma cells. In inflammatory processes known to be mediated by immune reactions this is easily understood, though the role of the lymphocyte and plasma cell are less easy to fathom in other instances.

The plasma cell

The plasma cell is a reliable marker of chronicity in inflammatory reactions. It measures 10 to 12 μm in diameter and has a single, slightly eccentrically placed nucleus in which the chromatin appears to be fragmented and concentrated at the nuclear membrane, giving a clock-face or cartwheel appearance. There is a prominent perinuclear halo which is the site of the Golgi apparatus. In sections stained with haematoxylin and eosin, the cytoplasm is markedly basophilic, an expression of the abundant secretion of RNA. This can be confirmed by treating sections with pyronin which stains the RNA red. Electron microscopically the structure mirrors the predominant secretory function of the plasma cell, much rough endoplasmic reticulum and a prominent Golgi apparatus being present.

The role of the plasma cell is to produce specific immunoglobulin (see Chapter 10); this can be confirmed using the appropriate fluorescein or peroxidase-linked antibodies which bind to the immunoglobulin in the plasma cell cytoplasm.

Some examples of non-specific chronic inflammation

Chronic osteitis

Acute osteitis occurs most often in children and usually involves the metaphysis of one of the long bones. Possibly because of the rather curious arrangement of the blood vessels in these areas, pyogenic microorganisms may localize here in the course of a bacteraemia. The presence of organisms such as *Staphylococcus aureus* elicits the usual acute inflammatory response, but the combination of the action of the necrotizing exotoxins secreted by the organisms and the rigid, unyielding nature of the bony tissue leads rapidly to necrosis and the accumulation of pus. This pus tends to track under the periosteum. The lifting away of the periosteum from the underlying bone further compromises the blood supply of the bone and may lead to more necrosis.

Early diagnosis and treatment can be of great benefit. If the presence of acute osteitis is recognized before there is any significant degree of pus formation, the administration of large doses of appropriate antibiotics may suffice to abort the inflammatory process. Once suppuration has occurred it is essential that the pus be drained and the increased tension within the bone relieved. If this is not done, extensive bone necrosis may follow and, ultimately, the dead bone may become separated from the viable neighbouring tissue to form what is known as a **sequestrum.**

This dead bone behaves as a foreign body and serves to keep the inflammatory process alight. Any pus formed within the bones may rupture through the periosteum and reach the skin surfaces through a number of sinus tracks which may heal and reopen many times in the course of the disease.

Meanwhile the persistence of the exudate and the presence of necrotic bone stimulates the formation of new bone by the periosteum. This new bone, known as the **involucrum,** surrounds portions of dead bone in a sleeve-like fashion. Since the inflammatory process still continues within the tissue deep to the involucrum, this too may become eroded and provide a passage for the discharge of deep-lying pus through a series of sinuses. Chronic osteitis, though now happily rather rare, is a classical example of an acute inflammatory reaction which becomes chronic through inadequacy of drainage of pus and the long-continued presence of foreign material in the form of the sequestrum.

Impaired drainage of normal secretions

It is wrong to think of adequate drainage in relation to chronic inflammation as applying only to removal of exudate. It is equally important for the normal flow of secretion from an organ to be maintained. Where such flow becomes completely or partially obstructed, the chances of an inflammatory process becoming chronic are greatly enhanced.

Three sites where chronic inflammation is not infrequently seen, and where such obstruction to normal flow probably plays a vital part, are the kidney, the pancreas and the salivary glands. Where there is actively secreting acinar tissue, as in the latter two, and the presence of chronic inflammation is associated with obstruction of the duct system, a marked degree of acinar atrophy is often seen.

Chronic pyelonephritis

Chronic pyelonephritis, a chronic inflammatory condition involving the renal pelvis as well as the parenchymal tissue, is common, being found to be present in some degree in about 2% of all autopsies on middle-aged and elderly adults. In its more severe form it constitutes an important cause of chronic renal failure and systemic hypertension. The chronic inflammation may follow one or more clinically obvious episodes of acute pyelonephritis, but in some cases it may be insidious in its origin.

Once the process has become chronic, it may be impossible to isolate pathogenic microorganisms from either the urine or the renal tissue. Nevertheless, it is likely that most cases are due to bacterial infection. There is no general agreement as to the routes by which invading organisms reach the kidney. The infections may be blood-borne, retrograde from the lower urinary tract, or may occur via the lymphatics. Most cases are associated with some obstruction to the normal outflow of urine. This may be due to a structural abnormality (e.g. the abnormal presence of valves at the vesico-urethral junction) or to vesico-ureteric reflux of urine. The importance of normal flow through the ureter in preventing infections of the upper urinary tract is shown by the frequent occurrence of acute pyelonephritis during pregnancy when the ureters are often partially obstructed and hence dilated.

In making the diagnosis of chronic pyelonephritis, macroscopic examination is often more reliable than microscopic. The kidneys are coarsely scarred, the scars often being U-shaped or 'saddle-shaped'. The scarring may lead to extreme shrinkage and distortion of the organ. Involvement of the calyces is an integral part of chronic pyelonephritis, and the cortical scars are usually related topographically to a distorted calyx.

On histological examination there is often a marked degree of lymphocytic and plasma cell infiltration in the interstitial tissue and in the subepithelial regions of the pelvis and calyces. Some of the glomeruli are completely replaced by scar tissue, while others show scarring at the periphery of Bowman's capsule. There is patchy loss of tubules. Some of the surviving tubules are enormously dilated and contain eosinophilic, colloid-like material which gives a pseudo-thyroid appearance to these areas. The blood vessels may show changes secondary to hypertension.

Chronic ulcerative colitis

This is a disease of unknown aetiology which is characterized clinically by bouts of dysentery (frequent passage of stools containing blood, pus and mucus). Ulcerative colitis may occur in all age groups. Occasionally it starts explosively and may pursue an acute fulminating course. Remissions are frequent and may last for long periods. Often the disease is insidious in its onset and chronic from the beginning.

The progress of the disease, in terms of structural changes in the tissues, can be studied by examining biopsies taken at sigmoidoscopy or colonoscopy. The earliest change is a marked degree of dilatation of blood vessels in the lamina propria of the rectal mucosa. This is followed by the appearance of an acute inflammatory cell infiltrate in the lamina propria and patchy loss of the columnar epithelium which lines the rectal and colonic wall. On sigmoidoscopic examination, the inflamed bowel wall is reddened and velvety in appearance and tiny ulcers may be noted.

The process then spreads to involve the crypts of Lieberkühn. Neutrophils collect within the crypt lumina and there may be loss of part or all of the epithelial lining of the affected crypt, this lesion being known as a **crypt abscess**. The epithelial cell destruction is probably mediated by neutrophil-derived lysosomal enzymes. Loss of the epithelial lining of the bowel wall may become quite extensive. The floor of such ulcerated areas can be seen to consist of inflamed granulation tissue which may stand proud of the surrounding surface in a polypoid manner. In other areas the lost epithelium is replaced by regenerated epithelium, but this is often less differentiated than normal.

In severe, long-standing cases the muscularis mucosae becomes thicker than normal and the inflammatory process may spread through it to involve the submucosal tissues. Eventually there may be a considerable degree of shortening of the colon, with loss of the normal pattern of taeniae coli. In long-standing colitis (more than 10 years) there is an enhanced risk of developing rectal or colonic carcinoma.

Chapter 10

The Immune System

It has been known for many centuries that a non-fatal attack of certain infectious diseases results in a diminution of the individual's susceptibility to that disease in the future. This degree of increased resistance against a specific infectious agent is known as **acquired specific immunity.** This phenomenon is the basis of many successful **immunization** programmes, some of which have led to the virtual eradication of some highly lethal infectious diseases such as smallpox.

While this has clearly been beneficial, the biological implications of acquired specific immunity are much more far-reaching. In most vertebrates there exists a system which is capable of :

1. **Recognition** of what is foreign to the host, i.e. the ability to distinguish between **self** and **non-self**
2. Mounting a highly **specific** response to what is recognized as foreign
3. **Memory**. The existence of memory in the immune system can be inferred since a **subsequent encounter** with what has previously been recognized as foreign evokes a response which is both greater in degree and much faster than that occurring on a **first encounter**.

Terminology

Some conceptual difficulties arise when we use the word **immunity** to cover the whole range of activities of the immune system since its commonly accepted meaning is of a state in which there is absolute or relative freedom from some harmful condition. There is no doubt that the altered reactivity of a host following an encounter with some foreign species is, on the whole, extremely beneficial to the host in that it constitutes a powerful defence against the effects of pathogenic microorganisms. However, the same mechanisms which operate to protect the host can be turned against it and cause serious damage to tissues. In this case, despite the dictum of Humpty Dumpty who declared that '**a word means precisely what I choose it to mean, neither more nor less**', the use of the word **immunity** seems less appropriate. Those events mediated through the immune system which are harmful to the host clearly need to be classified in some other way; this problem will be explored in later chapters.

Antigens

The genesis of an immune response requires contact of those cellular elements making up the immune system with a molecule which can be recognized as being of the 'non-self' variety. Those substances which are capable of inducing a specific response from these cellular elements are known as **antigens**. They are usually protein, polypeptide or polysaccharide in nature. The chemical sites on the cells of the immune system or on the specific globulins (antibodies) that are responsible for **recognition** of foreign chemical species are very small and will only bind to a few amino acids or sugar residues. This means that the part of an antigen eliciting specific recognition is correspondingly small. Most antigens in fact consist of many such areas, which are called determinants or **epitopes**. Each of these is capable of evoking a specific response.

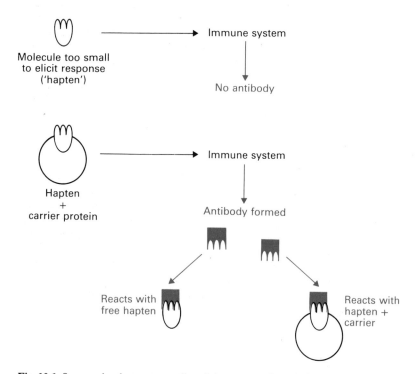

Fig. 10.1 Some molecules are too small to elicit a response from the immune system. Such molecules can bind to a carrier protein, which together can produce an immune response in which the endogenic determinant is the small molecule. Such small molecules are known as 'haptens'.

The ability of a chemical species to function as an antigen is related, in part, to its size. Most antigens have a molecular weight in excess of 10 000 and about 2500 seems to be the limit below which foreign substances cannot elicit a response on the part of the immune system. However, it is possible for certain small molecules, which cannot act as antigens by themselves, to bind to a carrier, usually a protein, and the complex formed by such binding can produce an immune response in which the antigenic determinant is the small 'passenger' molecule. These small molecules are known as **haptens**. The antibodies formed in response to the hapten/carrier complex can react specifically in solution with the free hapten (e.g. in sensitivity reactions to certain drugs) (Fig. 10.1).

Because of the 'foreignness' inherent in the concept of antigens, it is tempting to view them as chemical species derived entirely from the environment (**exogenous**). It is true that such antigens are involved in a wide spectrum of human diseases, including all infections and many hypersensitivity reactions such as asthma and hay fever. However, many antigens exist which are 'native' to the host; these **endogenous** antigens play an important part in many of the functions of the immune system both in health and disease. They may be classified as:

heterologous
autologous
homologous (iso-antigens)

Heterologous antigens

These are antigens which are common to species which are unrelated phylogenetically. The existence of such antigens can lead to curious cross-reactions which may be important in the genesis of certain diseases. One such example is the cross-reactivity that exists between the M proteins of certain strains of β-haemolytic *Streptococcus pyogenes* and determinants present in heart muscle and many other human tissues. Since there is a known association between infections with these streptococcal strains and acute rheumatic fever, cross-reactivity between the bacterial and human antigens has been implicated in the pathogenesis of this disease, though absolute proof that this is the mechanism responsible is still lacking.

Autologous antigens

These are the host's own normal constituents and under most circumstances are recognized as '**self**'. As a result of this they do not elicit an immune response from the host, a state which is known as

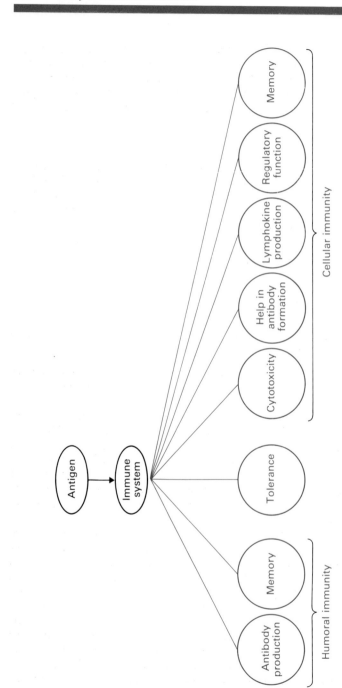

Fig. 10.2 The consequences of an encounter between antigen and host.

tolerance. There is a number of ways in which this state of tolerance can be broken down (see p. 169) and immune reactions can be mounted against one or more of the native tissue constituents. The disorders associated with this partial breakdown in the ability to distinguish between 'self' and 'non-self' are known as autoimmune diseases.

Homologous antigens

These molecules, also known as **iso-antigens**, are the determinants which distinguish the tissue components of one **individual** from another. Their expression is genetically controlled, as can be seen from the mode of inheritance of one important group of such antigens — the ABO blood group system.

Consequences of an Encounter Between Host and Antigen (Fig. 10.2)

The introduction of an antigen into a host may give rise to one or more of three basic reactions:

1. **Antibody formation**, i.e. the production of proteins of the globulin series which possess the ability to bind specifically to the antigenic determinant which has been introduced. The antibodies are produced by **plasma cells**, the fully differentiated form of one of the two major classes of lymphocytes. The essential role of antibodies in **defence** of the host is in defence against infections by extracellular, pathogenic microorganisms such as staphylococci and streptococci. In this type of response, known as the **humoral** type, bacterial toxins may be neutralized, complement-mediated cell lysis brought about, phagocytosis assisted through specific opsonization, and the entry of viruses to certain cells prevented.

2. The **clonal proliferation** of another class of lymphocytes which have a wide range of biological activities. These include the ability directly to lyse foreign cells, cells whose antigenic makeup has been modified by virus infections and certain tumour cells, and to release a range of **non-antigen specific** soluble products (known as **lymphokines**), some of which activate macrophages and others either 'help' or 'suppress' the function of one or both of the lymphocyte classes. The antigen-induced proliferation of this class of lymphocyte and the range of activities carried out by them is known as **cell-mediated immunity**, and insofar as defence against infection is concerned they are most effective against organisms which grow intracellularly such as viruses,

certain bacteria (e.g. the organisms responsible for tuberculosis and leprosy) and fungi.

3. The induction of a state of **specific tolerance** to a given antigen. This can occur when the antigen is introduced to the host during fetal or very early neonatal life. A second exposure to such an antigen is not followed by antibody production or proliferation of sensitized lymphocytes.

The Cellular Basis of Immune Reactions

In the previous section it has been stated that the response of the elements of the immune system following exposure to foreign molecules, to which the host is not tolerant, has a **dual nature**, expressed either by the production of immunoglobulins which react specifically with the antigen (**antibodies**) or by the proliferation of lymphocytes which have a variety of other functions, some of which have been listed above, or by both of these. The effector cell line in both reactions is the small lymphocyte; when an animal such as a rat is depleted of its small lymphocytes by repeated drainage of the thoracic duct, both sets of functions are lost.

Lymphocyte classes — T and B cells

The existence of functions as different as the production of specific antibody globulins on the one hand and the wide range of activities characteristic of cell-mediated immunity on the other suggested that these might be carried out by at least two distinct lines of small lymphocytes. The truth of this proposition began to emerge with the studies carried out by Miller in the mid-sixties on the role of the thymus, which up to that time had been regarded as a mysterious organ with no defined purpose. Miller found that if the thymus of a mouse was removed in the neonatal period the following events occurred:

1. There was a fall in the number of circulating lymphocytes.
2. The ability to reject a tissue graft from a different strain of the same species (an allogeneic graft) was lost.
3. There was a reduction in the antibody response to some antigens.
4. After three or four months the animals died of a wasting disease, probably related to an inability to resist infection since neonatally thymectomized animals kept under germ-free conditions did not succumb to this disorder.
5. They became particularly susceptible to virus infections.
6. The ability to mount an unimpaired antibody response to certain

antigens was retained and their plasma concentrations of immuno-globulins were not altered.

These data can be interpreted in the light of a series of elegant experiments in which immunological competence (e.g. the ability to reject allogeneic grafts) is first destroyed and then restored. For instance, if immunological competence is destroyed in an adult mouse by irradiation of the bone marrow it can be restored by transfer of bone marrow cells from an animal of the same species. If, in addition to irradiation of the bone marrow, the thymus is also removed, immunological competence cannot be restored by a transfusion of bone marrow cells, though it can be by a transfusion of adult spleen or lymph node cells. Thus the role of the thymus appears to be in the **processing** of a population of small lymphocytes derived from the bone marrow. In the absence of the thymus these cells cannot develop their normal range of functions. Small lymphocytes processed in this way are known as **T lymphocytes** or thymus-derived cells (Fig. 10.3).

While T cells clearly have a wide range of activities, they **cannot produce antibody**. Another lymphocyte population is the precursor for the mature, antibody-producing cell or **plasma cell**. The retention of the ability to produce antibody responses to certain antigens following neonatal thymectomy suggests that the bone marrow stem cells destined to become plasma cells and produce immunoglobulin are processed in some place other than the thymus. The only species in which such an organ has been identified with certainty is the chicken, in which there is a localized mass of lymphoid tissue in relation to an outpouching of the cloaca. This is known as the bursa of Fabricius and the small lymphocytes which are coded to transform into antibody-producing plasma cells on encountering the appropriate antigen are called **bursa-derived** or **B lymphocytes** (Fig. 10.3). It is still uncertain as to what tissues constitute the homologue in mammals of the bursa of Fabricius, but it has been suggested that the processing of B cell precursors takes place in the **gut-associated lymphoid tissue**, i.e. Peyer's patches in the intestine, pharyngeal tonsil, etc. However, recent studies suggest that the bone marrow is a more likely candidate.

T cell functions

Insofar as defence against infection is concerned, T cells function in two ways. On their own they act against those pathogens which can survive and grow intracellularly. In cooperation with B cells and with cells which present antigens to the immune system, they play a vital part in the up- or down-regulation of the immune response. In the former case the subset of T lymphocytes responsible is the **T helper cell** and in the

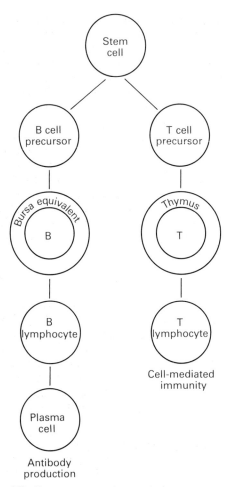

Fig. 10.3 The B and T cell compartments of the immune system.

latter the **T suppressor cell**. These subsets can be distinguished from each other by their possession of different antigens which can be shown to react with specific antibody globulins.

T lymphocytes also play an important part in the rejection of allogeneic grafts. There is a considerable amount of evidence that T cells may also recognize certain tumour cells as non-self and destroy them in the same way as the cells of an incompatible graft. This variety of **surveillance** may also serve to suppress cells which have not undergone malignant transformation but may have been altered by viruses or by spontaneous mutation.

T cells are responsible for a variety of inflammatory response occurring after second and subsequent exposures to certain antigens or haptens. The skin reactions, characterized by local redness and swelling occurring 24 to 48 hours after intradermal injection of antigens derived, for example, from the organisms responsible for tuberculosis or leprosy, are the archetype of this variety of T cell activity. This is known as **delayed hypersensitivity**, in contrast with the virtually immediate reactions due to antibody which, in sensitized subjects, may follow second and subsequent exposure to certain antigens. Delayed hypersensitivity can only be transferred from sensitized to normal individuals if lymphocytes are transferred, while the immediate type of hypersensitivity can be transferred via the medium of cell-free serum. While delayed hypersensitivity was originally defined in terms of the skin reactions described above, the process, of which the skin lesion is only one expression, plays an important part in the production of many serious pathological lesions, such as those of tuberculosis.

Mode of action of the T cell

The functions outlined above are carried out either through the medium of **cell-to-cell contact**, in the course of which allogeneic graft cells or transformed cells are destroyed by the T cells, or through the **synthesis** and **secretion** of a number of active compounds known as **lymphokines**. These are concerned primarily with mediating interactions between cells: T cells with B cells, and T cells with macrophages. It is worth noting that macrophages can also produce compounds which are capable of modulating the responses of the T cell. Included amongst the lymphokines are:

1. A factor **chemotactic** for macrophages
2. A factor which limits the mobility of the macrophages once it has arrived at the site from which the chemotactic signal was generated (**migration inhibition factor**)
3. A factor which **activates** macrophages and makes possible the intracellular killing of certain organisms. Action of this factor is accompanied by morphological changes in the plasma membrane of the macrophage, which becomes intensely convoluted or 'ruffled'.
4. A factor which increases the permeability of small vessels and makes it easier for macrophages to leave the microcirculation and travel to the point from which the chemotactic signal has been generated (**skin reactive factor**)
5. A factor which is **mitogenic** for T cells
6. A factor which inhibits proliferation of T cells
7. A factor which to a limited degree is capable of lysing certain cell

lines in culture. It has been suggested that this factor may have a role in suppressing tumour growth.

It is possible that the fifth and sixth factors may be related to up- and down-regulation of the immune response.

B cell function

As stated earlier, the B cell operates through the production of antibody, though before the synthesis and secretion of such antibody takes place the small lymphocyte must undergo a series of morphological and functional transformations and mature into the plasma cell. This cell possesses abundant cytoplasm and a well developed rough endoplasmic reticulum in which protein synthesis takes place. On light microscopy of sections stained with haematoxylin and eosin the large amounts of ribonucleic acid being produced are reflected in a marked degree of basophilia in the cytoplasm and there is a prominent Golgi apparatus which appears as a paranuclear clear zone.

Lifespan and circulation of small lymphocytes

The differing immunological roles of the T and B cells are also reflected in their other characteristics. The majority of circulating lymphocytes are T cells (70–80%) and this is likely to be an expression of their long life (a lifespan in man of five to ten years). It is presumably for this reason that thymectomy in adult life does not, as a rule, deprive the subject of immunological competence, since a long-lived population of memory T cells has already been established. B cells have a much shorter life span, though again, it seems likely that there is a fairly long-lived subset of memory B cells.

The differing immunological functions of the two sets of lymphocytes are also mirrored in terms of their relative mobility. The primary role of the B cell is to produce large amounts of specific immunoglobulin which can be discharged into the lymph and thence into the bloodstream from the secondary lymphoid tissue (lymph nodes and spleen) where there are large concentrations of B cells. Some aspects of T cell function require cell-to-cell contact, and lymphokine-mediated T cell/B cell interaction requires relatively close proximity of the interacting cells. Thus the T cell *must* be mobile and able to travel constantly between the blood and the secondary lymphoid tissue where antigens are trapped by macrophages. The bulk of this traffic occurs via the post-capillary venules in the lymph nodes. These venules can be recognized by their high, rather cuboidal endothelium. T cells emigrate via the inter-endothelial cell gaps from the blood into the lymph node

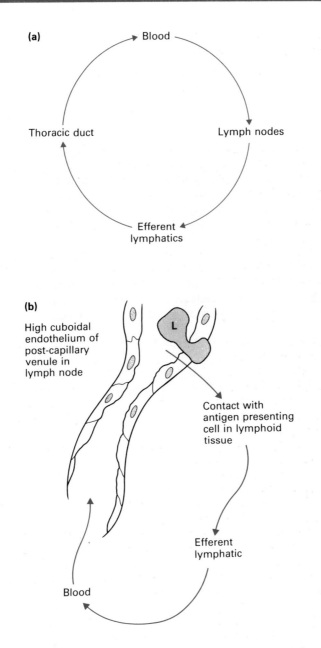

Fig. 10.4 (a) The main pathway for circulation of T lymphocytes. (b) Circulation of lymphocytes (L) within a lymph node.

tissue where they can come into contact with antigens processed by macrophages and other antigen-presenting cells, and thus become stimulated to divide and differentiate (Fig. 10.4).

Distribution of T and B cells within secondary lymphoid tissue

The functional anatomy of a lymph node can best be understood if one recalls that it contains two highly organized circulatory systems — one for blood and one for lymph. For maximum effectiveness of the immune response, the lymph circulation should be so designed as to provide the greatest possible opportunity for presentation of foreign antigens to the T and B cell population. Lymph from the tissues reaches the node via an **afferent** lymphatic which drains into a sinus ensheathing the outer margin of the node. From here the afferent lymph drains past both lymphocytes and the antigen-presenting cells, which either phagocytose or endocytose foreign antigens which require processing before presentation to the lymphocytes. The lymph then passes to the deepest portions of the node where it enters a series of **medullary sinuses** which join to form an **efferent** lymphatic channel.

Within the node the B cells are concentrated within the outer zone or **cortex** (Fig. 10.5). They are arranged in a series of localized aggregates

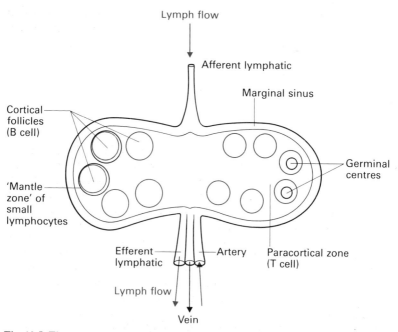

Fig. 10.5 The anatomy of a lymph node.

known as cortical follicles. In an unstimulated node the cortical follicles simply consist of spherical masses of small lymphocytes, but following stimulation their micro-anatomy changes. The centres of the follicles can now be seen to be occupied by numerous large, rather pale cells. Most of these are B cells which have been stimulated to proliferate, but intermingled with them are macrophages and some specialized antigen-presenting cells with long processes known as **dendritic cells.** Surrounding this zone of large, pale cells, which is called a **germinal centre**, is a **mantle** of small, darkly staining lymphocytes also belonging to the B cell series. In due time following antigenic stimulation some of the B cells differentiate into plasma cells. These are usually found in the portions of the node which lie between the medullary sinuses (the **medullary cords**).

The T cells are for the most part confined to a slightly deeper layer of the node known as the **paracortical** zone. Nodes from children with selective T cell deficiencies or from animals which have been thymectomized during the neonatal period show a virtual absence of lymphocytes from the paracortical area. Similarly the induction of a T cell response in animals, for example by grafting of allogeneic skin, will result in an expansion of the paracortical zone in the anatomically appropriate nodes.

The lymph node thus exemplifies a situation in which the two effector cell lines of the immune response are to a considerable extent separated. This separation is also seen in the white pulp of the spleen.

Identification of T and B lymphocytes

There are no morphological differences between lymphocytes of the T and B series. However, these cells possess a number of different surface markers and also respond to different sets of chemical species by polyclonal proliferation. These characteristics make it possible not only to distinguish between the two basic groups, but also to identify T cell subsets such as **helper** and **suppressor** cells. The outstanding feature of the B cell surface is the presence of immunoglobulin, which can be identified either by immunofluorescence or immunoperoxidase techniques using antibodies prepared against these immunoglobulins. Normally each lymphocyte is programmed to make immunoglobulin of only one specificity and it is this immunoglobulin on the B lymphocyte surface which acts as a specific receptor for antigen. T cells in the mouse carry a surface antigen known as **Thy 1**, which is also found on some brain and skin cells, and a set of three surface antigens (each of which can exist in one of two allelic forms) known as **LY 1, 2** and **3**. All of these are expressed on early T cells but with differentiation they tend

Table 10.1 The different properties of B and T lymphocytes.

Characteristic	B cell	T cell
Surface Ig	+	−
Erythrocyte rosetting	−	+
Surface receptor for C3	+	−
Surface receptor for Fc	+	−
Blast transformation induced by concanavalin A or phytohaemagglutinin	−	+
Blast transformation induced by pokeweed or lipopolysaccharide	+	−

to be lost. Most T cells have the interesting property of being able to bind untreated sheep red cells to form small 'rosettes' in vitro.

In addition to their possessing surface components which can be recognized by treating lymphocytes with appropriate antibodies linked to a fluorescent dye, T and B lymphocytes respond to different sets of stimulating agents which cause them to proliferate and become larger and more primitive in appearance (this response is known as **blast transformation**). The different properties of T and B cells are summarized in Table 10.1.

Antibodies

Antibodies can be defined both in operational and chemical terms. In the **operational** sense they are molecules which can bind specifically to the appropriate antigen and in so doing perform a range of tasks of great biological significance, though these are not all necessarily beneficial. Depending on the class of antibody involved, these operations include agglutination and lysis of bacteria (IgM), opsonization of such organisms and initiation of the 'classical' complement pathway through the ability to bind the C1q component of complement avidly (IgG_1), blocking of the entry of microorganisms from the respiratory tract, gut, eyes and urinary tract into the tissues which lie deep to the epithelia which line these areas (IgA), and binding to mast cells and basophils, which can have both helpful effects (e.g. in combating infestations by worms) and very harmful ones in which large amounts of histamine and leukotrienes are liberated from the mast cells, with the production of asthma, urticaria, hay fever and other manifestations of an overreaction to certain classes of antigen (IgE).

From the **chemical** point of view it has been known since the studies of Tiselius and his colleagues in the late 1930s that the antibody activity

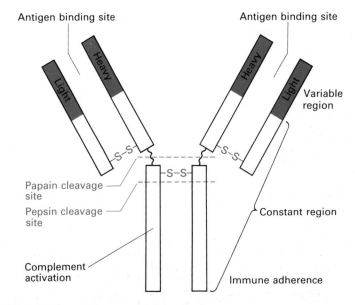

Fig. 10.6 A monomeric immunoglobulin molecule.

of the plasma resides in its **globulin** fraction, i.e. that group of plasma proteins which migrate most slowly on electrophoresis; antibodies are, in fact, also termed **immunoglobulins.**

Cleavage studies of immunoglobulins using various proteolytic enzymes led to the suggestion of a Y-shaped, four-chain model for immunoglobulin structure, which subsequent studies have confirmed. In the monomeric form which is characteristic of three of the five major classes of immunoglobulin, the molecule consists of four polypeptide chains which are held together by disulphide bonds (Fig. 10.6). Two of these chains have a molecular weight of 22 000 and are known as **light chains.** The other two have molecular weights ranging from 55 000 to 72 500 depending on the immunoglobulin class and are called **heavy chains.** Each monomer has a pair of identical heavy chains and a pair of identical light chains. The chemical and biological differences between the five classes of immunoglobulin are due to differences in their heavy chain structure and whether or not they exist as monomers (IgG, IgD, IgE), dimers (IgA) or pentamers (IgM). The heavy chain classes are designated as:

gamma	IgG	delta	IgD
alpha	IgA	epsilon	IgE
mu	IgM		

Two different classes of light chain exist and are known as kappa and lambda. Pairs of one or other of these are found in all five classes of immunoglobulin.

Relationship between structure and function in the immunoglobulin molecule

When a monomeric immunoglobulin molecule such as is illustrated in Fig. 10.6 is treated with the proteolytic enzyme papain, it is cleaved just above the disulphide bridges between the heavy chains and thus splits into three fragments. The two of these that contain the light chains are identical. Each possesses the ability to bind specifically to antigen and is known as the **Fab** (**fragment antigen binding**). When the appropriate antigen is in solution, the union between these fragments and the antigen leads to the formation of a soluble complex and this is due to the fact that binding is **univalent**. The third fragment has no power to bind to antigen, is easily crystallizable and is known as **Fc** (**fragment crystallizable**). It is, however, the site of important biological functions such as **complement activation** and **immune adherence** to receptors on the surface of neutrophils and macrophages. Treatment of an immunoglobulin molecule with another proteolytic enzyme, pepsin, cleaves the molecule below the disulphide bond, as shown in Fig. 10.6, with the production of a divalent $F(ab)_2$ fragment and a dimer consisting of only part of the Fc portion (pFc).

Diversity of antibody in relation to its structure

One of the most remarkable features of the antibody system is that each antibody has a combining site that matches with the epitope with which it binds specifically. Thus many thousand of such combining sites must exist. This diversity of antibodies is the expression of the great variability in the amino acid sequence which exists at the N-terminal or antigen-combining portion of both light and heavy chains; these portions of the chains are known as the **variable** regions. Both light and heavy chains possess units of about 110 amino acids which are known as domains. These portions of the chain are usually folded, the folded loops being bridged by disulphide bonds. When amino acid sequencing is carried out on a monoclonal immunoglobulin such as the proteins produced by myeloma cells, the light chain is shown to have two domains; a variable one at the amino terminal end (V_L) and a constant one (C_L), each occupying about half the length of the chain. The heavy chain also has a variable domain at its amino terminal end (V_H). Since this is about the same length as the variable domain found on light chains, only a quarter of the heavy chain is variable. The remaining three-quarters are divided into three constant domains (C_H1, 2, 3) (four in epsilon chains). To form the combining site, the polypeptide domains in the light and heavy chains are folded into their unique shape by weak non-covalent chemical forces **which are dictated by the amino acid sequences of each variable domain.** Since the amino acid sequence determines the shape of the combining site, it is necessary only to vary this sequence to create a specific antibody, and thus it is easy to conceive how a vast number of antibody molecules can come into being.

The genetic basis of combining site diversity

If we accept that a very large number of different combining sites can exist, does this mean that there is an equally vast array of genes to code for each of the possible amino acid sequences? Strict adherence to the one gene–one polypeptide view would mean just this, but in fact a quite different set of circumstances exists in relation to immunoglobulin chains. For each chain the variable and constant regions are coded for by a different gene. These genes are quite widely separated in the germ cell and are physically translocated and brought together in the course of B cell development. In the mouse it is possible to generate about 1200 variable regions in the kappa light chain and 9600 variable segments of the heavy chain are theoretically possible. The combination of these heavy and light chain variable segments in a single antigen-combining site means that the number of possible combining sites in a mouse system is the product of the number of heavy chain variables and the number of light chain variables, thus yielding the impressive number of 10^7 different combining sites from what is a comparatively small number of genes through the process of translocation of variable region genes during lymphocyte differentiation.

Immunoglobulin classes

Immunoglobulin G (IgG)

IgG is, in quantitative terms, the most important of the five main immunoglobulin classes, making up about 70–80% of plasma immunoglobulin. In structure it is monomeric and has the four-chain structure described above. It diffuses readily into the extravascular compartment and thus plays an important part in the neutralization of toxins and in opsonization of bacteria, though in order to accomplish this it is necessary for more than one IgG molecule to bind to a small area on the bacterial cell wall so that multiple Fc fragments may be presented to the receptors on phagocytic cells. The coating of certain target cells with IgG can also attract cells of the lymphoid system which have Fc receptors but which are not specifically sensitized to any epitope on the target. These cells can kill the antibody-coated targets and are known as **K** or **killer cells.**

Two molecules of IgG bound closely together on an antigenic surface can activate complement by the allosteric rearrangement of part of the Fc fragment. This particular form of expression of biological activity varies within the IgG class; variations in the C_H2 region and four subclasses of IgG have so far been identified. IgG_1 and IgG_3 molecules readily activate complement when bound to antigen; IgG_2 antibodies are less efficient in this respect, and IgG_4 does not activate complement at all.

Of all the immunoglobulins, only IgG can cross the placental barrier and thus is the most important of the antibody classes in protecting newborn infants against infections.

Immunoglobulin A (IgA)

IgA appears selectively in the seromucous secretions of the gastrointestinal and respiratory tracts, and in tears, sweat, bile and breast milk.

Basically it has the same four-chain structure as IgG, but the heavy chains have a higher molecular weight. IgA is dimerized by linkage to a small cysteine-rich protein known as the **J-chain** within the plasma cell where it is synthesized. This dimer is then released into the lamina propria of the gut mucosa or the subepithelial tissues of the respiratory tract and then transported across the surface epithelium into the lumen. While in transit across the epithelium the IgA becomes stabilized against proteolysis by attaching to a peptide known as the **secretory component**, which is secreted by the epithelial cells. The fact that dimerization takes place **within** the plasma cells ensures against the formation of dimers of **mixed specificity**, such as might occur if the process took place in the lamina propria. This avoids dilution of the antigen-combining efficiency of the molecule.

IgA is believed to act by inhibiting the adherence of coated microorganisms to mucosal surfaces and thus preventing them from entering the tissues. Both bacteria and viruses may be affected in this way; oral polio vaccines probably induce immunity by sensitizing the IgA-producing plasma cells in the mucosa of the gut. The role of the relatively large amounts of **monomeric IgA** in the plasma is still not clear.

Immunoglobulin M (IgM)

IgM is the largest of the immunoglobulins, with a molecular weight of 900 000. It consists of five basic four-chain units joined together to form a 20-chain molecule which is held together by disulphide bonds between the five Fc fragments and a J-chain identical with that involved in the dimerization of IgA. The mu chain of IgM is the heaviest of all the immunoglobulin chains and about 10% of its weight is accounted for by carbohydrate. Because of its pentameric structure, IgM has ten potential antigen-combining sites, but in practice, perhaps because of some inherent rigidity in the pentamer, only five of these are usually involved in antigen binding at any one time. The possession of multiple binding sites gives IgM the ability to bind with great strength to antigenic surfaces on which there is a repetitive epitope pattern.

IgM antibodies are the first ones formed after immunization. Once IgG synthesis starts, the level of IgM falls. When antibodies are made which react with the antigen-combining sites on IgM (anti-idiotype antibodies), they are also found to react with the IgG antibodies appearing later against the same antigens. These results have been interpreted as suggesting that the differentiating clone of lymphocytes responding to an antigen first uses a pair of V_L and V_H gene segments in combination with a pair of C_L and C_{mu} gene segments to produce the IgM antibody. Later the same variable gene segments are used with C_L and C_H segments to produce IgG antibodies which have the same specificity as the IgM.

Insofar as complement activation and consequent bacterial killing is concerned, IgM is the most effective of the immunoglobulins. Its very large size means that the molecule can cross capillary walls only with great difficulty and it does not cross the placental barrier in significant amounts. Thus if IgM is detected in cord blood or in blood taken from an infant within the first few days of life, it is reasonable to assume that it represents an immune response on the part of the child itself and that intrauterine or neonatal infection has occurred. This inability to cross the placenta has direct relevance to the rarity of haemolytic disease of the newborn due to ABO group incompatibility. Carbohydrate antigens such as A and B blood group substances elicit a prolonged response by IgM antibodies and the usual switch-over to IgG production does not occur. Most people produce antibodies to blood groups that are not their own as a result of stimulation by plant carbohydrates that strongly resemble blood group substances. If IgM antibodies crossed the placenta then incompatibility between the ABO blood groups of mother and baby would inevitably lead to immune haemolysis of the infant red cells.

Immunoglobulin D (IgD)

IgD is present in the plasma in only very small amounts. For a long time its function has been uncertain, but recently it has been found that about half of all B lymphocytes have IgD on their surface, often in association with monomeric IgM. Both the coating immunoglobulin molecules appear to have the same idiotypic determinants (i.e. they have the same V_H and V_L regions on their respective light and heavy chains). It seems likely that they function as mutually assisting antigen receptors for the control of B lymphocyte activation and suppression.

Immunoglobulin E (IgE)

IgE is normally present in only minute amounts in the plasma of most people. It has the ability to bind (via its Fc portion) to receptors on tissue mast cells, these cells having between 100 000 and 500 000 Fc receptors on their plasma membranes. When the appropriate antigen binds to the Fab portions of adjacent IgE molecules, a series of events is started which is not intrinsically different from that taking place when chemotactic signals bind to receptors on the neutrophil surface. In the case of the tissue mast cell, however, activation leads to a discharge of the contents of the cell granules, which include **histamine, leukotrienes** (products of arachidonic acid metabolism via the lipoxygenase

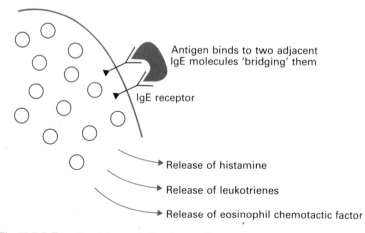

Fig. 10.7 IgE-mediated degranulation of mast cells.

pathway) and a factor chemotactic for eosinophils (Fig. 10.7). The release of these active compounds causes a local inflammatory reaction and, if the IgE antibody is bound to mast cells in the neighbourhood of bronchial smooth muscle, contraction of this smooth muscle. This reaction may be helpful in combating certain parasitic infestations. In some people there appears to be a genetically determined predisposition to produce large amounts of IgE-type antibody. This renders them more liable than others to a variety of unpleasant and even dangerous clinical expressions of large scale release of mast cell granule contents, such as asthma, hay fever and urticaria. The antigens that trigger these reactions are called **allergens**, and those with a constitutional predisposition to respond in this way are often spoken of as being **atopic**. This problem is explored at slightly greater length in Chapter 11.

The Immune Response

The induction of a response to any antigen on the part of the immune system depends primarily on the **recognition** of a specific epitope by genetically programmed lymphocytes. This is followed by a monoclonal form of **cell proliferation** and in turn by **differentiation**, which may lead to antibody production or to the initiation of one or more of the activities of the T cell system. In addition, there will be an increase in the number of cells programmed for recognition (or memory cells); this feature is responsible for the **increased speed** and **magnitude** of the reaction which takes place as a result of a subsequent exposure to the antigen concerned.

The functioning of such a system will depend both on the nature of the antigenic **signal** and of the mechanisms which exist for the **reception** of such a signal.

The signal

While both B and T cells may respond to the same antigen, the way in which this signal is presented is fundamental. B cells can recognize an antigen irrespective of the form in which it is presented. Thus these cells can bind free antigen in solution, antigens present on the membranes of cells, and antigens insolubilized in various ways. In contrast, the vast majority of T cells can only bind antigen which is associated with the surface of a cell. Helper T cells and those which secrete lymphokines recognize foreign antigens which have been processed and then presented to them on the surface of macrophages and, perhaps, other accessory cells such as dendritic cells. In addition, however, a second signal is required. This is provided by a glycoprotein on the surface of the presenting cell that is coded for by a gene sequence within the **major histocompatibility complex** (MHC). This is a set of genes responsible for the presence of a number of cell surface glycoproteins which are of great importance in cell recognition. Antigen-presenting cells such as the macrophage chiefly express MHC-coded surface glycoproteins known as class II histocompatibility antigens. However, in the case of **cytotoxic** T cells, which can eliminate cells infected by viruses, the cells of allogeneic grafts and certain tumour cells, the functions of this subset demand that recognition of self antigens associated with these targets can occur. All nucleated cells express another set of MHC-coded surface glycoproteins known as class I histocompatibility antigens (in man coded for by the HLA-A, -B and -C gene sequences), and in virally infected cells, for example, it is one of these self antigens together with new surface antigens coded for by the virus which is recognized by the T cell. Whether the foreign antigen which has been processed by the macrophage and the MHC-coded surface protein are physically associated with one another or whether they are separated is not known. If the former is the case, then one could postulate that the T cell has a single receptor for the antigen–MHC-coded protein complex; if the latter, then the T cell would have two separate receptors — one for the MHC-coded surface antigen and one for the foreign antigen.

In addition to their role in relation to antigen presentation, macrophages secrete a soluble factor which stimulates **helper** T cells and which is known as **interleukin 1 (IL 1)** (see Fig. 10.9, p. 126).

Receptors on B and T cells

Specific activation of B cells, with the resultant selection of a clone of antibody-producing cells, involves recognition of a homospecific antigen and, in the case of most antigens, assistance from the T cell population.

Some antigens seem able to trigger B cell responses in the absence of T cells and are called **thymus-independent antigens.** They are all polymers and include such molecules as pneumococcal polysaccharide, dextran, bacterial lipopolysaccharide, levan and others. The antibody response to these antigens is unusual in that it consists almost exclusively of IgM, very few memory cells are produced, and tolerance to these antigens is readily induced.

The actual recognition process is mediated by the presence on the surface of the appropriate B cell of immunoglobulins whose variable domains fit precisely with the antigenic determinant. Thus each

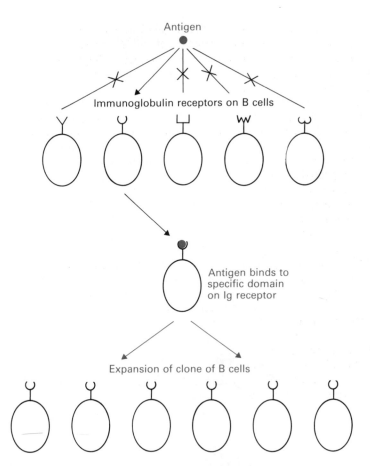

Fig. 10.8 Clonal selection in the immune response: result of the first exposure of B cells to antigen. Some of the clone will become memory cells and some effector cells.

lymphocyte is genetically programmed to bind one antigenic determinant. It is this specificity of the variable regions of the surface immunoglobulins which determines which clone of B cells will proliferate and differentiate (Fig. 10.8). All B cells express IgM on their surface and about 70% express IgD. Only a relatively small fraction of the B cell population express immunoglobulins of the other classes and on these cells IgM is expressed as well. The nature of the immunoglobulin receptors on the B cell surface has important implications in so far as the future production of the antibody classes is concerned. Those B cells bearing IgM or IgM and IgD on their surfaces, when stimulated by the appropriate antigen, give rise to clones of cells which, when differentiated into plasma cells, produce IgM only. If immunoglobulin of one of the other classes is present in addition to surface IgM, then class switching occurs and IgG, IgA or IgE antibodies will be produced depending on which of these is present on the unstimulated B cell surface.

Less is known of the T cell receptor, but it is now believed that it consists of a two-chain molecule (alpha and beta chain) with a molecular weight of about 40 000, each chain having one variable and one constant domain. While this molecule can discriminate between antigenic determinants much as an immunoglobulin does, it is not itself an immunoglobulin.

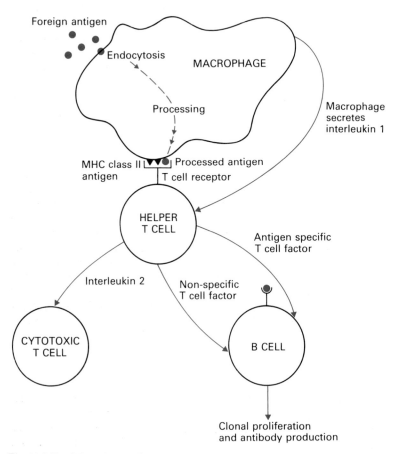

Fig. 10.9 Possible pathways of response to T-dependent antigen.

B and T cell cooperation (Fig. 10.9)

As already stated, most antigens fail to trigger proliferation and maturation of B cell clones without the active participation of helper T cells. Before cooperation between the helper T cell and the B cell can occur, the former must be stimulated. This stimulation is a dual process: first, specific stimulation in the form of antigen presented by macrophages together with MHC-coded surface proteins, and second, non-specific stimulation in the form of interleukin 1 released by the antigen-presenting cell. The stimulated helper cell then releases two soluble factors which cause B cells to which the **same antigens** have bound firstly to proliferate and secondly to mature, this latter process being associated with antibody production. It has also been suggested that an antigen-specific factor may be released from the stimulated helper T cell, but there is no unanimity on this point at present.

In addition to their role in respect of B cell activation, helper T cells, once appropriately stimulated, also act upon other T cells (both cytotoxic and helper subsets) through the release of a T cell growth factor known as interleukin 2. This substance stimulates the growth of T cells in culture and is also known to increase the rate of rejection of tumours in mice.

Summary

In summary, the mounting of an immune response requires, in most instances, the uptake and processing of antigen by an antigen-presenting cell such as the macrophage and the expression of the antigen or part of it on the surface membrane of this cell. This is followed by the clonal selection of B and T cells to proliferate and mature following the reception of appropriate signals. The signals are usually multiple and consist, in the case of the B cell, of the antigen itself, which binds to surface immunoglobulins, together with soluble factors released from helper T cells. In the case of the T cell, the signals consist of antigen expressed on the surface of the antigen-presenting cell, surface proteins coded by the MHC, and interleukin 1, a soluble product released by the macrophage (Fig. 10.9).

Complement

No account of the functional components of the immune response would be complete without some consideration of the role of complement. The complement system, which is involved in acute inflammation, phagocytosis and clotting, as well as in immune and hypersensitivity reactions, consists of at least nine proteins which, classically, become activated in sequence. Each activated component acquires the ability to activate several molecules of the next protein in line so that a marked amplification of the original step occurs, one activated molecule of C1 leading to a cascade in which thousands of molecules of the proteins 'further down the line' are activated. Each of the nine protein components is designated by a number prefixed by C. C1 consists of a trimolecular complex consisting of the subunits C1q, r and s.

The activation of the complement system takes place through the operation of one or both of two pathways, which ultimately converge after activation of C3. The first of these is known as the **classical** and the second as the **alternate** pathway of activation. For classical activation to occur (Fig. 10.10), bound IgG or IgM antibodies are essential, since C1q binds to the CH_2 of the Fc portion of these immunoglobulins. C1q has a collagen-like stem from which grow six peptide chains, each with a terminal subunit which binds to the Fc portion. For activation to occur, at least two of these subunits must bind to CH_2; this is much more easily accomplished with the pentameric IgM than with monomeric IgG. Thus IgM antibodies to red cells have a much greater haemolytic potential since 'one hit' will provide sufficient Fc binding sites to activate C1q. In the case of IgG, a greater number of 'hits' is required in order to have molecules of antibody bound close enough to each other to provide the dual binding sites required for C1q activation. C1q forms a calcium-dependent complex with the r and s components, and the whole, when activated, acquires esterase activity and binds first C4 and then C2. The C142 complex acts as convertase for C3. C3 activation leads to the production of C3a, which is chemotactic for phagocytes, and also causes the release of histamine from mast cells, and C3b, which is bound to the surface membrane of the cell to which the antibody is attached. C3b exhibits the phenomenon of **immune adherence** and binds to a receptor on the plasma membrane of both neutrophils and macrophages. In this way it acts as an **opsonin**. Thereafter, C5 is bound and then split to form C5a, which is strongly chemotactic for phagocytic cells, and C5b. C5b then forms a trimolecular complex with C6 and C7, which is also chemotactic for phagocytic cells. The final binding of one molecule of C8 with six of C9 leads to lysis of the cell membrane to which the antibody had originally bound.

The alternate pathway of complement activation (Fig. 10.11) can be stimulated by the polysaccharides of certain cell walls (e.g. bacterial endotoxins), by some aggregated immunoglobulins such as IgA which cannot bind C1q, and by a positive feedback mechanism from C3b formed in the course of classical activation. In the classical pathway, C3 is activated by the formation of the convertase C142. In the alternate

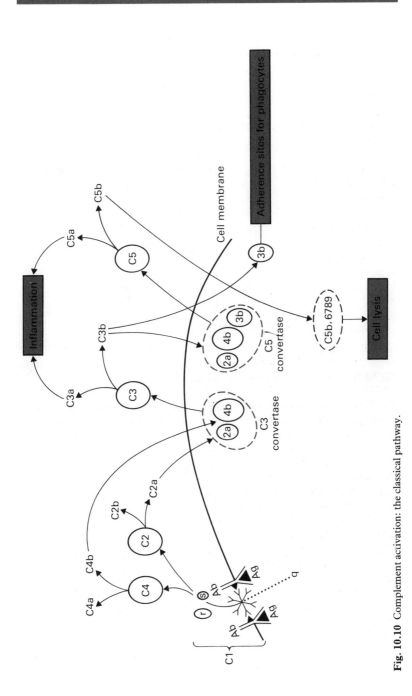

Fig. 10.10 Complement activation: the classical pathway.

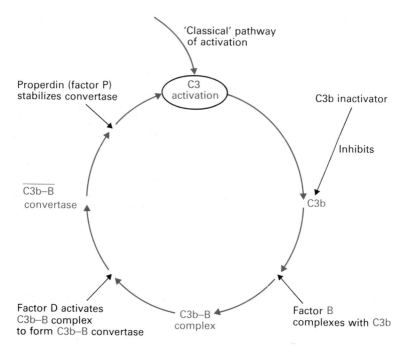

Fig. 10.11 Complement activation: the alternate pathway.

pathway, the convertase is formed by the action of certain proteins on C3b and factor B, a molecule with a molecular weight of 100 000 which complexes with C3b produced by either the classical or alternate pathways. Factor B has some similarities to C2 and, like C2, is coded for by the MHC. The C3b–B complex is activated by an enzyme known as factor D, and the active convertase is stabilized by factor P (properdin). The stabilized convertase can now act on C3 to produce more C3b, which together with factors B and D leads to the production of more convertase and still more activation of C3. Thus there is a positive feedback loop with tremendous amplifying potential, kept under control in normal individuals by a C3b inactivator. It is thought likely that, under normal circumstances, a small amount of C3b–B convertase is generated in the plasma, but the inherent lability of this convertase together with the action of C3b inactivator prevents a 'runaway' amplification occurring with ultimate depletion of C3. If this view is correct, one might regard the C3b activation pathway as 'ticking over quietly'. The importance of C3b inactivation can be seen in patients who lack the inactivator. Since C3b cannot be destroyed, there is continual activation of the alternate pathway through the feedback loop and this leads to very low plasma concentrations of C3 and factor B. Such patients suffer from repeated infections.

The immune response in defence against infection

The response of the immune system to invasion of the host by microorganisms is based entirely on recognition of the foreignness of the organisms and has nothing to do with their pathogenicity. Apart from such naturally occurring 'antibiotic' substances such as lysozyme (muramidase) and interferon 1, the mechanisms concerned initially with elimination of foreign microorganisms are **complement** and **phagocytic cells**, particularly in those instances when the cells of the immune system have not been 'primed' by previous exposure to the appropriate antigenic determinants. After several days, **antibody** and **cell-mediated responses** come into action, whereas complement and phagocytes can act within minutes.

Complement

Complement can act in a number of different ways in defence against infection. These are:

1. **Opsonization** through the adhesion of C3b to the bacterial surface
2. **Lysis** of bacterial cells through the activity of C8 and C9
3. Increasing the speed and magnitude of the **acute inflammatory response**

Antibody

As with complement, antibody can exert a protective effect in different ways (Fig. 10.12).

1. Neutralization of bacterial toxins (Fig. 10.12a). In some infections, such as tetanus, diphtheria and cholera, the most serious effects on the host are produced by the synthesis and secretion of powerful toxins (see Chapters 1 and 2). From a pragmatic point of view, in such disorders it is clearly more important that the toxins should be rendered inactive at the earliest possible stage than that the organisms should be eliminated. This function is served by antibodies, which can either combine with toxins near their biologically active site and stereochemically block their reaction with a specific substrate or, at a more distant point on the toxin molecule, cause some conformational change that can inhibit toxin activity. This mechanism will not act at its full potential at the time of a **first** infection and it is for this reason that **immunization** with bacterial

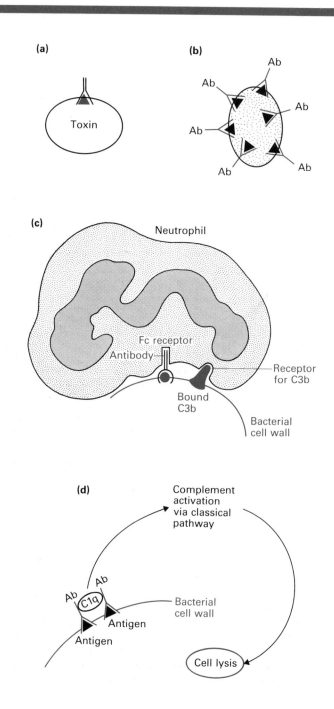

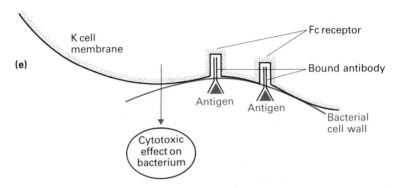

Fig. 10.12 The protective actions of antibody. (a) The neutralization of bacterial toxins: antibody binds with toxin near its biologically active site and blocks the toxin's reaction with its substrate. (b) Antibody can block the entry of viruses and bacteria into cells by coating them and preventing their adherence to mucosal surfaces. (c) Bound immunoglobulin acts as an opsonin and enhances phagocytosis. (d) Complement-mediated lysis of a bacterial cell. (e) Antibody-dependent cell-mediated cytotoxicity (ADCC): the role of antibody in the binding of 'killer' lymphocytes (killer cells) to a bacterial cell.

toxins altered, for example, by treatment with formaldehyde is undertaken in respect of a number of potentially lethal organisms (e.g. *Corynebacterium diphtheriae, Clostridium tetani*).

2. Preventing viral and bacterial entry (Fig. 10.12b). IgA antibodies, which are present in secretions such as saliva, tears, nasal secretions and those fluids bathing the gut surface, exert a protective effect by coating bacteria and viruses and thus preventing their adherence to mucosal surfaces and subsequent entry into the tissues. Again, in the case of first infections this mechanism may be relatively ineffective, but can operate powerfully in second and subsequent infections and in subjects who have been vaccinated with the appropriate antigen (e.g. oral poliomyelitis vaccine).

3. Opsonization (Fig. 10.12c). The presence of appropriate antibody has a dramatic effect on phagocytosis and hence on clearance of organisms from the blood, especially in those instances where the organisms concerned are encapsulated and resist adhesion to them by neutrophils or macrophages, or can elaborate antiphagocytic substances. Adhesion and subsequent phagocytosis are greatly enhanced by the coating of organisms by antibody, adhesion between the organism and the phagocytic cell being mediated through the Fc receptors on the surface of the latter. The antibody and C3b opsonins appear to act synergistically, and it is of advantage to the host that those immunoglobulin species (such as IgG1 and 3) which bind strongly to Fc receptors on phagocytes are also effective in fixing complement.

4. Complement-mediated cell lysis (Fig. 10.12d).

5. Antibody-dependent cell-mediated cytotoxicity (ADCC) (Fig. 10.12e). Apart from opsonization and complement-mediated lysis, antibody can help to bring about bacterial cell killing in yet another way. Cells coated with antibodies may bind lymphocytes, probably belonging to the 'null' group (i.e. those lymphocytes which have neither B or T markers), which are known as K or killer cells. These lymphocytes have surface Fc receptors through which binding to the surface of the antibody-coated cells occurs; once such binding has occurred, the K cells can produce a cytotoxic effect. In this situation there is no question of the K cells **recognizing** any antigenic determinants on the target cell — both binding and killing are non-specific.

Cell-mediated immunity

In defence against infection, apart from the role of helper T cells in relation to antibody production, cell-mediated immunity is of great importance, particularly in relation to those bacterial species which grow **inside** cells and which appear able to resist intracellular killing. Important examples include:

> *Mycobacterium tuberculosis*
> *Mycobacterium leprae*
> *Salmonella typhi*
> *Brucella abortus*
> *Listeria monocytogenes*

Cell-mediated immunity is also of great importance in the immunological response to viruses.

Cell-mediated immunity against bacteria. In relation to defence against facultative intracellular parasites such as the bacteria named above, cell-mediated immunity is expressed in the form of cooperation between appropriately stimulated T lymphocytes and macrophages (see Fig. 10.9). It is a process which is at once specific and non-specific. Its specificity resides in the fact that T cells must recognize their homo-specific antigen (in association with an appropriate MHC-coded antigen); this is supported by the fact that immunity against an organism such as *M. tuberculosis* can only be transferred from one animal to another through lymphocyte transfer. The non-specific part of the process is mediated through the activation of macrophages by the

lymphokines synthesized and released by activated T cells. Such soluble factors recruit macrophages to the site of infection, immobilize them at this site, increase their ability to kill intracellular organisms (possibly by enhancing the oxygen-dependent bactericidal function), and can even increase the number of C5a receptors on the surface of blood monocytes. Once macrophages have been activated as a result of the release of lymphokines by T cells in response to antigenic determinants on a specific organism, they acquire the ability to deal more effectively, not only with the organisms that elicited the T cell response, but with other bacterial species as well.

Cell-mediated immunity against viruses. The role of antibody in the prevention of viral infections by inhibiting the entry of viruses into the

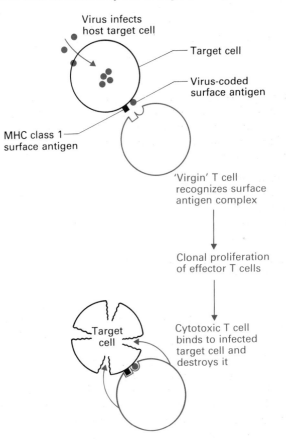

Fig. 10.13 Cytotoxic T cells in anti-viral immunity.

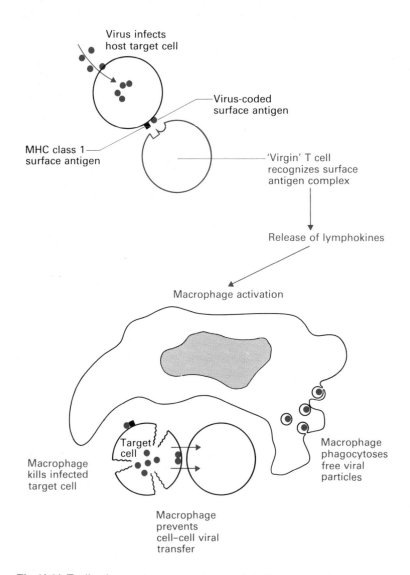

Fig. 10.14 T cell and macrophage cooperation in anti-viral immune reactions.

tissues has already been mentioned. Once such invasion has occurred, it is cell-mediated immunity which plays the dominant role in the modulation of recovery from viral infections. Specifically sensitized T cells may counter the effects of invasion of cells by viruses in a number of ways:

1. The most important of these is the direct destruction of infected cells by cytotoxic T cells (Fig. 10.13). Recognition of these infected cells by the T cells involves alteration of the normal surface antigens as a result of coding by the viral genome. In addition, as has already been mentioned, class 1 surface antigens coded for by the HLA A, B or C loci of the MHC are needed before recognition by the T cells can occur. The importance of the MHC-coded part of the signal can be shown in vitro, where T cells which are cytotoxic for cells of a certain strain infected by a virus will not kill cells of another strain infected by the same virus.
2. The release of lymphokines from activated T cells will attract macrophages to the site of infection (Fig. 10.14). These macrophages are activated by the lymphokines and may kill the infected cells, may phagocytose free viral particles, or may discourage the spread of virus from cell to cell which occurs as a result of the formation of intercellular bridges.
3. T cells may release type II interferon, one of a group of proteins which can block viral mRNA transcription and which render the cells adjacent to those that are infected unable to permit the replication of virus. Interferon II may also increase the non-specific cytotoxicity of killer cells to infected cells to which antibody has bound. This type of ADCC has been reported in cells infected with mumps and with herpes viruses.

Immunity against protozoal infections

In this group of infections it is quite common for elimination of the parasites by the immune system to be incomplete. Thus, while being able to resist a second infection, the host may at the same time still be harbouring a small number of living parasites. This state is known as **premunition.**

Both humoral and cell-mediated mechanisms may be involved in the immune reactions to protozoa. When the organisms are blood-borne, antibody and complement appear to play a dominant role, while parasites which develop in tissues usually elicit cell-mediated immunity.

Antigenic variation in evasion of the immune response. In the case of two important parasitic infections, **malaria** and **trypanosomiasis**, the

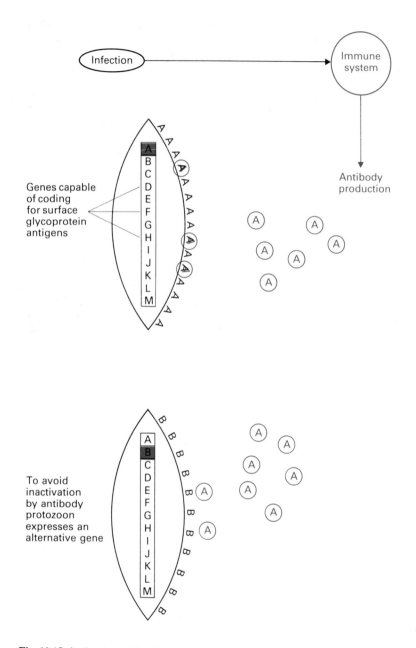

Fig. 10.15 Antigenic variation in a trypanosome.

effectiveness of antibody and complement in destroying the parasite may be overcome by the organisms varying their surface antigens into a form which existing antibody cannot inactivate. The trypanosome achieves this by expressing **in a constant sequence** alternative genes which code for surface glycoproteins (Fig. 10.15). When sufficient antibody is present in the plasma to bring about complement-mediated lysis of the organisms, the next gene in sequence is expressed and the surface antigens are altered. In due time, when new antibody has formed, the process is repeated; this can occur up to 20 times. Such a system clearly gives the trypanosome a very great advantage in terms of survival.

Immunity to helminths

Two striking features of the immune reactions elicited by helminths are the production of large amounts of IgE and a sharp rise in the number of circulating eosinophils. Degranulation of IgE-coated mast cells in the neighbourhood of the worm leads to the release of histamine (which can affect vascular permeability) and of a factor chemotactic for eosinophils. In in vitro culture systems, eosinophils can be shown to kill antibody-coated schistosomules, the cytotoxicity being associated with release of basic protein from the electron-dense core of the eosinophil granules.

Chapter 11

Disorders Related to the Immune System

All the biological mechanisms that make up the immune response may go awry in one way or another. The disorders which arise from such defects can be understood most easily if we classify them in relation to the individual functions which fail and, in the case of congenital immune deficiencies, in relation to the ontogeny of the immune system. Defective or harmful responses include the following:

1. The response to the introduction of an exogenous antigen may be inadequate. As a consequence, the host will be unable to mount an effective defence against infection. Such a defective reaction may be congenital or acquired (indeed is sometimes deliberately induced) and is known as **immune deficiency.**
2. The immune system may react to an inappropriate extent on encountering an exogenous antigen. Such a response may produce tissue damage by a variety of mechanisms. For this group of, on the whole, harmful reactions we use the term **hypersensitivity.**
3. The immune system may lose the ability to distinguish between self and non-self and as a result mount reactions against the antigens of the host. This process is known as **autoimmunity.**
4. Many **neoplastic** proliferations of the elements of the immune system can occur. Both the B and T cell systems may give rise to such disorders.

Immune Deficiency

Immune deficiency can involve either the **specific** afferent or efferent pathways of the immune system or the **non-specific** effector mechanisms such as the complement system and bacterial killing by phagocytes. Recognition that definite and measurable defects in the functions of the immune system can cause a reduced ability to combat infection dates back to 1952, when it was observed that a child suffering from repeated infections had no IgG in his plasma. Since then a wide variety of immune deficient states has been described.

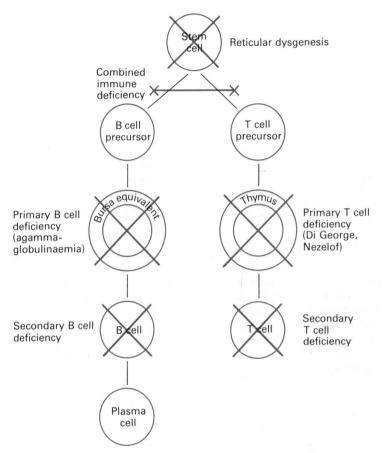

Fig. 11.1 The cellular components of the immune system and the sites of immune deficiency.

Disorders of specific immunity may arise at any point in the differentiation of the B and T cell system. The functional defect produced will depend on the point in the differentiation process at which a block occurs: the further back this point is, the broader the range of functions that is affected (Fig. 11.1)

Stem cell deficiency — defects arising before lymphoid cells are processed by either the thymus or the bursa equivalent

A deficiency in the number of stem cells produced leads to a deficiency or absence of the precursors of the B and T cells destined to undergo processing in the thymus or in the bursa equivalent. In its most severe form, known as **reticular dysgenesis**, there is a complete failure of development of other bone marrow cells in addition to the obvious gross defects in B and T cells. Such infants may die within the first week of life, usually due to overwhelming sepsis.

A more common variety of primary immune deficiency arising in the 'pre-thymus, pre-bursa' phase is severe combined immune deficiency (SCID). This may be inherited in an X-linked pattern or as an autosomal recessive. About half the sufferers lack the enzyme adenosine deaminase and these patients may be helped by blood transfusions, since the red cells contain this enzyme. The thymus is usually very small or even absent. When it can be found at post-mortem examination, there is a gross lack of thymic lymphocytes and complete absence of Hassall's corpuscles. Lymphoid tissue in the gut and other peripheral sites is also markedly atrophic. The combined defect, which affects both the B and T cell systems, is expressed by low immunoglobulin levels and a low blood lymphocyte count (fewer than 1.0×10^9/litre). These children can neither produce antibodies nor mount an effective cell-mediated reaction against intracellular bacteria or viruses. Normal immune function can be established by grafting bone marrow from a sibling with an identical or near identical major histocompatibility complex. Blood transfusion and treatment with thymic extracts may improve the situation, but many of these children die within the first year or two of life, often as a result of pulmonary infections caused by agents that are normally not particularly virulent (opportunistic infections). A common example of such an infection is that caused by the protozoon *Pneumocystis carinii*. This organism proliferates within the alveolar spaces, filling them with material that has a foamy appearance on microscopy and is eosinophilic in sections stained with haematoxylin and eosin. The use of special staining methods based on the use of silver shows the presence of many protozoa.

Other forms of combined immune deficiency

Two other forms of combined immune deficiency exist which are difficult to explain in terms of the development and maturation of the immune system. These are ataxia telangiectasia and Wiskott–Aldrich syndrome.

Ataxia telangiectasia

This fortunately rare syndrome, which is inherited as an autosomal recessive trait, consists of a triad:

1. Cerebellar degeneration and spinocerebellar atrophy, leading to the appearance of choreoathetoid movements early in life
2. The appearance at a somewhat later stage (between the ages of five and eight years) of leashes of dilated blood vessels, especially in the skin on the flexor surfaces of the forearms and in the conjunctiva (telangiectases)
3. Diminished resistance to infection. Plasma levels of IgE and IgA are lower than normal and there is also a depression of cell mediated immunity. The affected patients tend to have repeated infections of the sinuses and the respiratory tract and these may lead to the development of bronchiectasis

Ataxia telangiectasia is, in addition, one of a small number of syndromes associated with chromosomal breakages. Like the others in this group (Bloom's syndrome and Fanconi's anaemia), there is an increased risk of the development of malignant neoplasms predominantly derived from lymphoid cells. This is the commonest cause of death in ataxia telangiectasia sufferers.

Wiskott–Aldrich syndrome

This is a strange combination of clinical features characterized by a low platelet count, eczema and recurrent infection. The patients have low levels of IgM and, in keeping with this, a poor response to polysaccharide antigens. IgA and IgE concentrations are elevated and the IgG level is usually normal. In addition, some depression of cell-mediated immunity is also present. T cell numbers and effectiveness decline progressively and it takes a few years before the lymphocyte count is seriously diminished. Both the T cells and the platelets show absence of certain surface glycoproteins and it has been suggested that a defect in glycosylation, especially of sialidation, is present. As with ataxia telangiectasia, there is an increased risk of malignant neoplasms of the lymphoreticular system (5% of the patients die in this way).

The syndrome is inherited as an X-linked recessive trait and signs and symptoms of the disease usually appear in the first few months of life.

Primary deficiencies of T cell function

Should the thymus fail to develop, processing of the T cell precursors obviously cannot take place. The thymus is derived from the third and fourth pharyngeal pouches, as are the parathyroid glands. It is not surprising therefore that absence or inadequate development (hypoplasia) of the thymus may be associated with absence of the parathyroids and other anatomical abnormalities related to the pharyngeal pouches (DiGeorge's syndrome). In addition, anomalies in the cardiac outflow tracts are common. It has been suggested that these multiple organ defects may result from failure of the neural crest mesenchyme to migrate and to interact normally with pharyngeal epithelium. If only the thymus fails to develop and the parathyroids are normal, the condition is known as Nezelof's syndrome.

In the absence of the thymus, differentiated T cells are not produced and the T cell zones of lymph nodes do not become colonized. The primary B cell follicles are present, as one would expect, but if the degree of T cell deficiency is severe, the lack of helper T cell activity means that stimulation of the follicle centre cells and the development of germinal centres does not occur. This is reflected in an inadequate antibody response. Viral infections and infections with intracellular bacteria are particularly dangerous to these children and even the BCG vaccine used against tuberculosis may have very serious results.

Purine nucleoside phosphorylase (PNP) deficiency

A form of primary T cell dysfunction not associated with failure of the thymus to develop occurs when the enzyme purine nucleoside phosphorylase is absent from T cells. Nucleosides, especially desoxyguanosine, accumulate within the T cell and damage it. Suppressor T cells seem more sensitive to such metabolic damage than other T cell subsets.

Primary deficiencies of B cell function

Primary failure of normal B cell function may result from an absence of B cells, from the failure of B cells to differentiate into plasma cells, or from inability of the plasma cells to make one or other class of immunoglobulin. Any of these will be reflected in an absence of or very low plasma concentration of immunoglobulin. Children with this disorder show a tendency for repeated infections due to pyogenic organisms (such as *Staphylococcus aureus*, *Streptococcus pyogenes* and *pneumoniae*) and also fall victim to opportunistic infections (e.g. *Pneumocystis carinii*). Cell-mediated immunity is normal. Some cases are familial and sex-linked; others are sporadic.

Deficiencies related to non-specific immune functions

Phagocyte defects

These can be expressed as:

failure to respond to chemotactic signals
failures of lysosomal fusion
failures in bacterial killing

These have been discussed in some detail in Chapter 5 and further reference to them will not be made here.

Defects in complement function

Since each of the components of the complement sequence appears to be coded for separately, it is theoretically possible for any one of them to be absent from the plasma. In some instances, instead of a component being absent, it is present at a reduced level, suggesting that the fault lies in a regulatory gene rather than in the one coding for that specific component.

Difficulties may also arise if certain inhibitors of complement activity are absent. As pointed out in Chapter 10, absence of C3b inhibitor results in continuous high-level activation of the alternate pathway, with depletion of C3 and thus an ultimate decline in the efficacy of the complement system. Absence of C1 inhibitor, inherited as an autosomal dominant trait, leads to unfettered production of C2 kinin activity, which causes painful swollen patches in the skin and oedema in the gut and respiratory tract. This is known as **hereditary angio-oedema.** Sudden death from airway obstruction is a constant threat in these patients, and it has been suggested recently that the sudden deaths affecting the accursed Pyncheon family in Nathaniel Hawthorne's *House of the Seven Gables*, written in 1851, may be the earliest description of hereditary angio-oedema.

Secondary immune deficiency

Immune deficiency may occur in postnatal life as a result of the operation of a number of factors.

Age

Both in infancy and in old age there is a relative lack of effectiveness of the immune response. The transfer of maternal IgG across the placenta tends to compensate for this in infants.

Malnutrition

This may be associated with defective immunity in relation both to B and T cell function. It has been suggested that this may explain the relatively high mortality associated with diseases such as measles in underprivileged communities.

Neoplastic disorders of the immune system

Neoplastic B cell proliferations, such as the majority of the lymphomas, myelomatosis and chronic lymphocytic leukaemia, are associated with a decline in antibody responses. However, in Hodgkin's disease, which is believed by many to be related to proliferation of T cells, the patients exhibit various manifestations of a deficiency of cell-mediated immunity and are more susceptible to infections caused by mycobacteria, viruses and fungi.

Iatrogenic immune deficiency

Suppression of immune reactions may be produced **deliberately** under two sets of circumstances. The first of these is where an attempt is made to reduce the reaction to allografts. This will be discussed in more detail in Chapter 13. The second is in certain disease states such as systemic lupus erythematosus, where tissue damage is being caused by failure to distinguish between self and non-self antigens (autoimmune disorders). 'Damping down' the immune response by the use of appropriate drugs reduces the effects of the reaction and can improve the clinical state of the patient.

Iatrogenic immune suppression can also arise as a side-effect of treatments which are not primarily aimed at the components of the immune reaction. X-rays and cytotoxic drugs used in the treatment of malignant neoplasms may produce immune suppression, as may corticosteroids.

Infections

Good evidence exists that certain viral infections can cause immune suppression both in man and in other species. In some of these (e.g. measles), this effect has been ascribed to a direct cytotoxic effect on certain lymphocyte subsets. Malaria and the lepromatous form of leprosy are also associated with a decreased ability of the immune system to eliminate infecting microorganisms. In the latter, macrophages are seen to contain very large numbers of apparently healthy mycobacteria.

In recent years, increasing attention has been focused on a newly recognized form of acquired immune deficiency for which male homosexuals appear to be particularly at risk. This is known as the **acquired immune deficiency syndrome (AIDS)**.

AIDS is an extremely serious condition, with a high mortality rate, found chiefly in male homosexuals (especially those with multiple partners), in some natives of Haiti, in heroin addicts and in a few haemophiliacs who have received many transfusions of commercial Factor VIII. The patients often present with many enlarged lymph nodes which may show reactive changes in the B cell areas or, more rarely, atrophy of the B cell areas. This 'extended lymphadenopathy syndrome' may then be followed by recurrent opportunistic infections, which may be viral, bacterial or protozoal (*Pneumocystis carinii* being the protozoon most often implicated), and/or a rather curious malignant neoplasm of small blood vessels in the skin known as Kaposi's sarcoma.

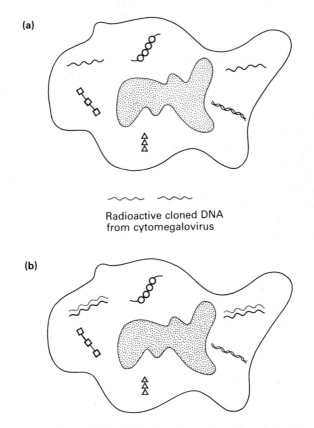

Radioactive cloned DNA
from cytomegalovirus

Fig. 11.2 In situ DNA–mRNA hybridization. (a) A cell from Kaposi's sarcoma. The cytoplasm contains many mRNAs. (b) Cloned DNA binds to the intracellular mRNA with complementary nucleotide sequences. Radioactivity in the tumour cell is detected using autoradiography.

Kaposi's sarcoma is one of the commonest malignant neoplasms in Africa, accounting for about 9% of all neoplasms in the indigenous population. In these African patients the neoplasm behaves in an aggressive fashion and often involves lymph nodes and internal organs. Kaposi's sarcoma also occurs in middle-aged and elderly Europeans, often of Eastern European origin, but in these patients the behaviour of the disease is much more indolent, and spread to distant sites is rare. In AIDS victims, the biological nature of the Kaposi's sarcoma resembles that found amongst Africans and is quite aggressive. It is not without interest that viral genetic material (**cytomegalovirus**) has been found in Kaposi's sarcoma using DNA hybridization techniques (Fig. 11.2). Patients with AIDS show a reversal of the normal helper/suppressor T cell ratio, the numbers of these subsets being determined by using monoclonal antibodies which can identify either helper or suppressor T cells, but not both. This decline in the population of helper T cells is believed to be the direct effect of an infection, the infectious agent being transferred from person to person through the medium of blood or plasma. Most recent evidence suggests that the infectious agent is a virus known as the human T cell lymphotropic virus type III (HTLV III).

Hypersensitivity

The introduction of a foreign antigen into an immunologically normal host induces a state of **altered reactivity** expressed by antibody production and/or the proliferation of sensitized T cells. In such a **primed** host, a second encounter with the same antigen will produce a reaction which is greater both in degree and in the speed of the response. On some occasions this second reaction may be inappropriate in degree and cause tissue damage. Such injurious reactions are subsumed within the term **hypersensitivity.**

Hypersensitivity reactions are best classified on the basis of the **mechanisms** involved in their production. This approach is embodied in the classification proposed by Gell and Coombes, in which four major types of immunologically mediated tissue injury are recognized.

Type I (immediate hypersensitivity, anaphylactic sensitivity, reagin-mediated allergy)

In this type of reaction a foreign antigen reacts with IgE bound to mast cells via the Fc portion. The bridging of the Fab portions of two adjacent IgE molecules by the antigen sets off a complex series of reactions which basically result in:

1. The release of preformed contents from the mast cell granules into the surrounding microenvironment

2. The synthesis of metabolites of arachidonic acid, which have powerful pharmacological effects, notably in relation to smooth muscle tone which is greatly increased

An IgE response to the introduction of, for the most part, harmless antigens lies at the heart of type I hypersensitivity. In those who suffer from this form of hypersensitivity there is, presumably, a failure on the part of suppressor T cells to inhibit responses of B cells to certain quite harmless antigens. Such people, who are spoken of as being **allergic**, make large amounts of IgE which is specific for some normally innocuous protein. This antibody then binds to the tissue mast cells, which are widely distributed in the skin, membranes of the nose, mouth, trachea, bronchi and bronchioles, gut and lymphoid tissues.

The surface of a mast cell is studded with between 100 000 and 500 000 receptors to which the inappropriately large amounts of IgE synthesized by allergic patients bind via the Fc fragment. At this point there is no functional disturbance. The latter only occurs on a second or subsequent exposure to the homospecific antigen, which reacts with the bound IgE and leads to degranulation of the mast cells. The sequence of events that follows binding of antigen to IgE is not dissimilar, in many respects, to that which occurs in the course of reception and transduction of chemotactic signals. Serine proesterase is activated and the resulting serine esterase causes changes in the fluidity of the cell membranes through methylation of phospholipids. The result is an influx of calcium ions through the membrane; this has two quite separate effects.

First, cyclic nucleotides increase and lead to the assembly of microfilaments and microtubules within the cell. Contraction of microfilaments causes the granules, which contain histamine, heparin, 5-hydroxytryptamine, platelet activating factor and eosinophil chemotactic factor, to move towards and then fuse with the plasma membrane of the mast cell, and to discharge their pharmacologically active contents (Fig. 11.3).

Second, the influx of calcium leads to the activation of phospholipase A_2 and the release of arachidonic acid (Fig. 11.4). With arachidonic acid as a starting point, a two-branched cascade occurs (Fig. 11.5). One pathway (the **cyclooxygenase** pathway) leads to the formation of prostaglandins via the endoperoxides PGG_2 and PGH_2. The second pathway, catalysed by the enzyme **lipoxygenase**, leads to the formation of powerful mediators known as the leukotrienes by converting arachidonic acid into 5-hydroperoxyeicosotetranenoic acid (5-HPTE). This molecule loses an hydroxyl group to become leukotriene A_4,

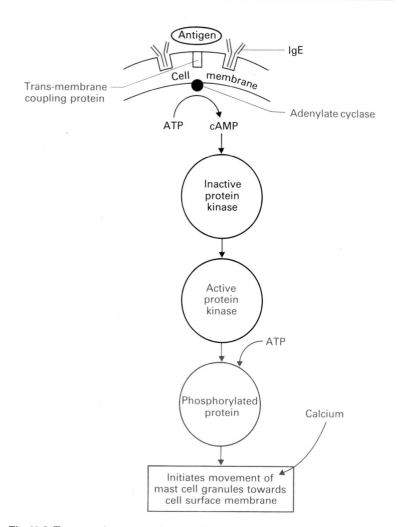

Fig. 11.3 Trans-membrane events in IgE-mediated mast cell degranulation.

which in turn can be converted to leukotriene B_4 by the addition of water or to leukotriene C_4 by the addition of glutathione. The loss of glutamic acid from C_4 converts the molecule into leukotriene D_4, and the loss of glycine from D_4 leads to the formation of leukotriene E_4. The mixture of C_4, D_4 and E_4 constitutes what was formerly known as **slow reacting substance A** (SRS A), a powerful and long-acting agent for the contraction of smooth muscle.

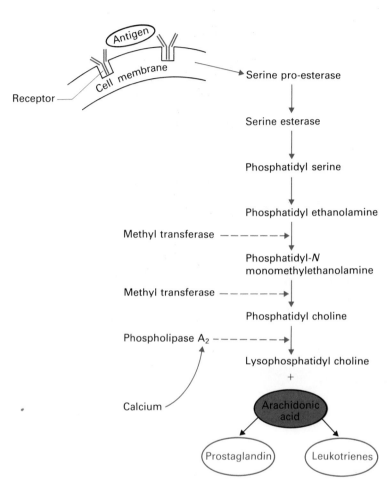

Fig. 11.4 Intramembrane events in IgE-mediated mast cell degranulation.

The release of these powerful agents leads to a number of different clinical expressions mediated, at least in part, by the route of exposure to the offending antigen and thus the location of the affected mast cells. These include:

1. Allergic rhinitis (hay fever)
2. Extrinsic allergic asthma, dominated by bronchospasm
3. Atopic conjunctivitis, caused by spores, danders and pollens
4. Atopic dermatitis resulting from a variety of allergens (e.g. penicillin, heavy metals, local anaesthetics, etc.)

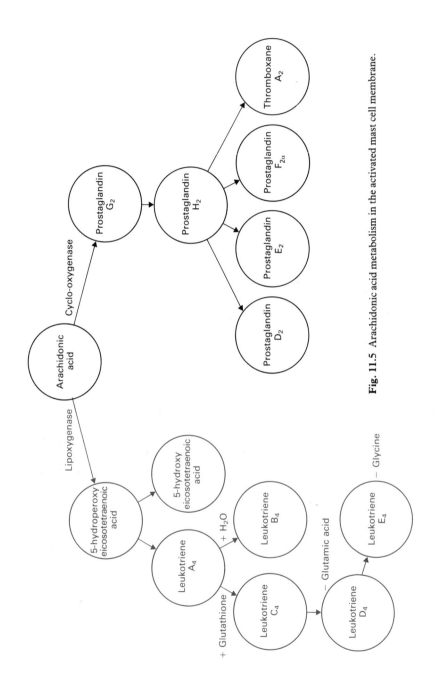

Fig. 11.5 Arachidonic acid metabolism in the activated mast cell membrane.

5. Urticarial angio-oedema characterized by intensely itchy skin papules and often related to insect bites or food allergies
6. Gastrointestinal disturbances such as pain, vomiting and diarrhoea, usually related to food allergies

The fact that hypersensitivity is related to a plasma component (IgE) can be demonstrated by the transfer of serum from an allergic to a non-allergic subject. If such serum is injected into the skin of the non-allergic person and this is followed by intradermal injection of the allergen at the same site, a characteristic wheal and flare reaction develops very quickly (the Prausnitz–Küstner reaction).

Treatment

Treatment of type I hypersensitivity is based on a number of factors which relate fairly logically to the steps involved in the development of the specific hypersensitivity:

1. The specific allergen can be avoided.
2. The tendency to react to the allergen can be reduced by giving repeated injections of small amounts of allergen.
3. The entry of calcium into the mast cell can be blocked by the administration of disodium cromoglycate.
4. The contraction of microfilaments, which is an essential precursor of mast cell degranulation, can be inhibited by the use of corticosteroids.
5. The effects of histamine can be blocked by administration of antihistamines.
6. Smooth muscle contraction can be inhibited by isoprenaline or adrenaline.
7. The cAMP/cGMP ratio can be increased by the use of theophylline or compounds that inhibit the enzyme phosphodiesterase and thus raise intracellular cAMP concentrations. As cAMP increases, the intracellular events described above are damped down.

Type II hypersensitivity (cytotoxic hypersensitivity)

In this type of reaction the tissue damage arises primarily from the presence of circulating antibody directed against some tissue component and the binding of that antibody to its specific epitope. Once such binding has occurred, damage to and death of the affected cells can come about through the operation of a number of effector mechanisms (see also Chapter 10).

1. Lysis of the cell membrane may occur as a result of activation of the complement system.

2. The cell to which antibody has bound may be phagocytosed by macrophages via the adherence mechanisms mediated through C3b or the Fc portion of immunoglobulin.
3. The antibody-coated cells may be killed by killer cells (antibody-dependent cytotoxicity).

Cytotoxic hypersensitivity is of particular clinical importance in relation to the cells of the blood.

Immune haemolysis is an archetype of a type 2 reaction. This may occur under three different sets of circumstances: incompatible blood transfusion, haemolytic disease of the newborn, and autoimmune haemolytic disease.

If the patient is given a blood transfusion incompatible for a major blood group system such as the ABO system (e.g. group A blood given to a group O recipient), the isoantibodies in the recipient (usually IgM) bind to the group A determinants on the donor red cell surface and cause severe reactions, including complement-mediated haemolysis and agglutination of the cells.

Another important example of haemolysis mediated via immune mechanisms is **haemolytic disease of the newborn,** which can arise as a result of incompatibility between mother and fetus in respect of the rhesus system, the baby being rhesus positive and the mother rhesus negative. Fetal red cells usually gain access to the maternal circulation only at the time of parturition and thus the mother only becomes sensitized to the fetal rhesus antigens at the end of the first pregnancy with a rhesus-positive child. This first child is thus usually unaffected. However, any subsequent rhesus-positive children show an increasing risk as the degree of maternal sensitization increases with each successive pregnancy.

Such maternal sensitization is dangerous to the fetus since the antibody elicited by the rhesus antigens is IgG, which can cross the placenta and enter the fetal circulation (Fig. 11.6). Affected children may be born dead and show evidence of severe anaemia, oedema thought to be due to cardiac failure, enlargement of certain viscera and, on histological examination of certain tissues, notably the liver, evidence of extensive extramedullary haemopoiesis. This, the most severe expression of rhesus incompatibility, is termed **hydrops fetalis.**

Less severely affected children may develop haemolytic anaemia of differing grades of severity and at different speeds. In addition to the obvious harmful effects of the anaemia, an additional danger is the large amount of bilirubin which accumulates in the plasma as a result of the intravascular haemolysis. Much of this bilirubin is not conjugated within the liver cells and, being lipid-soluble, accumulates within the central nervous system, especially in the basal ganglia. These

(a) First pregnancy

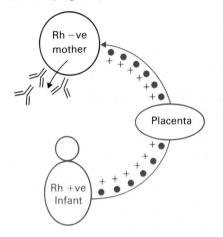

(b) Subsequent pregnancies

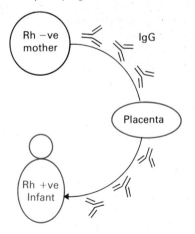

Fig. 11.6 Haemolytic disease of the newborn. (a) Rhesus (Rh) positive red cells from the fetus leak into the maternal circulation at the time of parturition and cause the mother to produce antibodies directed at the Rh antigens. (b) In subsequent pregnancies, if the infant is Rh positive, the IgG antibodies against Rh antigens cross the placenta and cause haemolysis of the fetal red blood cells.

accumulations of bile pigment lead to necrosis of neurons followed by reparative proliferation of glial fibres. The affected children often show mental retardation and may also suffer from spasticity and choreoathetoid movements. It is essential that unconjugated bilirubin levels in the plasma be monitored in infants with haemolytic disease of the newborn, since it is possible to prevent the bilirubin rising to dangerous levels by exchange transfusion. The sensitized fetal red cells are removed and replaced by fresh blood; this procedure can be repeated if necessary.

Clearly in all disease states, avoidance is more desirable than treatment, and in recent years a giant step has been taken towards eliminating the risk of haemolytic disease of the newborn due to rhesus incompatibility. This has been accomplished by the injection of anti-rhesus antibodies into the rhesus-negative mother just after parturition when rhesus-positive red cells derived from the fetus are present in her circulation. The rhesus-positive cells are eliminated by the antibody and thus sensitization of the mother is avoided.

Haemolysis also occurs in the course of certain autoimmune reactions, i.e. when there is a partial loss of the ability to discriminate between **self** and **non-self**. The red cells become coated with antibody and tend to be removed from the circulation as a result of immune adherence to macrophages which engulf the affected cells. The presence of the antibody coating on the red cell can be demonstrated by performing the Coombs' test (Fig. 11.7). Washed red cells from the patients are suspended in saline and a multivalent anti-human globulin is added to the suspension. The mixture is then incubated. If antibody is present on the red cell surface, the cells become agglutinated by the anti-human globulin (Fig. 11.7).

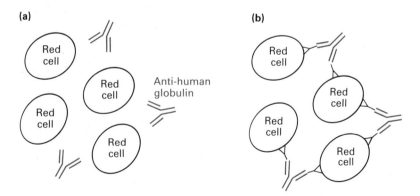

Fig. 11.7 The Coombs' test. (a) No antibody coating on red cells: there are no binding sites for anti-human globulin, therefore no agglutination of red cells occurs. (b) Red cells coated with antibody: anti-human globulin binds to the Fc portion, creating 'bridges' between the red cells, and agglutination occurs.

Autoantibodies directed against surface antigens of platelets have also been described in the condition known as **idiopathic thrombocytopenic purpura**. Most cases present under the age of 21 years. In its acute form, a common mode of presentation is with fever and a purpuric rash. Platelet destruction leads to a serious decline in the number of circulating platelets and this predisposes, not only to purpura, but also to bleeding in a number of sites, which may be serious or even fatal. Destruction of antibody-coated platelets is thought to be accomplished largely by macrophages in the spleen; this view is reinforced by the improvement that takes place after splenectomy.

Other examples of autoimmune type 2 hypersensitivity are considered in Chapter 12.

Drug-induced type 2 hypersensitivity

All the varieties of hypersensitivity can be elicited by drugs, but here only those operating through type 2 mechanisms are considered. Even in this restricted frame of reference, diverse mechanisms may be involved.

In one form, the drug or a part of it binds to a carrier (which may be a cell such as the red cell or platelet) and thus acts as a hapten. When binding takes place between the resulting antibody and the drug-related antigenic determinant, the carrier cell can be destroyed through one of the mechanisms already described. A classical example of such a reaction was the purpura which occurred in some people after taking the hypnotic drug Sedormid. The drug acted as a hapten bound to platelets, and the antibody formed in response bound to the drug and destroyed the innocent platelet by means of complement-mediated lysis. In vitro, the platelet lysis can be demonstrated only if the drug is added to a mixture of platelets and the patient's serum.

A totally different mechanism appears to operate in the case of a small number of drugs. Antibodies are formed which, instead of binding with the drug, react with **self** antigenic determinants and thus, by implication, are elicited by them. An example of this is the very widely used antihypertensive agent α-methyldopa. In a number of patients taking this compound, the red cells become coated with an antibody which binds with one of the antigens of the rhesus system (e). The reason postulated for these findings is that the interaction of the drug with the red cell membrane has revealed antigenic determinants which are normally masked.

Type III hypersensitivity (immune complex mediated hypersensitivity)

The union of antibody and antigen in very finely dispersed or soluble form is known as an **immune complex**. Such complexes are capable of eliciting an inflammatory reaction, usually by the activation of complement and the consequent attraction of neutrophils and platelets. While the tissue injury itself is largely due to the release of lysosomal enzymes from the neutrophils, the vasoactive amines released from aggregated platelets and the formation of platelet aggregates which can occlude vessels of the microcirculation, the role of the complement system in bringing about these events is a key one. The effect of immune complexes can be reduced greatly if the actions of C3 and later components of the complement sequence are inhibited. The **size** of the complexes is of considerable importance in determining the type of reaction which occurs. If the complex is large, it is usually phagocytosed, though phagocytosis may be preceded by an inflammatory reaction if the complex is localized within tissues. If the complex is very small, it may circulate in the plasma and pass harmlessly through the glomerular filter into the urine. The nature of the complex is, at least in part, governed by the relative proportions of antigen and antibody. If there is **antibody excess** or mild **antigen excess**, the complexes are rapidly precipitated and tend to be localized to the site of antigen introduction, thus giving local tissue reactions. If there is **moderate to gross antigen excess** the complexes formed are soluble. They can thus circulate widely and become deposited in relation to the basement membranes of small blood vessels (e.g. the glomerular capillaries), in the joints and in the skin. Immune complex localization in such sites can produce a spectrum of lesions. In small blood vessels there may be extensive necrosis of smooth muscle cells associated with deposition of fibrin and immunoglobulin. This type of reaction is called **fibrinoid necrosis**. When viewed microscopically in sections stained with haematoxylin and eosin, the necrotic portions of the blood vessel walls show a great affinity for the eosin and stain bright red with a curious 'smudged' appearance. These changes may involve the whole circumference of the vessel wall or only a segment of it. If sections containing such lesions are treated with the appropriate fluorescein-linked antisera, the presence of fibrin, immunoglobulins and, in most instances, C3 can be demonstrated.

Tissue reactions in response to the presence of immune complexes are influenced by whether the complexes are formed **locally** or are **within the circulation.**

Local formation of complex

For local complex formation the essential precondition is a **high concentration of circulating antibody,** leading to rapid precipitation of antigen at or near its point of entry to the tissues. The archetype of this situation is the Arthus reaction described by Maurice Arthus, who found that injection of antigen into the skin of hyperimmunized rabbits produced local reddening and oedema of the skin at the injection site within three to eight hours. In some instances the inflammatory reaction was so intense that local necrosis took place with the formation of a slough. Microscopically such a lesion is characterized by an intense neutrophil response, and the antigen is often precipitated by antibody within small venules. The Arthus reaction can be blocked by depleting the animal of complement or by the use of specific antineutrophil sera.

Arthus type reactions in human disease. Local formation of immune complex with a resulting inflammatory response is the pathogenetic mechanism operating in a number of human disorders.

In one of them, **rheumatoid arthritis**, which will be considered further in Chapter 12, immune complexes are formed locally within the joints as a result of the production of self-associating IgG–anti-IgG complexes by plasma cells within the synovial membrane.

Such local formation of immune complexes also underlies the pathological and clinical picture of a number of hypersensitivity disorders affecting the lung. In so-called **farmers' lung** the patients

Table 11.1 Some diseases of the lung caused by immune complexes.

Disease	Antigen
Pigeon fancier's disease	Serum protein in dust from dried faeces
Cheese washers' disease	Spores from *Penicillium casei*
Furrier's lung	Fox fur protein
Maple bark stripper's disease	Spores of cryptostroma

have been sensitized to components of thermophilic actinomycetes which grow in mouldy hay. When these patients, who have high levels of circulating antibody to the actinomycetes, are exposed to the dust from mouldy hay, they develop respiratory difficulties within a few hours. Intradermal injections of extracts of the offending organisms produce a classical Arthus reaction.

A similar situation arises in a number of other pulmonary disorders in which the inhalation of sensitizing dusts is followed by the local formation, within the lung tissue, of immune complexes which elicit an inflammatory reaction; these are listed in Table 11.1.

Immune complexes formed in the circulation

Soluble complexes within the circulation are usually formed under conditions of **moderate to gross antigen excess**. This results in the solubilization of the complexes which, if they are of appropriate size, can cause lesions in a wide variety of sites.

An interesting example of this type of immune complex mediated injury in man is so-called **serum sickness.** This is a syndrome which occurs in certain patients given large doses of foreign protein (most commonly derived from the horse) for various therapeutic purposes. The affected patients develop fever, joint pains and sometimes proteinuria about ten days after injection of the foreign protein. Since this occurs after only **one** injection, it is at first difficult to see how this reaction could be related to antigen–antibody binding. However, this

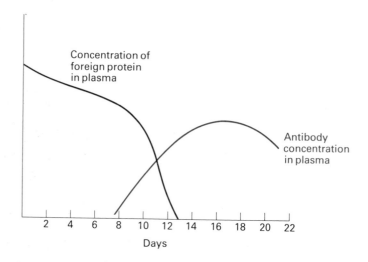

Fig. 11.8 Antigen and antibody concentrations in serum sickness. Pathogenic immune complexes are formed during the period of antigen excess.

conceptual difficulty can be overcome quite simply. After the injection of large amounts of foreign protein there is a slow fall in the plasma concentration of the circulating antigen. About eight days after the injection, the antibody formation elicited by the foreign protein leads to the appearance of circulating antibody in low concentration. A few days after this there is a sudden fall in the concentration of circulating antigen and a decrease in the level of complement. At this time the symptoms characteristic of serum sickness appear (Fig. 11.8). In animals in whom serum sickness has been induced, deposited immune complexes can be identified at various sites, notably in the glomeruli.

Eventually these complexes become phagocytosed by mesangial cells and the proteinuria gradually disappears.

Persistent circulating antigen and immune complex disease. The importance of the **persistence** of circulating antigen in the genesis of immune complex disease has now been demonstrated many times, notably by Dixon, who produced glomerular disease in rabbits by repeated injections of serum albumin from a different species, thus maintaining the presence of antigen in the plasma for a long time. If high titres of antibody were present, the glomerular lesions tended to be associated with proliferation of endothelial and/or mesangial cells. If the titres of antibody were low, the predominant morphological feature was thickening of the glomerular basement membrane. Both these morphological variants are present in human glomerular disease. Immunofluorescent and ultrastructural studies of renal biopsies from patients with glomerulonephritis have shown the presence of immune complexes from which, in some cases, the antigens have been eluted and identified (Figs 11.9, 11.10 and 11.11). A wide variety of such

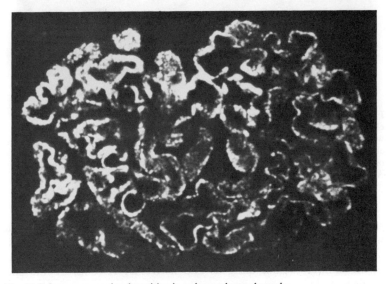

Fig. 11.9 Immune complex deposition in a glomerulus as shown by immunofluorescence. A frozen section from a renal biopsy taken from a patient suffering from immune complex mediated glomerulonephritis has been prepared. The section has been treated first with rabbit anti-human IgG and then with a fluorescein-linked goat anti-rabbit globulin. The granular fluorescent areas indicate where the IgG moiety of the immune complexes has been deposited in the glomerular capillary wall. (Photograph by courtesy of Dr A.J. Leathem.)

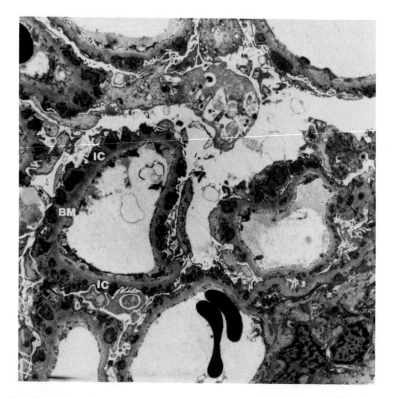

Fig. 11.10 Immune complex mediated glomerulonephritis. Low power transmission electron micrograph of portion of a glomerulus from a renal biopsy taken from a patient with immune complex mediated glomerulonephritis. The basement membranes (BM) are abnormally thick. Electron-dense immune complexes (IC) are present in large numbers on the subepithelial aspect of the basement membranes. (Photograph by courtesy of Dr A.J. Leathem.)

antigens, both exogenous and endogenous, have been implicated in human immune complex disease. They include streptococcal antigens, malarial antigens, the soluble antigen of hepatitis B virus, drugs such as penicillamine, tumour antigens and native DNA (both double and single stranded).

Type IV hypersensitivity (cell-mediated reactions)

Tissue injury resulting from the activities of sensitized T cells is common and includes some of the most widespread and serious

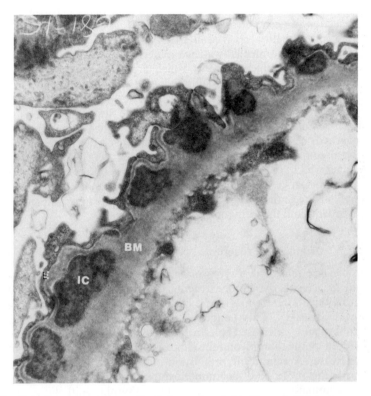

Fig. 11.11 Immune complex mediated glomerulonephritis. Transmission electron micrograph from the glomerulus shown in Fig. 11.10. This is a higher power view of a segment of the glomerular capillary wall showing the massive immune complexes (IC) on the outer aspect of the basement membrane (BM). E = epithelium. (Photograph by courtesy of Dr A.J. Leathem.)

disorders such as tuberculosis and leprosy. It is seen under three main sets of circumstances:

1. Hypersensitivity reactions elicited by a number of bacteria (tuberculosis and leprosy), viruses (smallpox, measles and herpes) and fungi (candidiasis, histoplasmosis). Of these, the **delayed** skin reactions induced by the injection of tuberculoprotein into the dermis of persons previously exposed to the mycobacterium, and hence with some degree of cell-mediated immunity, are highly characteristic. The interactions of sensitized T cells with macrophages, through the medium of lymphokine production have already been described (p. 137), and the tissue reactions characteristic of some of the pathological expressions of

cell-mediated reactions will be considered in more detail in Chapter 14.
2. Rejection of tissue or organ grafts
3. Contact dermatitis, as is seen after exposure to certain chemicals, plant products and metals (watchstrap dermatitis). Contact dermatitis is induced by complex antigens which are formed as the result of binding between the foreign substance and a carrier protein derived from the host's skin. The foreign substance acts as a hapten. The new complex antigen is presented to the immune system by specialized antigen-presenting cells in the epidermis which are known as Langerhans cells; it has been suggested that the carrier protein may be derived from surface components of these cells. A T cell reaction is mounted which, in histological terms, is expressed as a local infiltration of mononuclear cells, which reaches its maximum about 12 to 15 hours after exposure to the allergen. This cellular infiltrate is accompanied by local oedema and the formation of small blisters.

Type V (stimulatory) reactions

The concept that certain types of cell hyperfunction may be brought about as a result of immune reactions is a fairly new and obviously exciting one. The example more often cited is that of **thyrotoxicosis** (Graves' disease). This condition is characterized by an enlarged thyroid gland, increased plasma concentrations of the hormones produced by the thyroid, and the clinical features which arise from such an increase. A significant proportion of the patients show, in their plasma, the presence of an immunoglobulin which can be shown to have stimulatory effect on mammalian thyroid epithelium. Like thyroid-stimulating hormone (TSH), this immunoglobulin binds to the TSH receptor on the plasma membrane of the thyroid epithelial cell and, in the same way as TSH, produces sufficient change in the receptor or in the plasma membrane adjacent to it as to increase intracellular cAMP via activation of the adenylate cyclase system. Acting as a 'second messenger', the adenine nucleotide causes an increase in secretion of thyroid hormones. Other types of antibodies have been described which can also bind to the TSH receptor. One inhibits thyroid function and has been found in the serum of some patients suffering from **myxoedema**. Another promotes the growth of thyroid tissue but does not cause any increase in the output of thyroid hormones. The fact that three different antibodies exist, all binding to the TSH receptor and all producing different effects, suggests that the receptor itself is very complex in immunological terms. It is known that the TSH receptor consists of ganglioside and glycoprotein components. Antibodies that **block** thyroid function bind to the **glycoprotein** component of the receptor; those that **stimulate** thyroid activity bind to the **ganglioside** portion. Other models of antibody-mediated 'switching on' of cell functions have been described, but their relevance in clinical practice has yet to be established.

Autoimmunity

Fundamental to the successful operation of an immune system is the ability to distinguish between **self** and **non-self**. Not only does this discriminatory ability serve to protect against invasion by foreign species, but it prevents injury of the host organism's own tissues. If the immune system loses its normal unresponsiveness to self components, this state is known as **autoimmunity**.

Tolerance to self is normally induced in the perinatal period

Normally **tolerance** to self is induced during the development of the fetus and during very early neonatal life. The exposure of the immune system to potential antigens during the perinatal period, when that system is developing rapidly, leads to a failure to respond to those antigens when the animal becomes mature in the immunological sense. For instance, the injection of cells from one strain of mouse into newborn of another strain suppresses the ability of the recipient strain, in adult life, to reject a skin graft from the donor strain. It is possible that the exposure of immature lymphoid cells to a specific antigen might lead to the **deletion** of that particular clone and thus account for the immunological unresponsiveness in later life. Such tolerance is just as highly specific as any other aspect of immunological reactivity. If, for example, the pituitary is removed from a tree frog larva during the time when its immune system is developing and the excised tissue is kept alive by transplanting it into another tree frog larva, the animal from which the organ has been removed will be found to regard its own pituitary as **foreign** after the neonatal period.

Induction of tolerance in adult animals

Tolerance can be induced in adult animals as well as in neonates. This can be brought about under two sets of circumstances which, one might have imagined, would be mutually exclusive. The first of these, known as **low zone tolerance**, is induced when repeated **low** doses of certain antigens are used. Such tolerance is induced most easily by antigens which are weakly immunogenic, but can occur with strongly immunogenic antigens provided that antibody synthesis is inhibited during antigen dosage by the use of an immunosuppressive drug such as cyclophosphamide.

Tolerance can also be induced by the use of repeated **high** doses of antigen (**high zone tolerance**). The **state** of the antigen is also of some importance in experimental induction of tolerance. Proteins which are soluble rather than in a macromolecular or aggregated form are more easily able to induce tolerance. The avoidance of processing of antigen by macrophages before presentation to lymphocytes is also more likely to lead to tolerance of that antigen than to an immune response.

In low zone tolerance only T cells are unresponsive; in high zone tolerance both B and T cells are involved. Obviously **high zone tolerance** is a much more certain and secure method of maintaining immunological unresponsiveness to **self** antigens than the **low zone** variety, since it is quite easy to see how tolerant T cells could be bypassed by a change in one or more of the determinants in an antigen complex to which they had been made tolerant.

Another possible mode of maintaining tolerance to self antigens is via the operation of **suppressor T cell activity.** Any reduction in the population of suppressor T cells is associated with a tendency to form antibodies against self components. Neonatal thymectomy, which greatly reduces the population of suppressor T cells, exacerbates the autoimmune haemolytic anaemia which is characteristic of the New Zealand Black mouse. Similarly, the injection of thymocytes from young unaffected members of the same strain delays the appearance of the anaemia.

There are some self components to which tolerance does not normally develop but which do not elicit the formation of autoantibodies

It is quite possible that there is a small number of self tissue components to which the immune system has never been exposed and to which, therefore, tolerance never develops. Such antigens are spoken of as being **secluded** and probably include lens protein and the antigens of sperm.

Autoimmune disease is dealt with in Chapter 12.

Chapter 12

Autoimmune Disease

The concept that some diseases could be due to immune reactions mounted against self antigens stems from three very important sets of observations. The first was the recognition that certain haemolytic anaemias were associated with the presence of antibodies which could be shown to be cytotoxic to the patient's red cells. This was followed by the discovery, in 1956, that the sera of patients suffering from a disorder of the thyroid known as Hashimoto's thyroiditis contained antibodies which bound to thyroglobulin and to certain components of thyroid epithelium. At about the same time, workers in the USA produced an experimental thyroiditis in rabbits by injecting extracts of thyroid tissue. Since then autoimmunity has been invoked as the pathogenetic mechanism in a large number of diseases.

It is not always easy to establish absolute criteria which indicate that a specific disease has an autoimmune origin. Factors which suggest that this may be the case include the following:

1. **Indirect** evidence of immunological disturbance, such as increased levels of immunoglobulins in the plasma
2. **Direct** evidence of autoimmune reactivity as shown by the presence of autoantibodies in the plasma and blast transformation in vitro of lymphocytes exposed to self antigen
3. Tissue changes characterized by infiltration by lymphocytes, mononuclear phagocytes and plasma cells
4. Clinical and serological associations with other autoimmune diseases in either the patient or his family
5. The occurrence of a similar disease in animals that can be shown to be mediated by immune mechanisms

Do autoantibodies change tissue function and structure?

The effector mechanisms for the production of tissue damage in autoimmune disorders are essentially the same as those that operate in hypersensitivity. Many autoimmune diseases are associated with the presence of either circulating autoantibody or soluble immune complexes, and these can be grouped roughly into two divisions: **organ-specific** or **multisystem**. Organ-specific diseases can be still further subdivided into those in which there is a specific lesion in a target organ and the accompanying autoantibodies are directed against a specific component of that organ, and those where the lesions tend to be restricted to a single organ but the autoantibodies are not organ-specific and, indeed, sometimes not species-specific (e.g. primary biliary cirrhosis, where the target is intrahepatic bile duct epithelium but the antibody reacts in vitro with all mitochondria). The pattern of autoantibody production in such organ-specific diseases shows a considerable degree of overlap.

It should be clear from what has already been stated about the effects of the antibodies which bind to the TSH receptor in the thyroid (p. 164) and those which are implicated in autoimmune haemolytic anaemia that the features of certain disorders are directly due to the binding of autoantibody (Table 12.1). Another striking example of such a situation

Table 12.1 The pathogenic effects of autoantibodies.

Antigen	Effect	Disease
Platelet	Destruction	Idiopathic thrombo-cytopenic purpura
TSH receptor	Stimulation	Thyrotoxicosis
Glomerular basement membrane	Complement-mediated damage	Goodpasture's syndrome
Red cell membrane	Complement-mediated membrane damage	Autoimmune haemolytic anaemia
Acetylcholine receptor	Blocking/destruction of receptors	Myasthenia gravis
Intrinsic factor	Blocks absorption of vitamin B_{12}	Pernicious anaemia

is the disease **myasthenia gravis**, in which muscle contraction is impaired either by blocking of the acetylcholine receptors on the voluntary muscle or by actual destruction of the receptor, which can be shown to be stripped from the membrane of the muscle cells after they have been cross-linked by autoantibodies.

Some of the autoantibodies directed against acetylcholine receptors appear to be produced by the thymus. Thymocytes obtained at thymectomy from patients suffering from myasthenia gravis produced antibodies against acetylcholine receptors when cultured in vitro, and such antibodies have been shown to produce the muscle changes of myasthenia when injected into rats. The thymus contains a substance on some of its cells which resembles the acetylcholine receptor and this substance has been shown to be immunogenic in cell culture systems.

The presence of autoantibody need not indicate the presence of autoimmune disease

It is worth remembering that the presence of autoantibodies in the plasma does not necessarily signify the presence of autoimmune disease. Such antibodies are found in a number of healthy people and may well have no pathogenetic role. In addition, autoantibodies may occur as a *result* of tissue damage and not *cause* it. For instance, antibodies which react with human heart muscle are often found in the serum of patients who have undergone open heart surgery. Many autoimmune diseases exist in which autoantibodies are present in the patient's plasma, but for which no pathogenic role has as yet been identified. If autoantibodies are not responsible for the tissue damage which occurs in some autoimmune diseases, then it is necessary to invoke some other mechanism. It seems likely that the guilty party in these instances is either the T cell or the K cell. In Hashimoto's thyroiditis, where the antibodies reacting with thyroglobulin and thyroid microsomes can cross the placenta, there is no evidence of damage to the thyroid in children of sufferers from this disease, and in the experimental form of this disease caused by injecting thyroid extracts and complete Freund's adjuvant, the disease can only be reproduced in non-immunized animals by the transfer of lymphoid cells from affected animals, not by the transfer of plasma.

Possible mechanisms for the production of autoimmunity

Loss of tolerance to self components leading to autoimmunity could, theoretically, occur in a number of ways.

Exposure of previously secluded antigens

The possibility that tissue components exist which normally are not encountered by the immune system such as sperm and lens proteins has already been mentioned. Certainly some cases of open trauma to one eye may be followed two or three weeks later by a severe inflammatory reaction in the other eye. This has been termed **phacogenic ophthalmitis**. Similarly, some cases of male infertility are associated with the presence of antibodies directed against sperm, which are not normally encountered by the developing immune system. At one time it was thought that this secluded antigen situation existed in relation to thyroglobulin. This is incorrect; a small amount of thyroglobulin can be found in the lymph draining from the normal thyroid.

Alteration of self antigens so as to bypass tolerant T cells

Tolerance is due in many instances to failure of T cells to respond to a certain antigenic determinant and thus to help appropriate B cells to produce antibody. It is likely that this type of unresponsiveness can be overcome by some alteration in the **carrier** molecule. This might be accomplished by alteration of some of the determinants on the carrier or by addition of new ones.

In experimental autoimmune disease, extracts of **unaltered** tissue components do not, as a rule, elicit an autoimmune response. When such extracts are altered, either by treating them with certain chemicals or by incorporating them in Freund's adjuvant, autoantibodies are formed and the characteristic type of tissue damage occurs. However, there is no evidence that an such alteration of self antigens plays a role in *spontaneous* autoimmune disease.

Modification of self antigens can occur in association with the use of certain drugs and very likely as a result of some viral infections. One of the best known of the drug reactions (described on p. 157) is the autoimmune haemolytic anaemia occurring in some patients treated with the anti-hypertensive agent α-methyldopa. In affected patients, autoantibodies are produced against the e antigen of the rhesus system, presumably as a result of some modification of the red cell surface by the drug or one of its metabolites. The autoantigens may be directly modified and thus made immunogenic or, in some cases, there may be alterations in some molecule concerned in **associative recognition.** This is a phenomenon in which one membrane component provides help for the immune response to another. The appearance of a new helper determinant either by drug-related modification of an existing molecule or by the insertion of a new antigen as a result of viral infection may confer immunogenicity on a preexisting cell component.

Cross-reactions in bypassing tolerance

There is no doubt that certain exogenous antigens can be encountered by the immune system which share antigenic determinants with native tissue antigens. Normally one would expect tolerance for these determinants to exist. In just the same way as T cell tolerance can be overcome by some modification in the carrier molecule associated with an autoantigen, the presentation of one of these 'shared' determinants on a totally different carrier brings the normal immunological unresponsiveness for that antigen to an end. Rheumatic fever, a multisystem inflammatory disease which affects the heart most severely, follows an infection by certain strains of haemolytic streptococci. The antibodies which are produced as a result of such an infection also bind to antigenic components of heart muscle. Some patients may develop a neurological syndrome characterized by abnormal, involuntary movements (**Sydenham's chorea**). Their serum contains antibodies which can be shown by immunofluorescence to bind to neurons, and this binding can be inhibited by prior absorption of the serum by streptococcal cell membranes. A similar mechanism is believed to operate in the encephalitis which sometimes followed the use of rabies vaccine containing heterologous brain tissue.

Idiotype bypass

T helper cells with specificity for the idiotype on a certain B cell receptor play a role in the stimulation of that B cell clone. If, perhaps as a result of an infection, an antibody was formed which had an idiotype which cross-reacted with the receptor of a potentially autoreactive T or B cell, then an autoimmune response might occur. Cross-reacting idiotypes have been found in certain autoimmune diseases such as rheumatoid arthritis and systemic lupus erythematosus.

Inappropriate Ia expression

Most organ-specific antigens appear on the surface of the cells as class I but not class II MHC-coded molecules. As a result they cannot communicate with T inducers. It has been suggested that if class II genes could become derepressed, Ia molecules would be synthesized and appear on the surface of cells, thus rendering them immunogenic. Thyroid epithelial cells in culture can be persuaded to express Ia molecules (HLA-DR) on their surfaces after stimulation by phytohaemagglutinin, and the epithelial cells from thyroid glands of patients suffering from Graves' disease bind anti-HLA-DR antibodies, suggesting that such inappropriate expression of Ia can take place in 'real life' as well as in cell culture systems.

Impaired regulation of T cells

There can be little doubt that B cells from normal individuals have the potential to produce autoantibodies. It has been shown, for example, that normal lymphocytes in culture will produce IgM antibodies of the type seen in rheumatoid disease when stimulated with non-specific mitogens, and normal mice will also produce autoantibodies when they are injected with non-specific lymphocyte activators. In these situations the autoantibodies formed combine with antigens that are widely distributed. These include DNA, IgG, phospholipids, red blood cells and lymphocytes themselves. It has been suggested that these antibodies form a group whose production is an inherent property of the immune system.

Regulation of these potentially autoreactive B cells is probably one of the functions of the T cell population. One could regard the normal dormancy of autoreactive B cells as being the result either of the **action** of T suppressor cells, **lack** of activity on the part of appropriate T helper-inducer cells, or both. Certainly there is a reduction in suppressor T cells in a number of autoimmune diseases, and in one such disease — **multiple sclerosis** — clinical exacerbations and remissions parallel changes in the suppressor T cell population. We cannot be absolutely sure, however, that the decrease in suppressor T cells is responsible for the activation of autoreactive B cells. Indeed, it is possible that the reduction in the T cell subpopulation may be caused by the autoantibody; soluble immune complexes, for example, can impair both the function of suppressor cells and the expression of their markers. An **excess** of helper T cells has been recorded in a strain of mice prone to develop a disorder resembling lupus erythematosus in humans. This feature has not, as yet, been described in human autoimmune disease. However, increased helper T cell **activity** has been noted in procainamide-induced lupus. This may be due to an inhibition of cAMP formation by either the drug or its metabolites. A decline in intracellular cAMP stimulates helper cells. Methyldopa, on the other hand, which can cause autoimmune haemolysis, stimulates cAMP, an effect which inhibits suppressor cells. Thus autoimmunity could arise from either stimulatory or inhibitory effects on T cell subpopulations.

A possible role for anti-idiotype antibodies

Possible mechanisms for the activation of dormant, potentially autoreactive lymphocytes are discussed above. Such cells, as already stated, tend to produce autoantibodies that react with widely distributed antigens. In the case of those autoimmune states associated with the presence of highly specific autoantibodies, a normally regulated immune network seems essential. Examples include myasthenia gravis, in which there are antibodies directed against the beta subunit of the acetylcholine receptor, antibodies against the insulin receptor in type I diabetes mellitus, and the thyroid stimulating antibody found in primary thyrotoxicosis.

It has been suggested that the autoantibody binding to the acetylcholine receptor in myasthenia gravis may be an anti-idiotypic antibody. An **idiotype** is a serologically identifiable configuration in the antigen-binding region of an antibody. An anti-idiotype reacts specifically with this site (Fig. 12.1). Binding between idiotype and anti-idiotype can be inhibited by the antigen which originally elicited the formation of the first antibody, and, similarly, the anti-idiotype can inhibit binding between the antigen and the specific combining site on the first antibody.

In myasthenia gravis, acetylcholine plays the role of a ligand which binds both to its normal receptor and to its corresponding antibody.

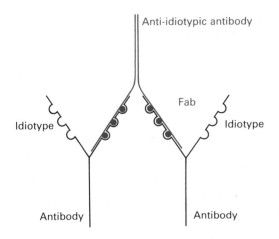

Fig. 12.1 Binding between idiotypes and an anti-idiotype antibody.

Thus both the receptor and the antibody must have similar ligand-binding structures. An anti-idiotype which combines with the ligand-binding structure in the variable region of the antibody can also bind to the corresponding structure in the receptor. Such an antibody has been described as 'a key which fits two similar but not identical locks'.

That this view is valid has been shown in a model system in which mice are immunized against a synthetic agonist of the acetylcholine receptor known as BisQ. Such mice make both antibodies against BisQ and anti-idiotype antibodies (anti-anti-bisQ). The anti-idiotype was shown to be able to bind specifically both to the anti-BisQ and to the acetylcholine receptor; its binding to anti-BisQ was stoichiometrically inhibited by purified acetylcholine receptors. In rabbits a similar experiment led not only to the production of autoantibodies but to a myasthenia-like syndrome in some of the immunized animals. Thus a normal immune response can lead to the production of autoantibodies and, under certain circumstances, to an autoimmune disease.

Some Examples of Autoimmune Disease

The clinical and pathological features of autoimmune diseases encompass a wide spectrum. As stated earlier, this ranges from **organ-specific disease associated with organ-specific antibodies** (such as is seen in Hashimoto's thyroiditis) through **disorders limited** to one organ or tissue but where the antibodies are not organ-specific (such as primary biliary cirrhosis) to the non-organ specific or system diseases where lesions may be found in many organs and a wide range of autoantibodies may be encountered (such as systemic lupus erythematosus and rheumatoid arthritis).

Hashimoto's thyroiditis

Hashimoto's thyroiditis was the first organ-specific autoimmune disease to be recognized and, in many ways, constitutes an archetype for this group of processes. It is the commonest cause of enlargement of the thyroid (goitre) associated with hypofunction in areas where iodine deficiency is not a factor. While hypothyroidism is the commonest functional expression of the disease, a proportion of affected patients present with evidence of hyperthyroidism, and for this variant the rather unhappy term 'Hashitoxicosis' has been coined.

Thyroiditis of this kind occurs most frequently in women (the female to male ratio being 10:1). In addition to this imbalance in the prevalence of the disease between the sexes, there are clearly some other genetic factors involved since thyroiditis appears to have a definite association with the histocompatibility antigen HLA-DR5.

Morphology of the thyroid

The gland is usually diffusely enlarged and its normal outline is preserved. Both capsular and cut surfaces show a marked accentuation of the lobular pattern. There is a striking change in the colour and texture of the gland substance. Instead of the normal reddish brown, the thyroid tissue is a pale yellowish or pinkish grey and is opaque, much of the colloid present in normal thyroid having been lost.

On histological examination, much of the normal thyroid is seen to be replaced by a florid cellular infiltrate consisting of plasma cells, large lymphocytes and macrophages. Not infrequently, lymphoid follicles with germinal centres can be seen, a feature which may also be present in the thyroid of patients with Graves' disease. Those thyroid follicles which remain are small and have lost most of their colloid content. Many of the remaining epithelial cells are larger than normal, are more eosinophilic than usual, and have a markedly granular cytoplasm, the granules representing a significant increase in the number of mitochondria, a characteristic feature of this disorder.

Antibodies found in Hashimoto's thyroiditis

Since the first demonstration by Roitt, Doniach and Campbell in 1956 that the sera of patients with Hashimoto's thyroiditis contained antibodies which reacted with thyroglobulin, a wide range of antibodies has been identified in these patients. Most have antibodies which bind to the TSH receptor, and these antibodies are of two types. The first stimulates **growth** of thyroid tissue, the second stimulates **hormone synthesis**. In addition, antibodies which 'block' the effect of these two types may also be present. Many patients have antibodies which bind to microsomes in the thyroid epithelium and the same antibodies also appear to react with antigens on the luminal surface of the thyroid epithelial cells. Roughly half the patients have antibodies which react with one or more components of thyroglobulin.

While the antimicrosomal antibody is cytotoxic for thyroid epithelial cells when they are dispersed and growing in monolayer culture, there is no good evidence that the damage to the thyroid parenchyma is directly due to these or other antibodies. As indicated previously, the transfer of these antibodies across the placenta does not appear to cause any thyroid dysfunction in the infants of mothers with Hashimoto's disease.

The relationship between Hashimoto's thyroiditis
and other autoimmune states

Generally there is a tendency for more than one autoimmune disorder to occur in a single patient. In such patients the overlap is usually between autoimmune states in the same part of the spectrum of autoimmune disease, i.e. patients with an organ-specific type of disorder may show evidence of another organ-specific disorder. Patients with Hashimoto's thyroiditis have a risk for developing pernicious anaemia which is 50 times greater than their age-matched peers, and autoimmune thyroid disease is frequently diagnosed in patients suffering from pernicious anaemia.

The degree of overlap between these two conditions is even greater in terms of the **antibodies** present in the plasma. Almost a third of patients with autoimmune thyroiditis have antibodies directed against the gastric parietal cells, and, in some series, half the patients with pernicious anaemia have been found to have antithyroid antibodies. There is no question of cross-reaction here; the antibodies are quite distinct.

Systemic lupus erythematosus

Systemic lupus erythematosus (SLE) is a multisystem autoimmune disease in which the lesions appear to be produced by immune complexes and which is characterized by a generalized excessive autoantibody production. There is a strong predilection for the disease to occur in females (female to male ratio = 9:1) and Negro females in the USA appear to be particularly at risk. An increased risk also seems to be conferred by the HLA antigens DR2, DR3 and BW15. Additional evidence of a genetic component comes from family clustering of cases and from a high degree of concordance in monozygotic twins.

The tissues most frequently involved are the **skin**, where there is a highly characteristic erythematous rash in the 'butterfly area' of the face, the **joints** (with the production of a polyarthritis), and the **kidney**, where a life-threatening glomerulonephritis may occur (Fig. 12.2). Other tissues such as the pleura and pericardium are not infrequently involved and increasing recognition has recently been paid to the effects

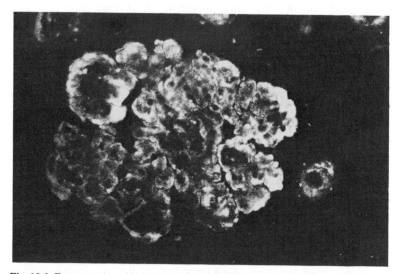

Fig. 12.2 Frozen section of kidney treated with rabbit anti-human IgG followed by goat anti-rabbit globulin linked with fluorescein. This patient had an immune complex mediated glomerulonephritis associated with systemic lupus erythematosus. The presence of fluorescent material in a so-called 'lumpy-bumpy' pattern indicates the sites of immune complex deposition.

of the disease on the central nervous system. In about half the cases, small warty excrescences may be seen on the heart valves (Libman–Sacks endocarditis).

Two views have been put forward to explain the hyperactivity of the B cells in SLE. The first of these postulates that there is a decline in suppressor T cell activity, thus allowing B cells an unfettered opportunity to produce large amounts of autoantibodies. Certainly a good number of patients with SLE do show evidence of decreased T cell activity, but this is by no means a universal phenomenon. The second suggestion put forward to account for the hyperactivity of the B lymphocytes in SLE is that some polyclonal activation of B cells has occurred directly, thus bypassing the need for a non-specific signal from the T helper cells. Such activation can occur when B cells are exposed to lipopolysaccharides such as bacterial endotoxins, and it has been suggested that similar lipopolysaccharides can be derived from cell membranes.

Antibodies found in systemic lupus erythematosus

Many antibodies can be produced in this condition, most, though not all, reacting with nuclear antigens. These antigens include:

1. **Double-stranded DNA.** The finding of antibodies directed against this antigen is virtually specific for SLE and the titre of these antibodies correlates well with the degree of activity of the disease.
2. **Deoxyribonucleoprotein.** Antibodies directed against this nuclear component are responsible for the LE cell phenomenon in vitro (see below).
3. **Single-stranded DNA**
4. **Nuclear ribonucleoprotein**
5. A nuclear antigen known as **Sm.** Antibodies binding to this are highly specific for SLE but do not correlate with the activity of the disease.
6. **Cardiolipins.** The presence of antibodies reacting with cardiolipins is the cause of the well recognized phenomenon of a so-called 'biological' false-positive Wasserman reaction.
7. **Red cells, lymphocytes and platelets.** Antibodies binding to surface antigens on these cells exert a cytotoxic effect, producing haemolytic anaemia, lymphopenia and thrombocytopenia.
8. **Factor VIII.** Antibodies elicited by this antigen may cause a bleeding disorder.

The LE cell phenomenon

In 1948, long before the concept of autoimmunity had been recognized, Hargreaves found that when blood is taken from patients with SLE, heparinized and allowed to incubate for between 40 and 60 minutes at 37°C, smears made from the buffy layer show the presence of phagocytic cells containing large basophilic masses which can be shown to be composed of nuclear material. It is now known that these phagocytosed nuclear masses arise as the result of interaction between nucleated blood cells and antibodies against deoxyribonucleoprotein. Healthy cells are not damaged by this antibody, but cells damaged during the taking of blood allow entry of the antibody and consequently its binding to its nuclear homospecific antigen. The damaged nucleus swells, is extruded from the cells and is then phagocytosed by a phagocyte, usually a polymorphonuclear leucocyte. There is no good evidence of significant damage being produced in vivo as the result of cytotoxic antibody, but occasionally the homologue of the nuclear material within the LE cell may be seen in the tissue in the form of amorphous masses which stain a purplish blue with haematoxylin and which are found in relation to the necrotic lesions characteristic of SLE.

The pathogenesis of the lesions

It is now generally accepted that the tissue damage occurring in SLE is the result of **immune complex deposition** with consequent activation of complement at the target sites by both the classical and alternate pathways, though the former seems to be by far the most important. The degree of activity of the disease correlates closely with the titre of antibodies against double-stranded DNA, and high titres of this antibody are themselves associated with a fall in the plasma complement concentration. The level of circulating immune complexes in the plasma also correlates with disease activity.

The presence of immunoglobulin (usually IgG_1 and IgG_3) and complement can be detected by immunofluorescence at the dermal/epidermal junction of the skin and in the glomerular capillary tufts in the kidneys of patients with lupus nephritis. A variety of glomerular lesions may be seen. In all affected tissues, as would be expected in a disorder characterized by immune complex deposition, necrotizing vascular lesions are present which chiefly affect the small vessels. Larger vessels in the kidney show a curious laminated intimal proliferation called, with some justice, 'onion skinning'.

Animal models of systemic lupus erythematosus

Our understanding of the processes involved in SLE has been improved by the finding of a number of animal models of the disease. Three of these exist in different strains of mouse (NZB/W, BXSB and MRL/1) and one in the dog.

The hybrid strain produced by mating New Zealand Black (NZB) with New Zealand White (NZW) mice has for many years been the classical model for SLE. The NZW parent produces large amounts of antibody when immunized with DNA, but does not develop the disease, and the NZB parent is similarly free from SLE, though it does tend to develop autoimmune haemolytic anaemia. Thus at least two genes must be involved in producing the greatly increased degree of susceptibility of the hybrid. This hybrid shows a decline in T suppressor cell activity fairly early in life. This is then followed by the appearance of antinuclear antibodies and the onset of autoimmune disease. The picture is complicated by the fact that both parent strains are infected with a leukaemia virus and there is similar evidence of viral infection in canine lupus and in some human patients. In the NZB/W hybrid, the predilection for females noted in humans is also present and 50% of the female mice are dead by the age of nine months. Males, on the other hand, usually live for 14 to 15 months before mortality on this scale occurs. Early castration and treatment with sex hormones can alter this state of affairs; an ovariectomized female given androgens will survive much longer than her untreated counterpart. In other murine SLE models, sex hormones do not appear to influence the situation. The MRL/1 mouse has a recessive gene which, when homozygous, codes for a tremendous degree of lymphocyte proliferation, and in the BXSB mouse the factor which accelerates the development of the lupus syndrome appears to be associated with the Y chromosome. Thus, even in the mouse, SLE appears to be a destination which can be reached by a variety of paths, some of which may involve infection.

Drug-induced SLE

A lupus-like syndrome, though usually without significant renal involvement, has been described following administration of a number of drugs including the antihypertensive agent hydralazine, procainamide and isoniazid. Withdrawal of the drug is usually followed by significant regression of the clinical and pathological features. Antibodies reacting with double-stranded DNA are not present, antibodies to nucleoprotein (which fix complement rather poorly) being most prominent. The risk of developing drug-induced SLE appears to be associated with the HLA antigen DR4 and it has been suggested that the basic defect in these patients is the inability to acetylate hydralazine or amine groups, thus leading to an accumulation of metabolites which might alter the antigenic properties of certain cell constituents as a result of covalent binding.

Rheumatoid disease

Rheumatoid disease is a chronic inflammatory disorder of unknown aetiology and incompletely understood pathogenesis which affects a number of tissues, most notably the joints. As with systemic lupus erythematosus, females have a higher risk of developing rheumatoid disease than male, the female to male ratio being of the order 3:1.

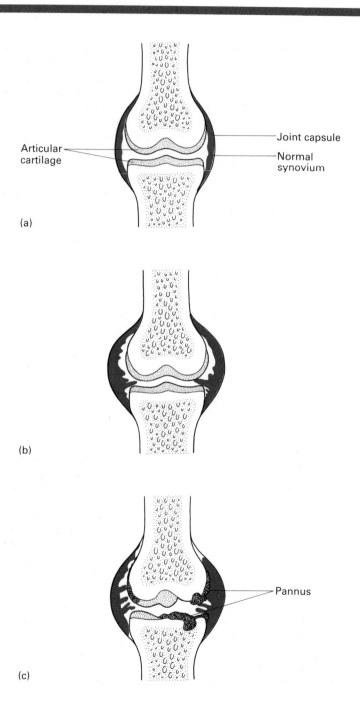

Involvement of skin, heart, blood vessels, eyes, lungs and voluntary muscles may occur, but the clinical picture tends to be dominated by a progressive and destructive arthritis. This usually starts in the small joints of the hands and feet, affecting these in a symmetrical fashion.

The early stages of the process are characterized by a rather non-specific, acute inflammatory process in the synovial membrane. The synovial blood vessels dilate, the tissue becomes oedematous and there is a mixed acute inflammatory infiltrate. This is followed by a massive infiltration of lymphocytes, plasma cells and macrophages. In many instances the lymphocytes aggregate into follicles and some of these may contain germinal centres. The synovial surface is partly covered by polymerized fibrin. At this stage the appearances of the synovium are still rather non-specific. The synovial fluid becomes cloudy due to the presence of large numbers of inflammatory cells and a high fibrinogen content may lead to the fluid clotting.

In most cases, this acute inflammatory process does not resolve and some sinister changes occur in the synovium (Fig. 12.3). The synovial lining cells, which share many of the characteristics of macrophages, proliferate and the synovial lining becomes hyperplastic. The tissue underlying the synovial cells becomes extremely vascular, taking on some of the characteristics of severely inflamed granulation tissue. The inflamed and hyperplastic synovium, now known as 'pannus' becomes adherent to the underlying articular cartilage and tends to spread across the whole articular surface. Pannus formation is associated with erosion of the underlying articular cartilage. In severe cases, the whole of the articular cartilage is destroyed with exposure of the underlying bone, which itself may show focal resorption. Eventually the joint space may become filled with scar tissue or even with some new bone, this obliteration of the space and destruction of joint function being termed **ankylosis**. The joint capsule, ligaments and tendons may also be affected, and tendon rupture is a well recognized complication of the rheumatoid process.

In about 20% of cases lesions in the subcutaneous collagen are associated with the arthritis. These are known as **rheumatoid nodules.** Each nodule consists of a central zone of necrotic collagen surrounded by a cellular infiltrate in which macrophages and some fibroblasts are prominent. These cells are arranged at the periphery of the necrotic collagen in a 'picket fence' fashion. Surrounding them is a zone of lymphocytes and plasma cells. Rheumatoid nodules occur most commonly on the extensor surfaces of the arms and elbows but many other sites have been recorded.

Fig. 12.3 Rheumatoid arthritis. (a) Normal joint. (b) The synovium becomes swollen and inflamed, there is a heavy infiltrate of lymphocytes and plasma cells, and the synovial lining cells become hyperplastic. (c) Vascular granulation tissue (pannus) forms, destroying the articular cartilage and the exposed bone.

The immunopathology of rheumatoid disease

Embodied in rheumatoid disease is an autoimmune response to the Fc portion of IgG, the antibodies directed against these antigens being known as rheumatoid factors (RF). The rheumatoid factors form complexes within the synovium and synovial fluid with the 'antigenic' IgG and these complexes are, at least in part, responsible for the characteristic pathological changes. Virtually all patients with rheumatoid disease can be shown to have formed rheumatoid factors which may be either IgM or IgG. When immunofluorescent methods are used in the examination of sections of inflamed synovium from patients with rheumatoid arthritis, few plasma cells can be shown to contain IgG. This apparent paradox can be resolved if one remembers that the nature of the association between the rheumatoid factors and the IgG (the Fab portions of the rheumatoid factor binding to the Fc portion of IgG) leads to a paucity of reaction sites for the fluorescent anti-IgG with which the section is treated. If the section is first treated with pepsin, the RF–IgG complex is broken by destroying the Fc region, and treatment of sections with fluorescein-labelled anti-IgG shows that 40–70% of the plasma cells contain immunoglobulin. In addition, immunoglobulin can be shown to be present in the synovial lining cells.

The immune complexes may mediate the destructive changes in the joint in a number of different ways. Binding of complement can initiate an Arthus-like response in the joint and the many acute inflammatory cells attracted in this way can release their lysosomal enzymes and thus contribute to the erosion of the articular cartilage. The immunoglobulin aggregates can also stimulate the macrophage activities of the synovial lining cells, either through reacting with receptors on these cells or by inducing the release of lymphokines from sensitized T cells. The activated synovial lining cells release lysosomal enzymes, most notably collagenase, which can be detected between the pannus and the articular cartilage using immunohistological methods. Activated macrophages can release plasminogen activator and the plasmin formed as a result of this can lead to the activation of latent collagenase in synovial lining cells. Another product of the activated macrophage, prostaglandin E_1 can lead to resorption of bone, as can the release from T cells of an osteoclast-stimulating factor.

These data make some contribution to understanding the pathogenesis of the joint changes, but the aetiology of the condition still remains obscure. There is clearly a genetic component since there is an association between risk for developing rheumatoid arthritis and the HLA antigens DW4 and DR4. Some variants of the disease have other HLA associations, suggesting that these may have some influence on the clinical and pathological picture in each of these variants.

What starts the autoimmune process off is unknown. Recently there has been some interest in the fact that many patients with rheumatoid disease have antibodies to a nuclear antigen in B cells which results from infection with the Epstein–Barr virus (the cause of infectious mononucleosis) but which is absent from normal lymphocytes. The interpretation of this finding is not easy and its relevance is not established.

Chapter 13

Transplantation and the Major Histocompatibility Complex

There are many situations in medical practice where it is clear that the gifts of prolongation of life and an adequate quality of life can only be conferred on a patient by replacement of a defective organ. Examples of this include chronic renal failure due to a variety of disorders, intractable cardiac failure secondary to ischaemia or one of the primary disorders of heart muscle, chronic respiratory failure due to widespread pulmonary fibrosis or widespread disease in the small pulmonary vessels, bone marrow failure and chronic liver failure. However, the transfer of a 'spare part' from one individual to another is not a simple matter and, unless the donor and the recipient are genetically identical or, at least, very similar, the grafted tissue undergoes a series of changes which result in its destruction as a functioning entity. This sequence of events is known as **rejection.**

Like every other branch of science, transplantation has its own vocabulary:

1. A graft taken from the patient himself is an **autograft.**
2. A graft where both donor and recipient are genetically identical (syngeneic) such as in the case of identical twins, is an **isograft.**
3. A graft where donor and recipient are of the same species but not identical in genetic make-up (allogeneic) is an **allograft.** The most common allograft is, of course, a blood transfusion.
4. A graft where donor and recipient are not of the same species (xenogeneic) is a **xenograft**, e.g. monkey to man.

The events which take place in allograft rejection can be studied easily in a model system where skin from one strain of mouse is grafted onto a mouse of another strain. The grafted skin becomes normally vascularized in a few days, but shortly after this it becomes infiltrated by lymphocytes and macrophages and the blood flow through the part begins to diminish. By 10 days or so after the transplant, the graft is necrotic and is sloughed off leaving a bare area of exposed dermis.

What is the evidence that the rejection is immunological in nature?

First and second set reactions

In granuloma formation, the second contact with the responsible antigen (such as schistosome ova) leads to an accelerated and increased tissue response, and this is a universal pattern in immune reactions. If graft rejection is mediated by immunological mechanisms, one would expect the rejection of a second graft from a given donor to a given recipient to be accelerated and this is indeed the case. Indeed, in the case of mouse skin, adequate vascularization of the graft may never occur and necrosis may be obvious within a few days. This very rapid rejection is known as a **second set reaction.** The **specificity** of this reaction is shown by the fact that if a graft from a donor of genetic make-up different from that of the first donor is transplanted into a previously skin-grafted mouse, a second set reaction does not occur and the graft is rejected at the same speed as would a first graft (**first set reaction**).

Cell-mediated reaction

Again, as in the case of the granuloma, the transfer of lymphoid cells from an animal which has had an allograft to an animal which has not results in the second animal showing accelerated rejection of a graft from the original donor animal. In animals which have been thymectomized during the neonatal period, allografts survive for prolonged periods. The ability to reject such grafts at a 'normal' speed is restored by an injection of lymphocytes from a genetically identical normal animal.

Antibody production

Humoral antibodies which react with the donor cells can be found in the blood of the recipient after rejection.

All these data indicate that **rejection is immunologically mediated.** The success of isografts between animals which have an identical genetic constitution suggests that the antigens responsible for rejection are genetically determined.

The major histocompatibility complex

The key to transplantation is the major histocompatibility complex (MHC). This has been extensively studied in mouse and man and in the latter is made up of a group of genes on the short arm of chromosome 6. In the mouse there are at least 20 transplantation loci, but the most important of these is the H-2 locus. This provokes intense allograft rejections which are difficult to suppress. The H-2 locus in fact consists of at least three loci, two of which code for the very 'strong' transplantation antigens H-2K and H-2D. The third locus codes for H-2L.

All lymphoid cells contain large amounts of the H-2K/D antigens, liver, lung, and kidneys have moderate amounts, and brain and voluntary muscle have rather little.

Antigens of this group have been termed **class I molecules** and can be identified on lymphoid cells by the cytotoxicity of antibodies which react with them. The mouse histocompatibility complex, however, also codes for another group of antigens which have been called **class II molecules** or **Ia antigens**. These antigens are recognized by T cells and are thus the signals which stimulate a variety of T cell functions. They cannot be identified using a panel of antibodies. However, when lymphocytes from animals which are different in respect of the genes determining Ia antigens are mixed together they will undergo 'blast' transformation and mitosis.

The major histocompatibility complex in man

As stated above, the MHC in man is located on the short arm of chromosome 6. The dominant group of antigens governing rejection reactions is spoken of as the HLA system. HLA stands for **H**uman **L**eucocyte **A**ntigen, since the class I molecules have been delineated through the effect of their homospecific antibodies against human leucocytes, which, of course, constitute an abundant source of nucleated cells.

The class I molecules are coded for at three major loci — A, B and C. HLA-A and -B probably constitute the homologues of the 'strong' transplantation antigens H-2D and H-2K in the mouse and readily induce the formation of complement-fixing cytotoxic antibodies which can be used for tissue typing. These antibodies can be found in the plasma of patients who have had blood transfusions and multiparous women who have become immunized against fetal antigens defined by paternally derived genes.

HLA typing in respect of these class I antigens is done by setting up an individual's lymphocytes against a panel of known antibodies in the presence of complement. Binding of antibody to its homospecific antigen on the surface of the lymphocyte leads to cell membrane damage; this is monitored by testing the cells' ability to exclude dyes such as trypan blue or eosin. A marked degree of polymorphism exists in respect of the major histocompatibility loci. There are 20 alleles for HLA-A, 42 for HLA-B and eight for HLA-C.

Class II antigens were originally defined by the HLA-D locus. This is now known not to be a single locus and has been split into DR and D, each of which code for class II molecules. There are 12 D alleles and 10 DR alleles. DR antigens are expressed on the surfaces of B lymphocytes, monocytes and macrophages. Another locus known as Sb which codes for class II molecules has been recognized. The combination of genes coding for transplantation antigens which is inherited from each parent is known as the **haplotype**.

The antigens coded for by the D genes are recognized by performing the **mixed lymphocyte reaction test** (MLR). In this test, lymphocytes, for example from a patient awaiting a renal transplant, are mixed with an equal number of lymphocytes drawn from a potential donor. The donor cells are pre-treated either by irradiation or with mitomycin, which prevents them undergoing blast transformation in response to the D antigens on the surface of the recipient's lymphocytes should these be different from the donor's. Blast transformation of the potential recipient's cells is detected by measuring their uptake of tritiated thymidine, which is greatly increased if blast transformation occurs. Unfortunately this test takes five days to perform and thus is of no practical use if transplantation of a cadaver kidney is being contemplated. Newer serological methods are now available, however, for the detection of D and DR antigens.

From the point of view of a surgeon wishing to undertake a transplantation procedure, the most important factor in predicting the success or otherwise of the outcome is the degree of matching between the HLA-A and HLA-B antigens of the potential donor and the recipient. When the donor is a sibling of the recipient with good HLA matching, the chances of 10-year survival in the presence of appropriate immunosuppression are now about 90%. However, if the donor and recipient are not siblings, the same degree of HLA-A and -B matching gives a success rate over a 10-year period of only 60–70%. The explanation given for this discrepancy is that when brothers or sisters share a common heritage of HLA-A and HLA-B antigens from one of their parents, they are likely to have inherited most or all of the genes which lie between these two loci. While individuals who are not related seem to be identical at their A and B loci, they may well have many genes in between which are not identical.

The mechanisms involved in allograft rejection

In man, the system which has been studied most extensively is the renal allograft. Here, rejection can be seen to occur at different times after transplantation and the events at these different stages probably mirror different mechanisms.

Hyperacute rejection

This takes place within minutes of the graft being inserted. It is characterized by the presence of small thrombi and of sludged red cells in the glomeruli. It is a classical example of a type II immunological reaction. Preformed antibodies, present either as a result of ABO incompatibility between donor and recipient or because the recipient has formed antibodies as a reaction to previous blood transfusions, bind to endothelial cells in the small vessels of the kidney and activate complement with all the consequences that this entails.

Early acute rejection

This takes place 7–10 days after transplantation. The affected donor kidney shows a dense infiltration by lymphocytes (Fig. 13.1) which, using appropriate markers, are shown to be T cells. Many of these are cytotoxic and damage peritubular capillaries. The presence of some antibody at this stage may be a help rather than a danger to the patient,

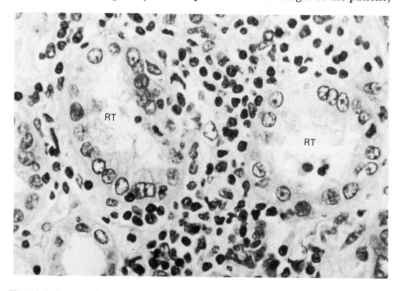

Fig. 13.1 Acute early rejection. This renal allograft was rejected 10 days after transplantation. The renal tubules (RT) and the peritubular blood vessels are surrounded by immunologically competent cells, the majority of which are T cells. These are exerting a direct cytotoxic effect on the constituents of the graft.

since these antibodies may bind to homospecific antigens on the donor graft and interfere with recognition of HLA antigens by the host T cells. This effect, which is known as **immunological enhancement**, may operate in the prolongation of graft survival which sometimes occurs in patients who have been given blood transfusions shortly before the grafting procedure.

Acute late rejection

This occurs in patients who have been immunosuppressed with prednisone and azathioprine. This regimen damps down the T cell response but is not completely effective in stopping antibody production. The rejection takes place between two and six weeks after the operation and is characterized by very florid vascular damage which appears to be mediated by antibody and complement (Fig. 13.2). The immunoglobulins and complement can be identified within the vessel walls by immunofluorescent techniques.

Late rejection

This can occur up to years after transplantation. The most prominent histological feature is fibromuscular hyperplasia of the intimal lining of

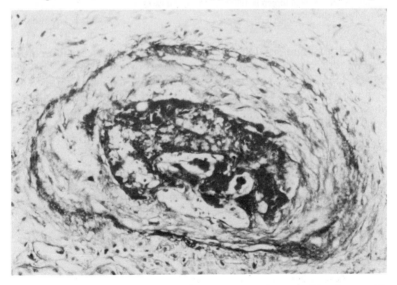

Fig. 13.2 Acute late rejection. The wall of the artery occupying most of the photographic field is severely disorganized and is infiltrated by a mixture of granular, lipid-containing cells and fibrin. The lumen is occluded by a darkly stained, fibrin-rich thrombus.

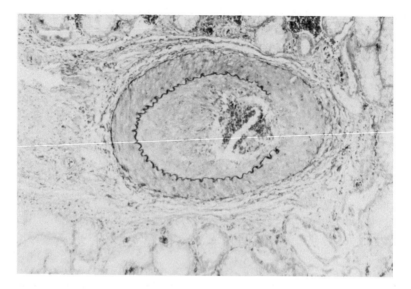

Fig. 13.3 Late rejection. In this allograft, removed from the recipient more than a year after transplantation because of a decline in renal function, the main structural change is vascular damage. There are obvious breaks in the wavy, darkly stained internal elastic lamina and the arterial lumen is markedly narrowed by fibromuscular intimal tissue which has proliferated.

small and medium-sized vessels in the kidney, with eventual occlusion leading to ischaemic necrosis of the glomeruli supplied by the affected vessels (Fig. 13.3). This too is thought to be mediated through the action of antibodies binding to HLA antigens on the endothelium of vessels in the donor kidney. Antibody and complement may also be seen to be deposited within the glomeruli.

The chances of rejection may be reduced essentially in two ways:

1. **Good matching between donor and recipient**
2. **Suppression of the immune responses of the recipient**

In so far as the first of these is concerned, the favoured priorities (in decreasing order) are stated by Najarian to be:

1. Monozygotic twin
2. Dizygotic twin
3. HLA-A and HLA-B identical sibling
4. HLA-one haplotype identical sibling

5. A sibling matched for less than two HLA antigens
6. A child identical for one haplotype
7. HLA-one haplotype identical parent
8. First order relatives (grandparents, uncles, aunts, cousins, etc.)
9. Cadavers with two or more matching HLA antigens
10. Cadavers with less than two matching HLA antigens

Immunosuppression

Azathioprine. This compound, which is broken down in the body to 6-mercaptopurine, is particularly helpful in inhibiting T cell mediated rejection. It interferes with enzyme systems involved in nucleic acid synthesis and is thus most likely to affect cells which are actively replicating. In the first days after transplantation, the cells most likely to be undergoing clonal expansion are the T cells and the drug thus inhibits lymphocyte proliferation. However, it is by no means specific for these cells and will affect other cell systems in which replication is a prominent feature.

Prednisone. This powerful steroid works in a different way from azathioprine and can thus have an additive effect in combating rejection. Like all corticosteroids, it has a strong anti-inflammatory effect and may also affect lymphocyte recirculation and the generation of effector T cells.

Cyclosporin A. This is a fungal product which, unlike azathioprine, has no effects on the replicating cells of the bone marrow. It selectively penetrates antigen-sensitive T cells in the G_0 to G_1 phase and inhibits an RNA polymerase. It has also been suggested that it can block the production of interleukin 2, which is required for the clonal expansion of cytotoxic T cells. It appears to be a most promising agent. At certain dose levels it is nephrotoxic and thus its blood concentration must be monitored carefully.

Antilymphocytic globulin. This means of immunosuppression was introduced in 1967. Essentially, it consists of the raising of antisera which, when injected intravenously, will cause complement-mediated lysis of the recipient's lymphocytes. In order to avoid the foreign IgG acting as an antigen, it is deaggregated before use, which seems to render it inactive in this restricted sense.

Bone marrow transplantation and graft versus host reactions

Thus far only the question of graft rejection by the recipient has been considered. Another aspect of the transplantation problem is what has been termed **graft versus host reaction.** This is a major factor in bone marrow transplantation, which is used in patients with aplastic anaemia, immunological deficiencies and those whose bone marrow has been ablated by therapy, e.g. for acute leukaemia.

The basis of a graft versus host (GvH) reaction is when competent lymphoid cells are transferred from a donor to a recipient who is unable to reject them. If the donor cells survive long enough to recognize the recipient's cells as 'foreign', they will mount immunological reactions against the recipient's cells, hence the term 'graft versus host'. In mice there will be inhibition of growth (so-called 'runting'), haemolytic anaemia and splenomegaly. In humans, GvH is characterized by fever, weight loss, a rash, splenomegaly, anaemia and diarrhoea. Cyclosporin A reduces the frequency of GvH and recently some success has been obtained by treating the bone marrow sample which is to be transplanted with monoclonal anti-T cell antibodies so that cells capable of responding to the recipient's antigens are removed.

HLA Relationships with Disease

Why do some people get certain diseases and others not? For many years geneticists have tried to answer this question. Apart from the various familial disorders for which the inheritance patterns have been worked out, some associations, though rather weak, were noted, for example the relationship between ABO blood groups and gastric carcinoma. In 1963 an association was noted between susceptibility to spontaneous murine leukaemia and certain antigens of the H-2 system, and in 1967 an association was described between certain HLA antigens in man and the risk of developing Hodgkin's disease. These early reports have led to a considerable degree of exploration of the relationships between human haplotypes and various diseases.

In considering this question, it must be remembered that there are a number of genes not directly concerned with transplantation reactions that are closely linked to the HLA complex on the short arm of chromosome 6. These include the gene determining properdin factor B (which is involved in the alternate pathway of complement activation), genes for controlling the production of the second and fourth components of complement, and a gene controlling the production of the enzyme 21-hydroxylase.

The distribution of HLA genes is non-uniform on a world-wide basis

The prevalence of various HLA determined antigens varies between populations. For instance, A30 is found in 28% of blacks, in only 5% of whites and not at all in Japanese. Aw24 occurs in 58.5% of Japanese, in 18% of whites and in only 6% of blacks. HLA-B8 occurs in 16% of whites, but in less than 0.5% of Japanese.

Linkage disequilibrium

Sometimes the alleles of two or more loci, for instance A1 and B8 or A1, B8 and DR3, occur together more frequently than would be expected if their association was only random. This is known as **linkage disequilibrium.**

Several explanations have been offered for this phenomenon. One suggests that at some point in the course of evolution, a certain combination of alleles may have conferred some selective advantage. This, while not provable, gains a little support from the fact that the frequency of certain alleles and haplotypes differs between populations living under different environmental conditions. Thus the haplotypes which show linkage disequilibrium in European whites are quite different from those occurring in West African blacks. The second suggestion put forward is that some haplotypes have arisen relatively recently (in evolutionary terms) and that there has been insufficient time for equilibration to occur by random recombination. The third possibility is that, as a result of migration, some 'foreign' haplotype or gene has been introduced into a population, leading to linkage disequilibrium in the genetic pool of that population. Many generations of random breeding may be required before this effect vanishes.

Linkage and association in human disease

The appropriate distinction between linkage and association should be made in considering genetic relationships in human disease. The term **linkage**, strictly speaking, applies to a situation where gene loci are close to each other on a particular chromosome. The presence of such linkage can only be recognized by carrying out family studies on more than one generation to see whether certain characteristics are indeed transmitted together. Not many human diseases have been shown to be linked to the HLA system in this way. Those which have been found include 21-hydroxylase deficiency, which leads to congenital adrenal hyperplasia (see p. 380), deficiencies of the second and fourth components of complement, and some cases of haemochromatosis.

The term **association** refers to a relationship between two separate characteristics, and this can be recognized by examining a large enough number of cases of a certain disease and controls. For example, HLA-B27 occurs more frequently in patients with ankylosing spondylitis than in a randomly selected control population.

The most striking association with HLA-determined antigens are to be found in disorders in which immune mechanisms are believed to be implicated — the rheumatic diseases and a group of diseases characterized by chronic inflammation and abnormal immunological reactions.

Family studies in autoimmune diseases suggest a genetic influence

Two striking family studies reported in 1982 can be quoted as strong support for the operation of genetic factors in autoimmune disease. The two families between them contained 70 relatives and 23 spouses. In one family the patient originally identified had autoimmune haemolytic anaemia and hypothyroidism. Five relatives had hyperthyroidism and three others had ulcerative colitis. In the second family, the proband had autoimmune thrombocytopenia. Four of her relatives had rheumatoid arthritis, systemic lupus erythematosus, autoimmune thrombocytopenia or asthma. There was no evidence of autoimmune disease in the spouses. Other studies also show evidence of this type of familial clustering. Even more suggestive is evidence obtained from studying identical twins. The concordance of systemic lupus erythematosus in identical twins ranges from 50 to 60%. In type I diabetes the concordance is also about 50% in so far as insulin requirement is concerned.

Ankylosing spondylitis

The most convincing of all HLA associations with disease is that between HLA-B27 and ankylosing spondylitis. It might be more correct to use the term preferred by some American writers, 'the spondyloarthropathies', because, while ankylosing spondylitis is the archetype, a number of other arthritides involving the spine, sacroiliac and axial joints have this association. This group of disorders includes:

1. Ankylosing spondylitis
2. Reiter's disease
3. Psoriatic arthritis
4. Post-shigella, post-salmonella and post-yersinia arthritis
5. Spondylitis associated with inflammatory bowel disease

The B27 antigen is found in more than 90% of white patients with ankylosing spondylitis and only in 10% of white controls. Possession of the antigen confers a risk of developing the disease which is 80–90 times greater than that in the control population. Even so, the individual with the B27 gene stands a change of only between 5 and 20% of developing ankylosing spondylitis. Fifty per cent of the first degree relatives of spondylitics with B27 also have the antigen, and 30% of them either develop ankylosing spondylitis or some other spondyloarthropathy.

The prevalence of B27 in different populations correlates quite well with the risk of developing the disease. B27 is virtually absent from Japan and ankylosing spondylitis is very rare among the Japanese. Conversely, there is a tribe of Indians in British Columbia (the Haidas) in whom the prevalence of B27 is more than 50%. This tribe also has a very high prevalence of ankylosing spondylitis. The presence of B27 in the haplotype confers a lower increment of risk relative to the control population in respect of the other spondyloarthropathies than it does in relation to ankylosing spondylitis (Table 13.1).

Table 13.1 The relative risks of various spondyloarthropathies in the presence of HLA-B27.

Disease	Relative risk
Reiter's disease	37.0
Post-salmonella arthritis	29.7
Post-shigella arthritis	20.7
Post-yersinia arthritis	17.6

One problem in relation to the association between B27 and ankylosing spondylitis is the different prevalence of the disease between the sexes. Males are affected five times as frequently as females, but the distribution of B27 is the same in both sexes.

Rheumatoid arthritis

Classic rheumatoid arthritis is associated with the class II antigens Dw4 and DR4. These are present in 25% of the control population and 45% of those with the disease. The DR4 association is strongest for those cases with severe erosive changes in the articular cartilage and underlying bone and who have rheumatoid factors in their plasma. Patients with rheumatoid arthritis who are treated with gold or D-penicillamine, and who develop an immune complex nephritis as a result, have an association with HLA-B8 and -DR3.

A group of other diseases, in all of which immune mechanisms appear to be implicated, have associations with antigens of both the class I and class II variety.

Coeliac disease

This condition is characterized by malabsorption associated with subtotal or total atrophy of the villi of the duodenum and jejunum. The patients are sensitive to the gliadin fraction of gluten and when this is withheld from their diet, their symptoms and the appearances of their gut mucosa both improve markedly. Such patients have a strong association with HLA-B8 (this being present in 60–81% of the patients and only in 16–22% of controls). DR3 is found in 79% of the patients and D7 in 45%. Small gut changes which are not dissimilar to those found in coeliac disease are also found in association with a bullous disorder of the skin known as **dermatitis herpetiformis**, 70% of patients having the skin lesions also showing the typical gut lesion. Eighty-five per cent of the group that have both the skin and small gut lesions are positive for B8 and Dw3. If only skin lesions are present, the proportion of patients having B8 and Dw3 falls to 30%. This strongly suggests that the association is with the gut lesion.

Myasthenia gravis

Myasthenia gravis, which has already been discussed previously in relation to anti-idiotypic antibodies, appears to exist in two forms so far as its genetic associations are concerned. The early onset type associated with thymic hyperplasia has an association with B8 and DR3. The adult onset type, which is usually associated with a tumour of the thymus (thymoma), does not show any strong HLA association.

Juvenile diabetes

So-called juvenile diabetes, which is usually early in onset and associated with a need for insulin, shows associations either for B8 and DR3 or B15 and DR4. The presence of DR3 increases the relative risk to 3.3 and that of DR4 to 6.4. Being homozygous for either of these antigens increases the relative risks to 10 and 16 respectively and if both DR3 and DR4 are present the relative risk rises to 33. The presence of an antigen coded for by an allelic variant of the factor B gene (BF1) is eight times more common in patients with juvenile diabetes than in the general population. It is not known whether DR3 and DR4 per se confer increased susceptibility to diabetes mellitus or whether they may be linked with some, as yet unknown, susceptibility gene.

Genes other than those coding for HLA antigens may show associations with certain autoimmune diseases

Correlations have been found between genes that specify certain phenotypic markers of immunoglobulins and some autoimmune diseases. One of these phenotypes called Gm is a polymorphic marker on the Fc portion of immunoglobulins. Its variants are associated with thyrotoxicosis (Graves' disease), myasthenia gravis and type 1 diabetes mellitus. The use of these markers, and of certain others as well, in association with HLA typing may greatly strengthen our recognition of a genetic component to certain diseases. For example, there is a recognized association between Graves' disease and HLA-B8/DR3. When Gm typing is added to the study of these patients, much stronger associations are found.

Possible mechanisms underlying the association with HLA type and disease susceptibility

Various explanations have been proposed to account for the associations between certain diseases and HLA type. The first of these has been called the 'molecular mimicry' hypothesis, according to which histocompatibility antigens might show partial homology with some of the determinants of certain microorganisms and that this might lead to cross-reaction phenomena. Another suggestion is that certain HLA antigens might be susceptible to alterations as a result of events such as viral infections, exposure to toxins and neoplastic transformation, and that this alteration might lead to a loss of tolerance of the HLA surface antigens. A third theory proposes that the Ir genes, which are associated with the HLA complex and which determine the degree of immune reactivity, are involved in the HLA-associated diseases and determine the immune overreaction which is a feature of many of the disorders.

A recent review suggests that the undoubted complexities in this area may be somewhat simplified if the genes associated with increased susceptibility to certain diseases are divided into two classes:

1. Those related to the regulation of the immune response
2. Those related to the effector arm of the immune system

In this scheme the former would determine whether or not autoantibodies were formed, and the latter would determine the development of lesions. The two varieties of gene would be unlinked in order to explain the presence of autoantibodies but the absence of the disease (such as may be seen in the relatives of some patients with autoimmune diseases). Only when **both classes** of gene are inherited does the disease develop.

Regulation of immune responses

An example which is cited to support this view is the frequent association between the HLA antigens B8 and DR3 and autoimmune disease. Both of these have independently been associated with abnormalities of immune regulation in individuals without any evidence of an autoimmune disorder.

Lymphocytes from normal individuals who have the HLA-B8 antigen respond less well to T cell mitogens such as phytohaemagglutinin than do the cells of those without this HLA antigen. Not all HLA-B8 subjects show this defect, which suggests that HLA-B8, by itself, may be insufficient to produce it. HLA-B8 is the commonest phenotype in the 'healthy', autoantibody-producing relatives of patients with autoimmune diseases.

Normal individuals with HLA-DR3 have lymphocytes which show some impairment of suppressor cell function when tested in vitro, and the number of immunoglobulin-secreting B cells is increased relative to DR3-negative persons. In vitro, possession of the DR3 allele is associated with abnormalities of phagocytosis by macrophages, and defects in Fc receptor function have been reported in normal individuals with the HLA-B8/DR3 haplotype. DR4, the allele which is associated with classical rheumatoid arthritis, is said to correlate with the ability of lymphocytes from normal persons to mount an immunological response in vitro when exposed to collagen.

In connection with some autoimmune disorders (systemic lupus erythematosus, primary biliary cirrhosis and type 1 diabetes), clinically healthy first degree relatives show impaired function of T suppressor cells, another indication of the influence of the genetic constitution of an individual on immune regulation.

The effector arm of the immune response in autoimmune disease

The elimination of immune complexes may well be mediated by the binding of C3b to its appropriate cell surface receptor, this being followed by binding and phagocytosis of the complex. The number of these receptors for C3b is genetically determined, and is reduced both in patients suffering from systemic lupus erythematosus and their clinically healthy first degree relatives. Thus one might possibly view systemic lupus as a disorder characterized by a genetically determined propensity to form autoantibodies in large amounts and a genetically determined inability to eliminate the immune complexes formed as a result of the presence of autoantibodies at appropriate concentrations. It is also not without interest that some relatives of patients with autoimmune diseases show mild changes in their tissues of the type which are characteristic of the disease process; for example, a moderate degree of villous atrophy of the small intestinal mucosa is found in about 10% of the asymptomatic first degree relatives of patients with dermatitis herpetiformis.

Chapter 14

Granulomatous Inflammation

Granulomatous inflammation is a special type of chronic inflammatory reaction which is characterized by the local accumulation of large numbers of macrophages, some of which may have undergone striking morphological and functional changes. The cell biology of the macrophage dictates many of the features of this type of inflammation, which is expressed in the form of some of the most widespread, common and serious infective diseases. At any given moment, just three of these — tuberculosis, leprosy and schistosomiasis (bilharziasis) affect more than 200 million people on a world-wide basis. Viewed superficially there are marked differences between many of the granulomatous disorders in respect of their tissue and clinical manifestations. Some, such as tuberculosis, may cause extensive tissue destruction if local, while others show only focal or more diffuse infiltration by macrophages. The common factor is, however, the macrophage, with its role in antigen presentation, its reactions to the soluble products secreted by sensitized T lymphocytes, and its capacity to function both as a phagocytic and secretory cell.

Cell Biology of the Macrophage

Ultimately the macrophage is derived from the bone marrow. A precursor cell in the marrow, the **promonocyte**, is released into the circulation as a **monocyte**. After 12 to 32 hours, this cell migrates into the tissues, where it undergoes maturation to form the **macrophage**. The tissues constitute the bourne from which, like the traveller in *Hamlet*, this cell never returns. The term macrophage was coined by Metchnikoff in the dying years of the nineteenth century. Its literal translation is '**big eater**' — a term which could refer equally to its large size, its ability to engulf large particles, and its great reserve capacity for phagocytosis. As pointed out in Chapter 5, the macrophage possesses certain inbuilt advantages over the neutrophil. It has a longer natural life span, it can resynthesize the membranes and the intracellular enzymes lost during phagocytosis (which the neutrophil cannot), it can ingest particles which are far larger than can be coped with by the neutrophil, and it can undergo mitotic division.

Phagocytosis and endocytosis

The macrophage can ingest a wide variety of substances which exist within its cytoplasm in membrane-bound vesicles (the phagosomes). Large particles are engulfed by phagocytosis — a process which is triggered by close contact between the plasma membrane of the macrophage and the object to be engulfed, this being aided by the process of opsonization. Like the neutrophil, the macrophage has surface receptors for the common opsonins IgG and the 3b component of complement. Binding to these receptors starts a series of membrane and intracytoplasmic events leading to the formation of pseudopodia, which surround the target particle. Other receptors have been described for activators of the alternate complement pathway and for **lectins**, a family of proteins which bind with exquisite specificity to a variety of sugars which are expressed on the surface of cells. The expression of some of these receptors can be profoundly influenced by factors external to the macrophage. Monocytes have hardly any receptors for the chemotactic C5a component of complement. However, if they are incubated in a medium containing lymphokines, expression of this receptor starts in a short time and eventually some 40 000 receptors can be found on the plasma membrane of each cell.

Bacterial killing

Just as with the neutrophil, ingestion of particles within phagosomes is associated with a respiratory burst and fusion of the phagosome with lysosomes. If the ingested particle is a microorganism it may be killed, the most important mechanism being the oxygen-dependent one described earlier (see p. 52). However, for some organisms, the mere fact that engulfment by macrophages has taken place is far from being a death warrant. Mycobacteria (including those responsible for tuberculosis and leprosy), brucella, listeria, salmonella, toxoplasma, leishmania, chlamydia, rickettsia and the agent of Legionnaire's disease are among those that maintain a symbiotic relationship with the macrophage unless the latter becomes activated, usually as a result of interaction with the soluble **lymphokines** released from activated T cells.

The Fate of Macrophages in Granulomatous Inflammation

Once a macrophage has migrated to a site of infection or tissue injury a number of possible fates await it. The material phagocytosed may prove toxic to the macrophage and the cell may die, with release of its intralysosomal contents into the surrounding extracellular milieu. If the inflammatory stimulus disappears, the macrophages which have gathered in response to its presence migrate from the site and the lesion resolves. Ingestion of non-toxic but undegradable material leads to conversion of the macrophage into a very long-lived form which persists in the tissue together with its intracytoplasmic load. The most striking changes, however, which macrophages can undergo are conversion into so-called **epithelioid cells** and fusion to form multinucleate giant cells or **macrophage polykaryons.**

Epithelioid cell transformation

In many granulomas (most notably in tuberculosis and sarcoidosis) some of the aggregated macrophages, which account for most of the bulk of the lesion, can be seen to have undergone a series of morphological changes which have led to them being called epithelioid cells. This is a rather unfortunate term coined by pathologists in the late nineteenth century who thought that there was some resemblance between these cells and squamous epithelium.

In essence the changes involved include elongation of the cells, which appear to be in close contact, the cell boundaries being very indistinct on light microscopy. When examined with the electron microscope, the plasma membranes of adjacent cells are seen to be closely applied to one another and often interdigitate. The epithelioid cell has much more rough endoplasmic reticulum, much more plasma membrane and a much more developed Golgi apparatus than the untransformed macrophage, features which suggest that the cell has become differentiated towards the **secretory** rather than the **phagocytic** end of the spectrum of macrophage activity. Indeed, epithelioid cells are only one-tenth as effective in phagocytosis as untransformed macrophages. There is less expression of surface receptors such as those for Fc and C5a. Phagocytosed material is seldom, if ever, seen in the cytoplasm and it would appear that in differentiating in this way the epithelioid cells have lost the normal ability of the macrophage to react with extracellular particles, though they retain the ability to express HLA-DR coded antigens on their surfaces and thus still have the potential to interact with T lymphocytes.

Histochemical studies have shown that the epithelioid cell contains the expected number of lysosomal enzymes, muramidase (lysozyme) and, rather surprisingly, angiotensin-converting enzyme. The role of this enzyme in granulomatous inflammation is not known, though it has been suggested, as a result of studies of schistosomiasis in the mouse, that it may inhibit further migration of macrophages and that its secretion may be controlled by T lymphocytes. Certainly there is much evidence to suggest that epithelioid cell formation is one of the expressions of cell-mediated immunity.

Multinucleated giant cell formation (macrophage polykaryons)

The long-continued presence of any foreign material, whether living (as in the case of the organisms responsible for tuberculosis or leprosy) or non-living, tends to elicit a response in which the macrophage in one or other of its functional and morphological forms is the dominant element.

The simplest example of this is the presence within the dermis of unabsorbed suture material. In this situation, as indeed in many other types of granulomatous inflammation, some members of the local macrophage infiltrate fuse to form multinucleated giant cells. Classic morphological pathology teaches us (quite wrongly) that there are two distinct forms of the multinucleate giant cell: the **foreign body giant cell** and the **Langhans' giant cell**. The former has its many nuclei dispersed more or less evenly through the cytoplasm. It commonly appears in response to the presence of exogenous foreign material such as sutures or to misplaced endogenous material such as hair, cholesterol crystals or keratin which have escaped from their normal confines and lie free in an inappropriate environment. The so-called Langhans giant cell has multiple nuclei which tend to lie at the periphery of the cell in a horseshoe pattern, leaving a clear zone of cytoplasm in the centre. The archetypal situation in which this variant is found is in chronic infective granulomas such as tuberculosis. In fact the Langhans' cell merely represents a later stage in the development of the macrophage polykaryon; it has a greater content of lysosomal enzymes and a more highly developed Golgi apparatus than the foreign body giant cell. If microtubule function in the latter is interfered with by adding colchicine, transformation into the Langhans' variant is blocked.

Formation of multinucleated giant cells

In certain experimentally induced chronic inflammatory lesions it has been shown that fusion of macrophages to form multinucleate giant cells only takes place when the population of macrophages first elicited by the injurious agent is reinforced by the arrival of new macrophages. If a glass coverslip is placed in the subcutaneous tissues of a mouse, within a very short time the glass becomes covered with macrophages. If the coverslip is removed at this time and placed within a diffusion chamber into which no further cell migration can occur and the whole apparatus returned to the subcutaneous tissue, no fusion of

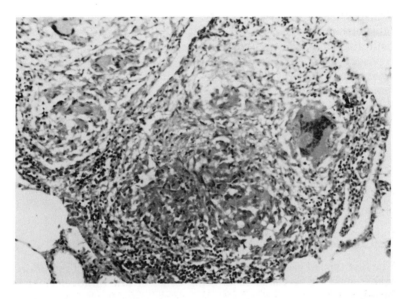

Fig. 14.1 Tuberculous granulomas. This photograph of lung from a child with miliary tuberculosis shows the presence of two granulomas. Rounded aggregates of epithelioid cells can be seen surrounded by a zone of lymphocytic infiltration. Some multinucleated Langhans' giant cells are also present. Central necrosis is not seen.

macrophages takes place, despite the fact that mitotic division occurs. If holes are made in such a diffusion chamber so that cells can gain access to it, macrophage fusion can be seen to occur. In addition to the recruitment of fresh macrophages, an additional factor which stimulates macrophage fusion and thus the formation of giant cells is the attempt by two or more cells to endocytose the same material. Once such fusion has occurred the resulting cell can fuse with other macrophages and hence acquire the impressive number of nuclei commonly seen in some granulomas (Fig. 14.1).

Role of the multinucleated giant cell

Giant cells in chronic inflammatory lesions behave like other multinucleated cells in that their nuclei enter the mitotic cycle in a near synchronous fashion. This is likely to lead to pooling of genetic material and some of the resulting chromosomes are defective. Polyploidy is present in some nuclei and this appears to shorten the lifespan of the cell. It has been suggested that the formation of the polykaryon, with the implication that its lifespan will inevitably be shorter than that of the unfused macrophage, is one of the ways in which the multiplication of macrophages in a chronic inflammatory focus can be controlled. It is probably unwise to accept too uncritically the thesis that the multinucleated giant cell merely constitutes a stage on the macrophage's path to oblivion. One recent study compares the bone resorptive activity of mononuclear and multinucleated macrophages derived from the rat. The polykaryon variants bound and degraded significantly more bone than the mononuclear cells, suggesting that, at least in the frame of reference provided by osteoclast formation, existence in a multinucleate form confers some advantage.

Classification of the Granulomatous Response

In terms of the processes involved, the question of how to classify granulomatous reactions has been considered in two ways.

Cell kinetics

The first type of classification is based on the cell kinetics of the lesion, granulomata being classified as being either of **low turnover** or **high turnover** type.

An aggregate of macrophages whose presence has been elicited by some persistent irritant will remain until the irritant is cleared (which may, of course, be never). The cell population is maintained firstly by continuing migration of macrophages to the site of the irritant. If this migration is balanced by death of macrophages within the lesion or emigration to draining nodes, then the lesion will remain more or less **constant in size.**

Another mechanism for maintaining the cell population within the lesion is mitotic division of the aggregated macrophages. The number of successful mitoses is usually restricted to two or three, so that in the long-term this mechanism cannot be very effective.

Lastly the macrophages which have aggregated at the site of the irritant may become immobilized and remain in situ for prolonged periods with few changes in the cell number due to either death or division.

In the so-called **low turnover** type of granuloma, the aggregated macrophages, as indicated above, remain for a long time within the lesion and there is little new migration of macrophages and little in the way of cell death or mitotic division. The irritant, which is typically non-toxic to the macrophage but poorly degradable by it (e.g. barium sulphate, carageenan), persists within the cells in relatively large amounts. Epithelioid cells are usually not present in such granulomas and the presence of lymphoid cells, which might suggest the involvement of immune mechanisms, is distinctly unusual.

In contrast, the macrophage population in the **high turnover** type of granuloma needs constant replenishment in order to compensate for the high death rate and the relatively short lifespan of the cells originally forming the lesion. The causative agents are usually highly toxic for the macrophages (e.g. mycobacteria, silica) and can be identified in only a small proportion of these cells. Such granulomas show evidence of functional heterogeneity within the macrophage population and epithelioid cell transformation is a common phenomenon. Some of the most important disorders affecting humans are characterized by this high turnover type of granulomatous inflammation, amongst them tuberculosis and leprosy.

Involvement of immunological mechanisms

Since most granulomas of clinical significance are of the high turnover variety, some additional ways in which they could be classified would be useful in understanding their pathogenesis. Recently some writers have attempted to divide up the granulomas on the basis of whether or not immune mechanisms are involved in their formation.

Granulomas without evidence of immunological mechanisms

The major feature of such granulomas is the lack of specific recognition of the irritant by the immune system and, therefore, the lack of an enhanced response on a second exposure to the irritant. Thus no matter how great the frequency of exposure, the lesions always appear at the same time after the irritant has entered the host and the size of the lesions is the same on each occasion. It is impossible to transfer reactivity from one animal to another either with serum or cells, and immunosuppressive measures do not affect the development of the lesion.

An experimental model of this type of reaction which has been studied extensively is the granuloma which follows the injection of small plastic beads into the tissue. In vitro the beads activate Hageman factor and generate kinin activity in normal human and mouse plasma. When such beads are injected into pigeons, which lack Hageman factor, no granulomas are formed. Agents such as talc and silica which cause granulomas of this type are believed to operate through similar mechanisms.

Granulomas in which immunological mechanisms are involved

The fundamental difference between granulomas in which immune mechanisms play a part and those which have been described above is that in the former case the first exposure to an irritant induces an altered state of reactivity. This expresses itself in the form of an accelerated and more severe reaction on second and subsequent exposures to the irritant. The formation of the granuloma can be inhibited by measures designed to suppress immunity and the altered reactivity can be transferred from animal to animal by either cells, serum or both.

Mechanisms underlying the induction of 'immunologically mediated' granulomas. Much of the basic knowledge relating to immunologically mediated granulomas has been derived from studies of the tissue reactions to infestation by the helminth *Schistosoma* (bilharzia), which is a parasite affecting more than 100 000 000 people. The worms themselves induce no lasting tissue response, but many of the eggs they lay do not escape from the body of the host and it is these eggs which induce granuloma formation. When eggs of *Schistosoma mansoni* are injected into the tissues of a mouse, no inflammatory response is seen for 48 hours (a fact possibly related to the presence of anti-Hageman factor activity in the eggs). Macrophages and eosinophils start to accumulate round the eggs about 60 hours after injection; this occurs at much the same time as delayed hypersensitivity can be demonstrated in the mouse foot pad following injection of soluble schistosomal egg antigens. Priming of the mouse host by prior intraperitoneal injection of *Schistosoma mansoni* leads to faster and more severe granuloma formation. A similar enhancement of the reaction can be seen on first exposure to *Schistosoma* in mice who have received injections of spleen or lymph node cells from an animal with schistosomal granulomas (**passive transfer**).

It is possible to culture living granulomas isolated from the livers of infected mice. These studies have demonstrated the secretion from the cells of the granuloma of two lymphokines: **macrophage migration inhibiting factor** (MIF) and a factor which promotes the activity of eosinophils. In addition, lysosomal enzymes and a factor which stimulates fibroblast proliferation and the synthesis of collagen can be identified in the culture fluid. Very little antibody globulin can be isolated from these lesions. These data indicate the importance of cell-mediated immunity, at least in this model, and also show that such a granuloma carries within itself the means by which both necrosis and scarring can be brought about.

Scar tissue formation in granulomas. The formation of scar tissue in and around granulomas is probably largely controlled by the secretion of the cells which make up the lesion. The degree of such scarring is determined by the balance between factors which stimulate fibroblasts and hence collagen formation and those which work in a contrary way and lead to collagen breakdown. Both these sets of factors are governed, at least in part, by the macrophage. The macrophage can secrete substances which stimulate fibroblast division (interleukin 1 is probably one such substance) and fibronectin, which it also secretes, is chemotactic for fibroblasts. On the other hand, macrophages can secrete enzymes which break down collagen, and fluid in which macrophages have been cultured has been described as being able to inhibit collagen synthesis.

This brief general account of the nature of immunologically modulated granulomatous reactions sets the stage for the consideration in Chapter 15 of some of the serious human disorders in which the development of such lesions is a dominant feature.

Chapter 15

Some Specific Granulomatous Disorders

Tuberculosis

Tuberculosis is a disease of great antiquity, diagnosable lesions having been found in Egyptian mummies dating back as far as 3400 BC. Hippocrates knew tuberculosis in its pulmonary form and the great Persian physician Avicenna, who died in 1037 AD recognized that it was contagious. The term 'tubercle' was first applied to the pulmonary lesions in the seventeenth century by Sylvius. The fact that tuberculosis is an infective disease was confirmed roughly 100 years ago by the great bacteriologist Robert Koch. In doing so he put forward three postulates, fulfilment of which is still regarded in many instances as being essential in ascribing the origin of a disease to an infective cause.

Koch's postulates

1. The suspected organisms must be present in the lesions in all cases of the disease.
2. It must be possible to isolate the suspected organisms in pure culture from the lesions.
3. It must be possible to reproduce the disease by injecting or otherwise introducing the organisms into a healthy animal.

Some epidemiological considerations

The mortality and morbidity due to tuberculosis have decreased so sharply in the affluent countries of the West that it is difficult now to conceive of its overwhelming importance as a cause of death and misery even as recently as 40 years ago. In the USA at the beginning of this century, tuberculosis was the premier cause of death, being responsible for the death of 200 per 100 000 population annually. By 1965 it had dropped to eighteenth place and killed only 4.1 per 100 000 each year. Similarly, in Scotland, male mortality ascribable to tuberculosis decreased from 58 per 100 000 in 1938 to 4 per 100 000 by 1972.

However, in countries which are less privileged economically, the prevalence of tuberculosis remains much as it was half a century ago, and it has been estimated that, on a world-wide basis, three to five million people die each year from this disease.

When there is a sharp decline in mortality and morbidity from any disease there is a natural temptation to regard this as a triumph for the art of medicine. In the case of tuberculosis this is true to only a very limited extent and much of the credit for the great improvement must go to socioeconomic factors. These include:

1. Improved housing with less overcrowding
2. Improved nutrition
3. Improved sanitation
4. Effective chemotherapy for sufferers from the disease
5. Early detection by mass miniature radiography and hence early treatment
6. Pasteurization of milk and tuberculin testing of dairy cattle leading to the virtual elimination of primary intestinal tuberculosis

It is important to recognize that there are certain segments of the population who have a higher than average risk of developing tuberculosis. These include diabetics, patients on immunosuppressive treatment, patients with silicosis and, in Britain, Asian immigrants, who are many times more likely to develop the disease than indigenous Britons.

The organism

Tuberculosis is caused by **Mycobacterium tuberculosis.** This is a slender, slightly curved, rod-shaped organism which can be stained only with some difficulty and which has the remarkable property, once it has been stained, of resisting decolorization by acid and alcohol. This 'acid fastness' is related to the presence of large amounts of complex lipid substances (neutral fats, phosphatides and various long chain fatty acids) in the capsule of the bacillus. The organism is stained by the Ziehl–Neelsen method (hot carbolfuchsin followed by decolorization in acid and alcohol, and counterstaining with methylene blue or malachite green). The bacilli may also be stained with auramine, a dye which exhibits yellow fluorescence when exposed to ultraviolet light; it is often easier to identify the mycobacteria in material treated in this way than by conventional light microscopic methods.

Mycobacteria are aerobic and grow slowly in culture. They are extremely resistant to drying and this means that infection can follow inhalation of dust in which infected dried sputum is present. At least five strains of the organisms exist:

human
bovine
murine
avian
reptilian

In humans the infection may be acquired in three ways:

inhalation
ingestion
inoculation

In communities where the dairy herds are free from mycobacterial infection, only the first of these is at all common or important.

Tuberculous granulomas

The essential lesion of tuberculosis is the **tuberculous granuloma**. The development of tuberculous granuloma, or follicle as it is sometimes called, is the archetypal response of all tissues to the presence of the *Mycobacterium tuberculosis*. The extensive tissue destruction which may be found in this disease depends on the number of such granulomas, their growth and confluence, the degree of the characteristic **caseation necrosis** which occurs, and the attempts at repair which the long continued presence of the lesions ultimately stimulates.

Unlike organisms such as *Clostridium welchii* or *Staphylococcus aureus* which produce toxins directly damaging to the tissues, the mycobacterium has not, as yet, been shown to have any direct cytotoxic effect. Indeed, it survives and multiplies within macrophages in cell culture without any harm coming to the cultured cells. The tissue damage which is so prominent a feature of tuberculosis is largely, if not entirely, mediated by the **specific altered reactivity of the immune system which occurs as a result of introduction of the mycobacterium into the host**. This altered state of reactivity expresses itself in two ways: first, by enhanced resistance to infection and more effective **clearing** of the mycobacteria from the tissues of the host, and second, by the appearance of hypersensitivity through which tissue damage is caused.

The evolution of a tuberculous granuloma (Fig. 15.1)

Following the introduction of the bacilli into the tissues, there is a very mild, transient, acute inflammatory reaction in which neutrophils participate. The organisms are presumably engulfed by the local macrophage population and, in association with class II MHC-coded membrane proteins, the mycobacterial antigens are presented to

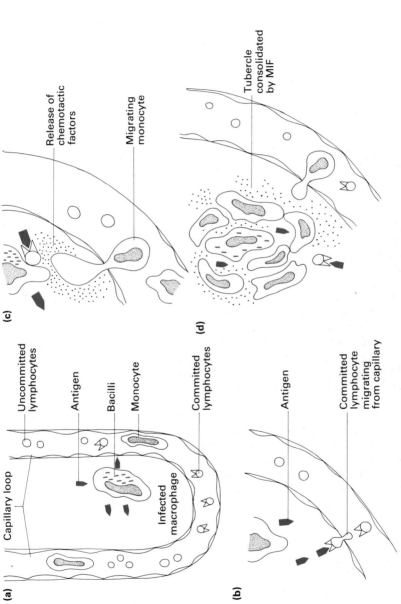

Fig. 15.1 The formation of a tuberculous granuloma. MIF = macrophage migration inhibiting factor.

appropriate T helper cells. The interaction between these two groups of cells leads to the proliferation of specifically coded T cells and to the release of lymphokines from them.

This is followed by an infiltration by macrophages which group together to form focal accumulations at the site of infection and then become immobilized at that site. The whole process is subtly modulated by the immune system. One lymphokine is **chemotactic** for the macrophages, while another (MIF) renders them relatively **immobile**. The fact that, in an **unprimed host**, bacillus-bearing macrophages travel from the site of infection in the tissue to the draining lymph nodes suggests that the full action of MIF takes some time to express itself in vivo. In addition, the stimulated T cells also secrete a **gamma interferon** which increases the expression of class II MHC-coded proteins on the macrophage membrane and thus can increase the ability of the local macrophages to present antigen.

Many of the macrophages then undergo **epithelioid cell** transformation. This, as described in Chapter 14, is associated with loss of the ability to phagocytose foreign particles. Some of the macrophages fuse, with the formation of multinucleate giant cells which mature and acquire the characteristic 'horseshoe' arrangement of nuclei found in the Langhans giant cell. This mass of epithelioid cells becomes

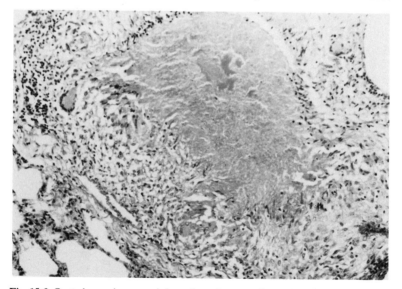

Fig. 15.2 Central caseation necrosis in a tuberculous granuloma. The central portion of this granuloma, which at an earlier stage was rich in epithelioid cells, is replaced by an area of coagulative necrosis which is rich in lipid and which has a marked affinity for eosin.

surrounded by a mantle of lymphocytes which can be shown, by use of appropriate antibodies, to be T cells.

Within 10 to 14 days, evidence of necrosis begins to appear in the centre of the lesion. The necrosis is coagulative in type and is characterized by the appearance of firm, allegedly cheesy material (hence the name **caseation** necrosis). On histological examination, caseation necrosis shows virtually complete obliteration of normal cell and tissue outlines, all the tissue elements being merged into an amorphous mass of material which appears bright red in sections stained with haematoxylin and eosin (Fig. 15.2). What determines the central necrosis is not well understood. Presumably one of the important effector mechanisms is release of lysosomal enzymes from dying macrophages, which, of course, disappear from the centre of the lesion as the necrosis develops. It is believed that caseation necrosis is the morphological expression of a marked degree of delayed hypersensitivity, though evidence gained in experimental studies of mycobacterial infections in rats suggests that humoral factors also have a part in the induction of the necrosis. In this situation it has been suggested that the local formation of immune complexes in the centre of the lesions, where antigen is in excess, is a powerful influence in modulating the degree of necrosis. Such complexes are said to form if cell-mediated immunity declines thus allowing the mycobacteria to proliferate. If complexes form under conditions of *antibody* excess, epithelioid cell transformation rather than necrosis tends to occur.

The sum of all these events constitutes the basic tissue response in tuberculosis.

The natural history of the tissue response

Experience has shown that different tissues and different individuals may react very differently to the presence of *Mycobacterium tuberculosis*. Some lesions are small and heal readily, some may cause extensive local tissue destruction and others may release organisms which can spread throughout the body. These differences are probably accounted for by interactions between the virulence of the organisms and the size of the dose, local and general resistance, which may be either innate or acquired, and the type and degree of hypersensitivity.

Some of the factors believed to be associated with variations in host response are discussed below.

Innate immunity

This is difficult to disentangle from factors related to exposure to the organism and to unfavourable socioeconomic circumstances. However, it appears that certain groups are inherently more susceptible to tuberculosis, notably North American Indians and the Negro races. At an experimental level, where conditions are much easier to control, there is no doubt that strains of certain species of animals can be bred which differ markedly in their degree of resistance to infection by *Mycobacterium tuberculosis.*

Age

In communities where there is a high prevalence of tuberculosis, the very young (under five years) and elderly appear to be more at risk for developing overt tuberculosis. In the UK, where the incidence of tuberculosis has been falling steadily, the increased risk in young children appears to have been eliminated and those at greatest risk are socially and economically deprived middle-aged and elderly men, many of whom are poorly nourished and unsatisfactorily housed.

Immunosuppression

Immunosuppression associated either with certain disorders or with certain treatments (such as prolonged administration of high doses of corticosteroids) increases the risk of tuberculosis, as do certain occupational hazards such as silicosis, which may be contracted in coal mining, sand blasting and quarrying.

Previous exposure to mycobacteria

Previous exposure to mycobacteria is one of the most important factors in modulating the natural history of a tuberculous infection. Certainly a second infection produces tissue reactions which differ markedly from those seen after a primary infection. This was first explored by Robert Koch in the course of studies of experimental tuberculosis in the guinea pig. His observations have a significant bearing, not only on the natural history of the disease, but also on the evolution of the basic pathological unit — the tuberculous granuloma.

The Koch phenomenon. If *M. tuberculosis* is injected subcutaneously into a guinea pig which has not previously been exposed to the organism, no reaction is seen at the injection site for the first 10 to 14 days. Then a nodule develops and if this is excised and examined histologically, tuberculous granulomas are seen. Meanwhile mycobacteria have been transported by macrophages to the regional draining nodes and in due time cause enlargement of these nodes and caseous necrosis within them. In time, infected macrophages escape from the nodes and the inoculated animals usually die from disseminated disease.

If the size of the initial dose has been such that the animal survives at least four weeks and a second subcutaneous injection of *M. tuberculosis* is given at that time and at a different site, a nodule forms rapidly (within a few days), ulcerates and then heals. **No regional lymph node involvement occurs.**

These observations indicate that:

1. The local tissue response to the second infection is much more rapid than to the first.
2. Local clearance of organisms by activated macrophages following a second infection is much more effective than after a first infection since the inflammatory process resolves quite rapidly.
3. Macrophages containing viable organisms are immobilized at the site of the local infection since there is no evidence of spread to the draining lymph nodes in the second infection.
4. Local hypersensitivity is increased after a second infection since rapid central necrosis leading to ulceration may occur.

These events have been interpreted as being due to the development of altered reactivity on the part of the host immune system. This leads to an increased ability to clear the infecting organisms from the tissue and thus to an enhanced resistance to the infection (immunity), and to an increased tendency for tissue damage, probably also mediated by immune mechanisms, to occur (hypersensitivity). It must be said, however, that in light of the failure of certain large scale trials of the efficacy of vaccination using attenuated strains of *Mycobacterium tuberculosis*, some workers have challenged this view of the Koch phenomenon.

Favourable aspects of the altered reactivity of the immune system. The altered reactivity that occurs after infection by *Mycobacterium tuberculosis* is largely, but not entirely, expressed in the form of cell-mediated reactions (delayed hypersensitivity). Committed T cells encounter bacterial antigens expressed on the surface of macrophages or other antigen-presenting cells and proliferate. Helper T cells release lymphokines which include factors chemotactic to the macrophage and factors which tend to immobilize them at the site of bacterial lodgement (MIF). The macrophages become better able to kill intracellular organisms, and the symbiotic relationship which can exist between mycobacteria and virgin macrophages is largely ended. This aspect of the altered immune state is obviously favourable for the survival of the infected host, though the enhanced resistance to the mycobacteria is not nearly as effective as that seen, for example, after smallpox or diphtheria.

Hypersensitivity to components of the mycobacterium

Most people now agree that the chief factor modulating the degree of tissue destruction in tuberculosis is hypersensitivity to some antigenic components of the bacillus. In addition to its role in causing caseation necrosis, hypersensitivity is probably also associated with the very severe constitutional effects that accompany the lodgement of large numbers of the bacillus. The liquefactive necrosis that tends to occur when there is active local proliferation of mycobacteria may well be associated with the formation of immune complexes in a zone of antigen excess (see p. 213). Such liquefied tissue debris usually contains very large numbers of mycobacteria and shows a marked tendency to rupture into adjacent tissue planes or into bronchi, lymphatics and blood vessels. Sometimes such debris tracks down through a tissue plane and may present as a soft mass at a point some distance away. Such a lesion is spoken of as a '**cold abscess**' since it consists of a localized mass of what looks like pus but lacks the heat and redness normally associated with abscess formation.

The relationship between immunity and hypersensitivity. The relationship between enhanced resistance to infection by the mycobacterium and the tissue damaging hypersensitivity reactions is one of the most difficult questions to answer satisfactorily. Is the difference between these two expressions of altered reactivity (allergy) merely a quantitative one or is the 'protective face' of altered reactivity distinct from the 'tissue damaging' hypersensitivity?

At present there is no definite answer to this problem but there is evidence that suggests that the second of these possibilities is the correct one:

1. The degree of **protection** produced by vaccination with an attenuated strain of the organism (BCG vaccination) is not related to the degree of **hypersensitivity** produced. For example, a guinea pig immunized in this way and reacting to a skin dose of tuberculin (mycobacterial protein) at a titre of 1/10 000 is likely to survive an intramuscular challenge with live mycobacteria for about 99 days. An animal treated in the same way but reacting to tuberculin at a titre of only 1/10 is likely to survive a subsequent challenge for 250 days.

2. It is possible to induce protection against a challenge with live bacilli by injecting a guinea pig with bacilli extracted using methyl alcohol without hypersensitivity developing.

3. Hypersensitivity can be induced without any protection against live bacilli being conferred at the same time. This can be accomplished by injecting mycobacterial protein together with some of the bacillary lipids.

4. Both in mice and in man two types of response can be seen following exposure to mycobacteria. In humans showing the first of these responses, the injection of tuberculoprotein is followed by a fairly rapid reaction which peaks at 48 hours, resolves rapidly, itches but is not painful, and is often seen in recipients of BCG vaccine in the UK. The other pattern of response develops a little more slowly, peaks at 72 to 96 hours, lasts for two to three weeks, often shows evidence of necrosis and is often seen in those with a history of previous tuberculosis. The first pattern is believed to be associated with a higher degree of resistance to infection, the second with a greater degree of hypersensitivity. The basis for an individual developing one or other of these responses may well be previous exposure to mycobacteria other than the major pathogens *M. tuberculosis* and *M. leprae*. There are some 30 species of mycobacteria. The two major pathogens are usually encountered only when contact with patients who have open tuberculosis or leprosy takes place. Many of the other species are very common in the environment and may be encountered very frequently. It has been suggested that when there has been 'moderate' exposure to such more or less harmless mycobacteria via the oral route, that the first type of skin response is likely to develop. Where there has been 'excessive' exposure to these mycobacterial species, a high degree of hypersensitivity is found and BCG vaccination confers little protection.

First infection type pulmonary tuberculosis (childhood tuberculosis)

The lodgement of *M. tuberculosis* in a child's lung is usually followed by the development of a small lesion, often measuring not more than 1 cm along its longest axis. This lesion is almost always situated just beneath the pleura either in the basal segment of the upper lobe of the lung or in the apical segment of the lower lobe. Classically this parenchymal lesion is known as the Ghon focus. As might be expected in a primary infection, macrophages laden with organisms travel to the draining hilar lymph nodes and, just as in the guinea pig experiments described by Koch, these nodes become enlarged and show caseation necrosis. It is a characteristic feature of childhood infections that, irrespective of the site of the lodgement of the organisms, there is a relatively inconspicuous local tissue response which tends to be overshadowed by the involvement of the draining lymph nodes. The combination of this inconspicuous parenchymal lesion and the prominent lymphadeno-pathy is known as the **primary complex** or **Ghon complex** (Fig. 15.3).

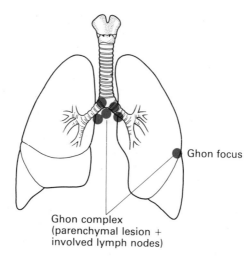

Ghon focus

Ghon complex
(parenchymal lesion +
involved lymph nodes)

Fig. 15.3 Primary infection with *Mycobacterium tuberculosis*.

The natural history of the primary complex

Healing. Most lesions, both in the lung parenchyma and in the hilar nodes, will heal. This may be brought about by complete replacement of any areas of caseation necrosis by fibrous tissue or, more often, by the local walling off of the necrotic area by scar tissue followed by the deposition of calcium salts in the caseous material (**dystrophic calcification**). Organisms may survive in these calcified foci and, even years later, if immune regulatory mechanisms become less efficient may start to proliferate.

Exudative responses. If the degree of hypersensitivity that develops following infection is of high grade, a severe exudative type of response, characterized by the outpouring of a fibrin-rich exudate in which epithelioid and giant cells are scanty, may be found. This type of reaction may also manifest in the form of a large pleural effusion with a massive accumulation of serous fluid in which the cell population is scanty and the number of organisms that can be isolated is very small.

Spread. If the primary reaction is dominated by caseation and softening of the necrotic material, then spread to distant areas may occur. Such spread may take place via the bronchi or via the bloodstream (**haematogenous spread**). It occurs most often after softening of the caseous lymph node component of the primary complex. The organisms may reach the blood either by direct involvement of small blood vessels or via thoracic duct lymph.

If the number of organisms released into the circulation is large and the host resistance is low, the systemic spread of the mycobacteria is expressed by the development of very large numbers of small granulomatous lesions, more or less equal in size, which stud the kidneys, spleen, brain, meninges, adrenals and, to a lesser extent, the liver. The rather distressing habit of pathologists of an earlier day of describing lesions in terms of food led to these lesions being compared with millet seeds, hence the term **miliary tuberculosis.**

Classically we tend to associate miliary tuberculosis with infections in childhood, but it is far from uncommon in the elderly, especially in those receiving immunosuppressive therapy. These patients show both diminished resistance to the infection and diminished hypersensitivity, the latter being expressed in terms of negative skin reactions to intradermal injections of tuberculoprotein. Bone marrow or liver biopsy may be useful diagnostic procedures in such cases since the lesions are so widespread that the chances of obtaining a positive result on biopsy are quite high.

If the dose of mycobacteria reaching the bloodstream is small, a different result may be seen both in children and in adults. Disseminated organisms may lodge and cause lesions in only one organ or tissue and the clinical picture will be determined by the site of such lesions. For example, a patient with tuberculous granulomas in the brain might present with the clinical features of a space-occupying lesion. Many tissues can be involved in this way, some of the most commonly affected being the kidneys, adrenals, fallopian tubes, bones, joints and tendon sheaths.

Adult type pulmonary tuberculosis

In adult pulmonary tuberculosis the parenchymal lesions usually start in the subapical region of the upper lobe, where they are known as **Assman foci** (Fig. 15.4). Apart from the fact, which may well be quite irrelevant, that the bacilli are obligate aerobes and that the ventilation in this part of the lung is said to be greater than in other segments, the reason for this localization is not known. The prominent lymph node involvement seen in primary infections is not present, though microscopic lesions may be seen.

The origin of adult-type infections is still poorly understood and controversial. The lesions might arise from:

1. A primary infection which, due to reasons unknown, has elicited a tissue response which differs from that seen in childhood

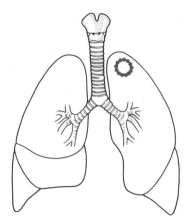

Fig. 15.4 Secondary infection with *Mycobacterium tuberculosis*.

2. A second infection in someone previously exposed to *M. tuberculosis* and who has, as a result, developed some degree of both immunity and hypersensitivity
3. A reactivation of a previous infection due to a decline in the efficiency of cell-mediated immunity as a result of malnutrition, overindulgence in alcohol, immunosuppression, etc.

The natural history of adult type pulmonary tuberculosis

Healing. As with childhood lesions in the lung, if the host has a high degree of immunity the lesions may heal with some scarring and calcification. Appropriate antimicrobial therapy reduces the amount of scar tissue formed and if there has been cavitation (see below) the end result may be a smooth-walled cavity with very little peripheral fibrosis.

Softening and cavitation. Softening of caseous material may occur and if this is associated with erosion into a bronchus a **cavity** develops. Apart from the destruction of lung tissue that this entails, cavitation is an extremely unfavourable development. Direct communication of the lesion with a major airway increases oxygen tension and thus favours multiplication of the bacilli since they are obligate aerobes. The patient will cough up infected material and thus be a danger to those in contact with him, and a natural pathway will have been created for spread within the patient's own lung via the ramifications of the bronchial tree. Blood vessels in the cavity walls are frequently involved in the inflammatory process; sometimes they become blocked by small thrombi but not infrequently they become eroded and this is followed by bleeding, which may be massive.

Caseating lesions within the lung parenchyma are sometimes associated with involvement of the **pleura**. This may be expressed in the form of a **serous effusion** or a persistent **fibrinous exudate** which may lead to obliteration of the pleural cavity by the processes of organization and repair. Occasionally the affected pleural cavity contains abundant, partly liquefied, caseous material; this situation is known as a **tuberculous empyema**.

Spread. In addition to spread via the bloodstream which can follow the same patterns as described for childhood infections, an important aspect of spread in adults involves natural anatomical pathways. If a bronchus is eroded, spread of infected material may occur by inhalation, with distal extension of the inflammatory process within the lung. This usually leads to a patchy tuberculous bronchopneumonia, but if the number of bacilli is very large and there is high grade local tissue hypersensitivity, a massive degree of caseation can take place which may involve several segments of lung tissue or even a whole lobe.

Spread of infected caseous material can also occur in a proximal direction with involvement of the larynx. The patient may swallow some of the infected material and tuberculous involvement of the bowel may follow. The ulceration chiefly affects the small intestine. The sites of predilection are the Peyer's patches, the ulcers tending to spread round the circumference of the bowel wall in a napkin-ring pattern. When they heal, fibrous strictures may form and lead to chronic or subacute intestinal obstruction. It is not without interest that the ulcers of typhoid fever also involve the Peyer's patches but tend to lie parallel to the long axis of the bowel.

Leprosy

Leprosy is a chronic infectious disease of humans caused by *Mycobacterium leprae* (one of the first bacterial pathogens to be recognized). It affects principally the skin, the nasal mucosa, the peripheral nerves and the testes, having a predilection for tissues that are relatively cool. The organism has much the same morphological features as any other mycobacterium, but is more easily decolorized by acid than *M. tuberculosis*. Thus a modification of the Ziehl–Neelsen method is used which takes account of this. Also, unlike *M. tuberculosis*, the leprosy bacillus is an obligate intracellular parasite and cannot be cultured in any known medium. However, it does survive and proliferate in the footpad of the mouse and in the nine-banded armadillo.

Leprosy is a rare disease in Western communities, but on a world-wide basis it is estimated that there are more than 11 million sufferers, 60% of these being found in Asia. In India alone there are 3.5 million lepers.

Transmission of leprosy is from person to person. The infectivity rate is low, only 5 to 10% of contacts actually developing the disease. The period between exposure to the organism and the first appearance of tuberculoid lesions is about three to six years, though much longer incubation periods (10 to 20 years) have been reported in relation to the lepromatous form of the disease.

Local tissue responses in leprosy depend on the degree of cell-mediated immunity

The tissue responses of the host to infection with *Mycobacterium leprae* cover a wide spectrum. At the two extremes of this spectrum are the types of response which have been characterized as **lepromatous** and **tuberculoid** leprosy.

Lepromatous leprosy

In the lepromatous form of leprosy there are widespread lesions in the skin and mucous membranes. The lesions consist of poorly organized infiltrates comprising very large numbers of macrophages, which look foamy, and smaller numbers of lymphocytes, plasma cells and mast cells. When sections of such lesions are stained appropriately, acid- and alcohol-fast bacilli can be seen in enormous numbers within the macrophages, being arranged either in compact masses or in bundles, somewhat similar to a cigarette pack. Ultrastructural studies show that the organisms are also contained within the Schwann cells ensheathing the cutaneous nerves. One gram of tissue from a lepromatous area may contain as many as 10^7 bacilli.

Tuberculoid leprosy

In this form of the disease the lesions are far scantier and involvement of peripheral nerves is quite common. On histological examination, in contrast to the lepromatous form, there are tightly packed and well-organized macrophage granulomas with no evidence of caseation. Lymphocytes are numerous, the macrophages have often undergone epithelioid cell transformation, and occasional multinucleate giant cells may be seen. Acid-fast bacilli are extremely difficult to find in these lesions; it may be impossible to see any on light microscopic examination, though electron microscopy may reveal some bacterial remnants.

Intermediate forms

Between these two poles a large number of intermediate forms of tissue response exist. The more closely they resemble the lepromatous type, the more bacilli can be identified in sections, the reverse being true the more closely they resemble the tuberculoid type.

Lepromatous and tuberculoid leprosy represent two extremes of the cell-mediated response

In tuberculoid leprosy, the type of lesion present and the fact that cutaneous hypersensitivity can be demonstrated by the use of antigen extracted from leprous tissue suggests that some cell-mediated immunity is present, though not to a degree sufficient to eliminate the mycobacteria from the host. In lepromatous leprosy, the absence of well-formed epithelioid cell granulomas, the absence of skin hypersensitivity, and the absence of effective microbicidal function on the part of the infiltrating macrophages all suggest the opposite — poor or absent cell-mediated immunity. This impression is strengthened by the observation that lymphocytes from patients with lepromatous leprosy fail to respond by undergoing blast transformation in the presence of *M. leprae* in vitro while those from patients suffering from the tuberculoid form of the disease respond strongly. The relative failure of T cell directed microbial elimination seen in the lepromatous form of leprosy may be due to a local change in the relative proportion of T cell subsets in the lesions themselves. The T cells in lepromatous lesions consist almost entirely of **suppressor cells** (OKT8/Leu2a-positive) while, in contrast, those in tuberculoid lesions are mainly **helper cells** (OKT4/Leu3a-positive). No marked differences were noted in the blood of these groups of patients in respect of the T cell subsets.

Interestingly, while patients with lepromatous leprosy exhibit impaired cell-mediated immunity, at least in relation to *M. leprae*, they are capable of making large amounts of antibody directed against determinants of the leprosy bacillus, though autoantibodies may be formed as well, suggesting some fault in B cell regulation. In some patients, immune complexes are formed and these occasionally deposit in small subcutaneous blood vessels giving rise to slightly tender nodules (**erythema nodosum leprosum**). The killing of organisms in patients with lepromatous leprosy by appropriate antimicrobial agents can lead to an increase in cell-mediated immunity, and there may be a change in the character of the lesions with some progression occurring towards the tuberculoid type. This suggests that the local T cell deficiency may be related in some way to the antigen load.

Sarcoidosis

Winston Churchill once wrote of Russia that it was 'a riddle, wrapped in a mystery, inside an enigma'. The same might be said of sarcoidosis.

It is a disease of unknown aetiology which is fairly common in Northern Europe, with the highest incidence in Sweden. It is characterized morphologically by the presence of well-formed epithelioid granulomas which show little or no central necrosis. These may be present in any organ or tissue. Multinucleated giant cells in the granulomas often show the presence of calcified bodies within the cytoplasm. These are sometimes star-shaped (hence the name **asteroid bodies**) or rounded and basophilic. Their presence is not diagnostic of sarcoidosis. The granulomas are often very sharply demarcated from the surrounding tissue and are cuffed by a mantle of lymphocytes which is much less conspicuous than that seen in relation to tuberculous lesions.

Distribution of the lesions

Sarcoidosis is a systemic disease in that most organs and tissues may be affected. The lung is the most frequently and prominently involved target. Chest x-ray shows the presence of widespread miliary mottling associated with enlargement of the hilar lymph nodes. The pulmonary symptoms are usually much milder than the radiological appearances would suggest.

Other lymph nodes, liver and spleen are also frequently involved. In the skeleton the small bones of the fingers are most conspicuously affected; x-ray examination shows the presence of small cyst-like lesions.

A variety of skin lesions may be seen as well as involvement of the uveal tract in the eye, the lacrimal gland and the salivary glands. When all the last three are involved at the same time, the triad is spoken of as Heerfordt's syndrome. On rare occasions sarcoidosis has been reported as affecting the neurohypophysis, with the production of diabetes insipidus. Hypercalcaemia is not uncommon in these patients, but the origin of this phenomenon is still not clear.

Aetiology and pathogenesis

Both the aetiology and the pathogenesis of sarcoidosis are poorly understood. One of the major difficulties is obviously the fact that the basic pathological unit, the epithelioid granuloma, is non-specific and, as described previously, is a tissue reaction found after exposure to a large number of irritants, both living and non-living. While it is likely that the tissue response in sarcoidosis is an expression of cell-mediated immunity, we cannot be sure of this. In this connection it is not without interest that patients usually show diminished skin hypersensitivity as judged by their lack of response to tuberculoprotein.

Suggestions have been made that sarcoidosis may be:

1. The result of a mycobacterial infection in a patient with altered cell-mediated immune reactions
2. The result of a non-specific reaction to a wide variety of irritants. This would account for the histological features but would not explain the peculiar clustering of lesions which constitutes the clinical syndrome of sarcoidosis
3. The result of an infection by an agent not as yet identified. Evidence which might be interpreted as supporting this view is derived from experiments in immunologically deficient mice. If such animals are injected with material from the lesions of a patient with sarcoidosis, the animal will develop large numbers of epithelioid cell granulomas. Material from these can then be transferred to another immunologically deficient mouse with the same results.

Syphilis

Syphilis is an important member of the group of sexually transmitted diseases. It is alleged that the disease was unknown in Europe until the last decade of the fiteenth century when Columbus's sailors were said to have introduced it on their return from the first voyage to the Americas. A large scale outbreak was recorded after the siege and capture of Naples by Charles VIII of France in 1495–1496. The French called syphilis 'the Italian disease' and the Neapolitans dubbed it the 'French Pox'. This episode tells us more about people than it does about syphilis. The name syphilis is derived from a poem by Girolamo Fracastoro, who died in 1533, in which an amorous and presumptuous shepherd boy named Syphilus was visited with the disease as a punishment for having taken his pleasure with the goddess Aphrodite. The poem, now entitled 'Syphilis or a Poetical History of the French Pox', was translated into English in about 1680 by Nahum Tate, the poet laureate of the day, who is perhaps better known for having provided Shakespeare's *King Lear* with a happy ending in which Cordelia marries Edgar and lives contentedly ever after.

The organism

Syphilis is caused by a spirochaete, *Treponema pallidum*. This is a corkscrew-shaped bacillus which is resistant to ordinary staining methods and which, as yet, cannot be cultured in artificial media or in tissue culture systems. It can be maintained in the tissues of living animals and the rabbit testis is most frequently used for this purpose. The spirochaetes can be seen in fluid taken from ulcerated lesions in the early stages of the disease either by using darkfield microscopy or by impregnating the organisms with certain silver salts. *Treponema pallidum* spreads widely throughout the body of infected subjects and this is aided by its invasive properties. These probably derive, in part, from the mucopolysaccharide capsule which is antiphagocytic and may also down regulate the T cell response. In addition, the treponema possesses enzymes which attack the constituents of the intercellular ground substance. The organism is very sensitive to heat and drying; stories of syphilis having been acquired via the medium of 'cracked tea cups' and the like are thus inherently improbable. Other than in congenital syphilis, where the infection is transplacental, direct contact is required.

Treponema pallidum shows considerable ability to **adhere** to the surface of a number of cell types. Only the tapered end of the organism adheres to subjacent plasma membranes, suggesting the presence of a receptor in this part of the bacterial cell wall.

The immune response to infection

Within one to three weeks of the first lesions of syphilis appearing, an immune response in the form of antibody production can be demonstrated. Two interesting groups of antibodies have been identified. The first of these forms the basis for widely used diagnostic tests — the VDRL (Venereal Disease Research Laboratory) and Wasserman reactions.

Wasserman antibodies (anticardiolipin)

The Wasserman antibody is an IgM molecule which reacts with a constituent of the lipid membranes of many cell organelles, notably mitochondria. The antigen is diphosphatidylglycerol, often called **cardiolipin** since a common source is an alcoholic extract of beef heart. The presence of this antibody in serum is not an absolutely reliable indicator of syphilis since biological false-positive reactions may occur in association with a number of non-treponemal and non-venereal diseases, including:

malaria
leprosy
glandular fever
trypanosomiasis
some other treponemal disorders (e.g. yaws, pinta and bejel)
mycoplasmal pneumonia
some autoimmune haemolytic anaemias
systemic lupus erythematosus
after some Coxsackie B virus infections

Initially this wide range of disorders capable of eliciting the presence of the anticardiolipin antibody and the wide distribution within tissues of cardiolipin suggested that antibody formation was secondary to tissue damage and was not related to any specific antigen associated with *Treponema pallidum* itself. Cardiolipin has, however, now been shown to be present in *Treponema*, and it may well be that it is this bacterium-associated cardiolipin that acts as the antigen. Anticardiolipin antibodies do not react with intact organisms and the case must still be regarded as not proven.

Antibodies binding specifically with intact Treponema pallidum

These antibodies can be detected in two ways: (a) by the **immobilization** of organisms in suspension, or (b) by the **fluorescent antibody** technique. In this group there are antibodies which react with all treponemas and others which react only with *Treponema pallidum*.

The natural history and lesions of syphilis

As already stated, apart from the congenital form of the disease, syphilis is contracted as a result of direct sexual contact with an infected person. Minute abrasions of the skin and mucous membranes in those areas making such contact facilitate the entry of the organisms into the tissues. After a three- to four-week incubation period the primary lesions appear at the site of infection. Such a lesion is usually situated in the genital region, but in those who prefer the more recherché forms of sexual congress they may be found on the lips, tongue, finger or anus. In at least half the patients, the disease will follow a course lasting many years if untreated. The natural history in these cases appears to fall into three clearly defined and separable stages which have been termed primary, secondary and tertiary.

Primary syphilis

The primary lesion usually occurs within a month of infection; occasionally the incubation period may be longer. The lesion, an indurated papule which is usually painless but often ulcerates, is known as a **chancre**.

In microscopic terms the tissue response is that of a localized inflammatory reaction characterized by a dense cellular infiltrate in which plasma cells, lymphocytes (both T and B cells) and macrophages are prominent. The endothelial linings of small blood vessels in the affected areas show a marked degree of swelling. This, if extreme, can lead to virtual obliteration of their lumina and patchy local ischaemia which may contribute to ulceration of the chancre. The draining lymph nodes are usually enlarged.

Organisms are usually plentiful in the tissues at this stage and can be found in the fluid which oozes from ulcerated chancres. Local clearance of organisms appears to be effective since the chancre heals spontaneously. In about half the patients the disease progresses no further, but in the others widespread dissemination of the treponema occurs and within a few weeks to a few months the next stage of the disease appears.

Secondary syphilis

This stage commonly occurs within two to three months after exposure to infection. A generalized skin rash appears, the face, palms and soles being particularly likely to be involved. The rash usually consists of many reddish or copper-coloured papules, but other types of lesion have been described.

The mucous membranes of the mouth and pharynx show the presence of whitish patches, some of which break down to give the lesions known as 'snail track' ulcers. In the moist cutaneous and mucocutaneous areas of the anus, vulva and perineum, flat papules develop which are known as **condylomata lata**. These contain large numbers of organisms and are very infectious. Generalized slight enlargement of lymph nodes is common, those in the epitrochlear region and those related to the posterior border of the sternomastoid being most frequently involved. Immune complexes may be formed which can give rise to lesions in a number of different places, the most noteworthy being the kidney where glomerulonephritis may occur. Fever, muscle pains and a general malaise occur quite commonly.

Both these symptoms and the various lesions disappear spontaneously after a few months and such patients no longer constitute a hazard to their sexual partners. A fairly high grade of immunity has now been established, but complete clearance of organisms usually does not take place. The treponemas appear to enter a latent phase which may last for many years. Presumably this latent period is brought to an end when some diminution in cell-mediated immunity occurs, though it is not known how this comes about.

Tertiary syphilis

Unlike the tissue responses seen in the primary and secondary stages of syphilis, the lesions which occur when the latent period comes to an end are very destructive and may lead to situations which can be crippling or even life threatening.

Two basic tissue responses are seen in the tertiary stage of syphilis. These are (a) a special type of coagulative necrosis known as **gummatous necrosis**, and (b) inflammatory damage to small blood vessels in a wide variety of sites. This may lead to necrosis of the areas of tissue which they perfuse. Affected vessels show a severe degree of endothelial thickening with reduction of the lumina, and are cuffed by plasma cells and lymphocytes.

Gummatous necrosis. A gumma may occur anywhere in the body. The clinical features which arise from their presence will depend on their anatomical situation. The gumma is an area of rubbery coagulative necrosis which bears some superficial resemblance to caseation necrosis. However, the centre of a gumma does not show the complete obliteration of cell and tissue outlines that is so characteristic a feature of caseation. The borders of the gumma show the presence of plump fibroblasts, macrophages and lymphocytes. Blood vessels at the periphery show narrowing of their lumina and this may contribute to the necrosis. Treponemas are very scanty and are difficult to demonstrate in lesions. Healing of the gummas differs from the healing seen in tuberculosis. Fibrous bands criss-cross the necrotic area and coarse scarring results. Sites of predilection for such necrosis to occur include the liver, testis, subcutaneous tissue, and bone (especially the tibia, ulna, clavicle, skull, nasal and palatal bones). The resulting lesions, especially in bone, can lead to bizarre and striking clinical and pathological pictures.

The pathogenesis of gummatous necrosis is still unknown. It has been suggested that it is a hypersensitivity phenomenon.

Small blood vessel disease. Small blood vessels in a variety of sites show periadventitial cuffing by lymphocytes and plasma cells. Endothelial cells swell and may proliferate and this can lead to obliteration of the lumina.

Such changes in the small blood vessels have a particularly baneful effect on the cardiovascular system. The ascending and thoracic parts of the aorta are the chief targets. The vasa vasorum in the adventitia and their extensions into the outer tunica media become cuffed by inflammatory cells. This is followed by destruction of both the elastic laminae and the smooth muscle cells in the media and this inevitably leads to loss of the normal recoil of the aortic wall. The weakening of the aortic wall can lead to local dilatation of the vessel or **aneurysm** formation. The intimal surface of a vessel affected in this way often shows a curious wrinkled pattern which has been likened to the appearance of tree bark. Any destructive process associated with scarring in the media of large elastic arteries shows this feature, which is therefore not diagnostic of tertiary syphilis. Not infrequently the weakening process in the aortic media extends proximally to involve the aortic root, which becomes dilated as a result. This will give rise to incompetence of the aortic valve with consequent regurgitation of blood during diastole. Apart from the obvious dilatation of the aortic ring, the commissures between the valve cusps are widened and the cusps themselves show a characteristic cord-like thickening along their free edges which, presumably, is due to the alteration in haemodynamics. As with the wrinkling of the intimal surface mentioned above, these appearances of the aortic valve can occur in any condition giving rise to dilatation of the aortic root (e.g. ankylosing spondylitis) and are not diagnostic of syphilis. Before the introduction of penicillin treatment for syphilis, aortic valve disease of this type was a common cause of both left ventricular failure and sudden death. Its frequency in Western countries has declined very steeply.

Syphilis and the central nervous system. The lesions of tertiary syphilis occurring in the central nervous system fall into two distinct groups:

1. Those lesions which involve the meninges and their small blood vessels lead to a chronic meningitis, patchy gummatous necrosis and severe narrowing of arterial lumina as a result of swelling of endothelial cells. Lesions tend to occur early in the tertiary stage and have even been recorded in the secondary stage of the disease.
2. So-called **parenchymatous neurosyphilis** occurs late in the tertiary stage and involves degeneration of the neuronal elements themselves.

Meningovascular syphilis. Syphilis may involve either the leptomeninges or the pachymeninges, the former being more frequently affected. Leptomeningitis occurs most often at the base of the brain; the meninges become swollen and thickened and occasionally small patches of gummatous necrosis may be seen. Cranial nerve involvement is not uncommon and the process may also obstruct the foramina of the fourth ventricle and thus cause hydrocephalus. Pachymeningitis may occur over the surface of the cerebral hemispheres and also in relation to parts of the spinal cord, where the blood vessel involvement can cause patchy necrosis. These conditions are now very rarely seen.

Parenchymatous neurosyphilis. Two quite distinct sets of lesions and clinical syndromes can be encountered.

The first of these is termed **tabes dorsalis**. This is characterized by degeneration of certain sensory fibres in the posterior nerve roots and in the posterior columns of the spinal cord. This leads to atrophy, the posterior columns are seen to be shrunken and greyish in colour (instead of white) at post-mortem examination. The overlying leptomeninges are thickened and the posterior nerve roots are also atrophic.

On microscopic examination the posterior columns show fibre loss and demyelination. Similar changes may occur in more proximally situated parts of the nervous system (e.g. the optic discs and the third cranial nerve). The degeneration leads to severe loss of function, especially in relation to deep pressure sensation, vibration sense, position sense and coordination. The patients may develop a characteristic unsteady and 'stamping' gait since they cannot feel the ground beneath their feet. Deep tendon reflexes disappear and there may be episodes of very severe shooting pains in the limbs, these being known as 'lightning pains'. The lack of sensation may lead ultimately to disorganization of large joints such as the knee (Charcot's joints).

The pathogenesis of tabes dorsalis is still unknown. It is not likely to be related to proliferation of the organisms at a time when cell-mediated immunity is deficient, since organisms are very scanty indeed in the lesions.

The second type of parenchymatous lesion seen in neurosyphilis is known as **general paresis of the insane.** It was once one of the commonest causes of long-term admission to mental hospitals.

General paresis of the insane is a chronic treponemal inflammatory disorder in which, in contrast, to tabes dorsalis, it is reasonably easy to identify the organisms. The brain becomes shrunken and the cerebral cortices are disorganized, the graphic term 'windswept cortex' being applied by some writers. The structural changes in the brain consist essentially of degeneration of nerve cells and their fibres, especially in the grey matter, with an associated proliferation of astrocytes and glial fibres. The small intracerebral blood vessels show the expected perivascular cuffing by lymphocytes and plasma cells and swelling of the endothelial lining.

In the early stages the clinical picture is characterized by deterioration in personality and changes in mental function. This may express itself in the form of delusions which may be at once bizarre and grandiose. If unchecked by treatment, the mental changes may proceed inexorably to a complete dementia. Disturbances related to other functions may also be seen. These include tremors of the lips and tongue, general weakness, minor convulsive seizures and disturbances of finer movements.

Congenital syphilis

The presence of treponemas in the blood of a pregnant woman exposes the fetus to the hazard of transplacental infection. This usually occurs at about the fifth month of pregnancy. Depending on the degree of maternal spirochaetaemia, the fetus may be aborted or the child may die at birth, the lesions of congenital syphilis may appear early in the neonatal period, or the infection may remain latent for quite long periods.

If the infection is sufficiently severe to cause lesions in the perinatal period, the clinical picture tends to be dominated by skin and mucous membrane lesions in which severe loss of surface epithelium may occur. These lesions are intensely infective and contain relatively vast numbers of organisms. Typical inflammatory changes are seen at the growing ends of bones and in relation to the periosteum. Severe deformities of bone may result, including the formation of periosteal new bone over the anterior surface of the tibia giving rise to a **sabre-like** appearance.

The **liver** may be diffusely affected by the syphilitic inflammatory reaction and this leads to an equally diffuse form of scarring where individual liver cells or small groups of such cells are surrounded by fine trabecula of fibrous tissue. Severe interstitial fibrosis may be seen in the **lung**, leading to a marked narrowing of air spaces and, in the most severe examples, to a relatively airless lung. The **cornea** is very often the seat of an inflammatory reaction and the **teeth** can show a characteristic deformity, the incisors being 'screwdriver' or 'peg' shaped (Hutchinson's teeth).

If the congenital infection manifests itself after a prolonged latent period the features are usually similar to those seen in the tertiary stage of an acquired infection, though the presence of inflammation of the cornea together with these features should suggest the possibility of transplacental infection.

Chapter 16

Amyloid and Amyloidosis

Amyloidosis is a set of disorders characterized by the extracellular deposition of one of a group of fibrillar proteins. This may occur under a wide variety of different pathological circumstances. This infiltration, which imparts a waxy quality to the affected tissues, was first recognized by Rokitansky in the mid-nineteenth century, but the term 'amyloid' (starch-like) was coined by Virchow. He used this term because of staining reactions of the infiltrating material which he associated with the presence of a starch-like material (amylum).

Identification of amyloid in tissue

In general terms, any organ in which a large amount of one of the amyloids is deposited is larger and paler than normal. A somewhat waxy appearance may be noted and the consistency is firmer than normal, so that the cut edges of the organ are very sharp instead of having the usual slight bulge. Macroscopically, amyloid can be demonstrated by treating the affected tissues with Lugol's iodine and then washing them. The amyloid deposits stain a rich brown colour.

Microscopically, the protein can be recognized by:

1. Its eosinophilia and apparent homogeneity in haematoxylin and eosin stained sections
2. Its ability to bind the dye Congo red, which stains amyloid an orange-red colour. When such positively stained material is examined in polarized light, a characteristic green/yellow birefringence is seen which is termed dichroism. This is a fairly sensitive method and, apart from ultrastructural examination, is the most reliable one available to the diagnostic histopathologist.
3. Its ability to exhibit metachromasia when sections are stained with methyl violet, the amyloid staining red. This is not a very satisfactory method since the dye tends to leak out into the mounting medium and it is thus unsuitable for making permanent preparations.
4. Its ultrastructural appearance. Amyloid consists of bundles of wavy fibrils varying in width from 7 to 14 nm, and up to 1600 nm in length. Often these fibrils are seen to be arranged in parallel bundles, which was at one time believed to account for their birefringence in polarized light. In addition to the filaments which can be seen to form the fibrils,

curious pentagonal subunits can be seen which, chemically at least, do not appear to be related to the fibrillar proteins.

We now know that there are several distinct chemical varieties of amyloid, yet all of these share the histological and ultrastructural characters described above. The unifying feature of all these molecules is the possession in every instance of a beta-pleated sheet structure — a structure not normally found in this almost pure conformational state in mammalian tissues or, so far as we know, in tissues other than those of invertebrates. Thus the amyloidoses do not constitute a single disease entity, but are a variety of widely differing disease processes which result in the deposition of twisted beta-pleated sheet fibrils. On this structure depends the reaction with Congo red and also a relative resistance of the fibrils to solution in physiological solvents and to normal proteolytic digestion. These last features are of great importance in terms of the natural histories of the disease processes, since the accumulation of the fibrillar protein may continue relentlessly, leading to pressure atrophy of the normal elements of the tissue in which the amyloid deposition has occurred.

Classification of amyloids and amyloidoses

Older classifications are based on clinical and pathological criteria and are riddled with inconsistencies. For instance, **primary amyloidosis** was defined by the presence of a tendency to nodular deposition of amyloid with a predilection for mesenchymal tissues (e.g. the cardiovascular system) and, most important of all, an **absence** of any recognizable preceding or concurrent disease. The only distinction between this and the entity known as 'amyloidosis associated with multiple myelomatosis' was the presence in the latter of the osteolytic lesions which are characteristic of myeloma. The **secondary** form of amyloidosis was so called because it followed or coexisted with a wide variety of disease processes, most of which were inflammatory in nature. In this type the amyloid shows a predilection for parenchymal tissues such as liver, kidney and spleen.

Now that we know that the only unifying feature of the amyloids is their structure, it seems more appropriate to classify the amyloidoses on the basis of the chemical nature of the amyloid protein or of its precursor where this is known, on whether the disorder is acquired or inherited, and on the distribution pattern of the fibril deposition.

Acquired Systemic Amyloidosis

Amyloid of immune origin

In one group of amyloid fibrils (isolated in the first instance from patients with the 'primary' form of amyloidosis), the major protein component has been found to be either an intact light polypeptide chain from an immunoglobulin, the N-terminal fragment of such a light chain, or both an intact light chain and its homologous N-terminal fragment. The majority are lambda light chains or fragments thereof. Anti-idiotypic antibodies raised against this type of amyloid protein in an individual patient do not react with other light chain derived amyloid proteins but seem specific for that patient. Such antisera react not only with the amyloid fibril proteins, but also with a soluble protein in the patient's plasma; this plasma component is an intact circulating light chain (i.e. a serum Bence Jones protein).

Thus the cellular source of amyloid fibril protein of this type is almost certainly an immunocyte-derived clone of cells whose protein products circulate in the plasma in the form of a Bence Jones protein and undergo an alteration which converts them into beta-pleated sheet fibrils which are then deposited in the tissues. The question which immediately arises from these data is how the soluble light chains undergo this change. Investigators have used methods which progressively cleave lambda and kappa Bence Jones proteins into their Vl and Cl portions. In the course of enzymatic digestion of the lambda light chains, precipitates form which, when examined by light microscopy, are seen to be stained positively by Congo red and show dichroism when examined in polarized light. Studies with the electron microscope show that these precipitates consist of fibrils which are morphologically indistinguishable from amyloid fibrils. Not all lambda light chains behave in this way and we have to conclude that inherent in the structure of the variable region of some light chains is a capacity to form beta-pleated sheet fibrils when this portion of the light chain is enzymatically cleaved from the rest. What this quality is that separates so-called 'amyloidogenic' light chains from those which will not form amyloid fibrils is not known. However, what is certain is that the characteristic properties of the amyloid fibril proteins of this or any other subclass are directly related to the beta-pleated configuration, since both naturally occurring beta-pleated fibrils (such as the silk of the egg stalk of the *Chrysopa* moth) and synthetically created ones like the beta form of poly-L-lysine behave in exactly the same way as amyloid fibrils. This type of amyloid fibril is found in patients with what Glenner has described as 'immunocyte dyscrasias', i.e. abnormal monoclonal proliferations of cells of the B lymphocyte series. Sometimes the processes are overtly neoplastic, as in the classic example of plasma cell myeloma.

Amyloid of immune origin is also found in patients with Waldenström's macroglobulinaemia, heavy chain disease, other monoclonal gammopathies which are not obviously neoplastic, and, interestingly enough, even in some patients with agammaglobulin-aemia.

Amyloidosis associated with monoclonal protein production is a disease of middle life and old age and affects males more frequently than females. Nearly all the patients show the presence of a serum or urinary monoclonal immunoglobulin with a Bence Jones protein or sometimes only a Bence Jones protein, and the bone marrow contains an excessive number of plasma cells. While the clinical expressions of this form of amyloidosis are very large in number, certain symptom complexes strongly suggest its presence:

1. Peripheral neuropathy. This resembles that seen in diabetes mellitus and autonomic manifestations such as impotence, disturbances of gastrointestinal motility, orthostatic hypotension and dyshidrosis may be prominent. The patient may complain of painful sensory disturbances usually in a 'glove and stocking' distribution.
2. Restrictive cardiomyopathy. This is caused by infiltration between the heart muscle fibres, with a marked increase in the stiffness of the myocardium and, among other problems, a lessening of diastolic compliance. Signs and symptoms of right-sided heart failure tend to dominate the clinical picture and an erroneous diagnosis of constrictive pericarditis is not infrequently made in the first instance. Patients with cardiac amyloidosis are exquisitely sensitive to digitalis and fatal arrhythmias have been recorded following its administration. These patients may also have pulmonary infiltration by amyloid; while cardiac amyloidosis may occur in other amyloidosis syndromes, involvement of the pulmonary parenchyma is invariably a manifestation of the immune-mediated form.
3. Skin manifestations. Patients with this type of amyloidosis may show 'pinch purpura' or waxy nodules of amyloid infiltration in the skin. Baldness and patchy areas of thickening such as are seen in scleroderma may also occur.
4. Polyarthropathy. A distribution pattern of polyarthropathy similar to that seen in rheumatoid arthritis may be a sign of this variety of amyloidosis. Large joints are particularly frequently affected.
5. Macroglossia (enlargement of the tongue). This may be the initial sign of this form of amyloidosis.
6. Isolated factor X deficiency leading to a haemorrhagic state
7. Idiopathic carpal tunnel syndrome

Reactive systemic amyloidosis

The amyloid fibril protein found here has been called protein AA. It has no chemical resemblance to the amyloid of immune origin. Unlike the proteins in amyloid of immune origin, which appear to be specific for each patient, the N-terminal fragments of the various AA proteins found in reactive systemic amyloidosis (secondary amyloidosis) show a striking degree of homogeneity, most of them having the sequence Arg-Ser-Phe-Phe-Ser-Phe-Leu-Gly-Glu-Ala. Similar AA proteins have been found in amyloid fibrils deposited in animal tissues as a result of certain experimental manoeuvres and this gives support to the use of such animal studies as models of reactive systemic amyloidosis. As in the case of amyloid of immune origin, a soluble serum precursor has been found. It has been suggested that the structure of this serum AA is similar to one of the apoproteins of high density lipoprotein, but this is still uncertain. A rather similar AA protein has also been found in familial Mediterranean fever, one of the heredofamilial amyloidoses.

Clinical and pathological features

The sites of predilection for amyloid deposition of this type are the liver, kidneys, spleen and adrenals. However, many other tissues may be involved and the diagnosis may be made by biopsying one of these, such as the rectal mucosa or the gum.

The conditions with which this form of amyloidosis is believed to be associated causally are:

1. Chronic inflammatory diseases in which infection is **known** to play a part, the most common being tuberculosis, leprosy, syphilis, chronic osteomyelitis and bronchiectasis
2. Chronic inflammatory diseases in which infection **may** play a part, e.g. Reiter's syndrome and Whipple's disease
3. Chronic inflammatory diseases of uncertain aetiology such as rheumatoid arthritis and its variants, other connective tissue diseases, Crohn's disease and ulcerative colitis
4. Long-standing paraplegia (probably because of the risk of recurrent renal infections)
5. Neoplasms, especially carcinoma of the kidney. Amyloid is found in association with other neoplasms, as already indicated, light chain derived amyloid being found in some examples of neoplastic proliferations of the lymphoreticular system, notably myeloma, and amyloid protein related chemically to the specific peptide product being found in some tumours of the endocrine system, notably medullary carcinoma of the thyroid.

Chronic inflammatory diseases constitute the major causal association of amyloid deposition of the AA type. However, with the advent of antibiotic therapy, the incidence of diseases such as chronic osteitis and bronchiectasis has fallen sharply, and the introduction of successful methods for the treatment of tuberculosis has meant a marked decline in the frequency of tuberculosis-associated amyloidosis. Nevertheless, in those parts of the world where tuberculosis still occurs on a large scale, it remains a far from negligible cause of amyloidosis.

Leprosy, because of the very large number of sufferers world-wide, probably ranks high as a cause of reactive systemic amyloidosis. In a study carried out in the USA in 1967, the major cause of death in 30% of those dying of leprosy was amyloidosis. In this country the most common disease causally associated with reactive systemic amyloidosis is rheumatoid arthritis. There is some controversy as to the precise frequency with which it occurs and there is also some variation encountered in patients with this disease in so far as the distribution pattern of the amyloid is concerned. Amyloidosis of this type is also an important cause of morbidity and death in patients with juvenile rheumatoid arthritis; of the deaths that occurred in a ten-year follow-up period in one series, amyloidosis accounted for one-third.

The association between paraplegia and a high risk of amyloidosis has been known for many years; in one series of paraplegics coming to necropsy, 40% were found to have amyloidosis.

Some specific patterns of organ involvement. The **spleen** is enlarged and firm and the cut edges are much 'sharper' than usual. The distribution

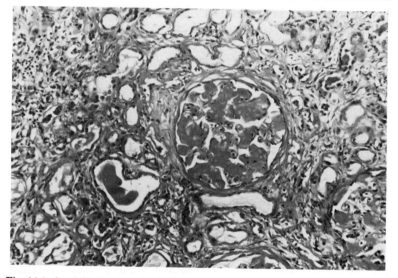

Fig. 16.1 Amyloid deposition in the kidney. The bulk of the glomerulus shown in the centre of the field has been replaced by material which is apparently structureless. This stains positively with Congo red and shows dichroism when examined in polarized light. This material is amyloid, in this case the reactive type (AA). This material can also be seen to be deposited in relation to the basement membranes of small blood vessels and renal tubules.

of the amyloid protein is usually focal, the walls of the arterioles of the malpighian corpuscles being particularly affected. As the degree of deposition increases, so the malpighian corpuscles become completely replaced by the protein; at this stage the cut surface of the spleen shows numerous small, translucent nodules scattered against the background of red pulp. This appearance has been given the somewhat unfortunate name of 'sago spleen'. Sometimes, however, the distribution pattern is a diffuse one.

The **liver** is also enlarged, sometimes hugely so, and is firm and pale. The amyloid protein is usually deposited in the walls of the sinusoids in the spaces of Disse (between the liver cells and the endothelium). Eventually the cords of liver cells undergo atrophy but, because of the large functional reserves of the liver, the clinical effects of such infiltration are slight as a rule.

In the **kidney** the amyloid is seen to be deposited in the glomeruli, the arterioles, and in relation to the basement membrane of the tubules (Fig. 16.1). In most instances the kidney is enlarged, pale and firm, but in a few cases secondary ischaemic changes dominate the picture and may lead to scarring and shrinkage of the organ.

Other chemical types of amyloid fibril

The amyloid protein associated with familial Portuguese polyneuropathy appears to have a structure closely resembling that of prealbumin (see below).

Medullary carcinoma of the thyroid is invariably associated with the presence of amyloid in the tumour stroma. Analysis has shown this to contain a polypeptide, the amino acid sequence of which is identical with that found in positions 9 to 19 of thyrocalcitonin. Amyloid may occur in the stroma of some islet cell tumours of the pancreas, and has been found to have some chemical relationship to insulin in those tumours which secrete insulin.

Heredofamilial Systemic Amyloidoses

These exist in two basic forms — a neuropathic and a non-neuropathic variety. In one of the neuropathic forms the amyloid protein has been characterized as being closely related to prealbumin. This form of amyloid protein has been termed AFp. Interestingly, antibodies raised against this protein react with guanidine-denatured fibrils from nerve, meninges, thyroid and kidney of patients with deposition of this amyloid protein.

Systemic AFp deposition, which was first described in Portugal (hence the name 'Portuguese polyneuropathy'), expresses itself clinically in the form of the insidious onset of a progressive, often symmetrical, polyneuropathy, affecting principally the lower limbs. It has an autosomal dominant pattern of inheritance. Amyloid deposits are found in most of the organs including the meninges, spinal and cranial nerves, heart, vessels, testes and ovaries. The brain and spinal cord are usually spared. Other varieties of neuropathic amyloidoses have been described, including one in which a peripheral neuropathy, and heart, liver and eye dysfunctions are present. This type has been traced to a Swiss family which emigrated to the USA in 1883. Of the 66 members of the family thus far investigated, 29 have been found to have amyloidosis.

Other forms of heredofamilial amyloidosis include a curious syndrome in which affected subjects develop urticaria associated with fever during adolescence and this can be followed by deafness, glaucoma and death from renal failure secondary to deposition of amyloid. Familial cardiac failure due to amyloid deposition in the heart has also been described. This occurred in a Danish family in which five of the twelve members presented in their 40s with cardiac failure.

Acquired Organ-Limited Amyloidosis

The type of amyloid protein may be of immune origin. Deposits have been recorded as isolated instances in the larynx, bronchi, lung, urinary tract, bone marrow and lymph nodes.

Amyloid deposition in the heart may lead to senile cardiac amyloidosis. The reported overall incidence of predominant or isolated cardiac amyloidosis is about 2%, with the frequency increasing to 50% after the age of 90. In this condition the atria are usually first affected, with the process extending to the ventricles, aorta and pulmonary artery at a later stage. The amyloid protein deposited appears to be distinct from those already described and, for the present, has been termed ASC_1. Cardiac hypertrophy is a prominent feature and the majority of the patients have some form of arrhythmia.

Deposition of amyloid in the brain is quite common. It occurs in a number of different forms and may be found both in relation to blood vessels or within senile plaques. One morphological form appears to be confined to cases of **spongiform** encephalopathy such as kuru and Creutzfeldt–Jakob disease.

Amyloid deposition in the skin occurs in a number of different forms and in association with a number of different disorders of the skin.

Chapter 17

The General Pathology of Viral Infection

Viruses are obligate, intracellular parasites and account for 60% of all infectious illnesses. The spectrum of disease caused by viruses ranges from trivial disorders to lethal or crippling situations, and the range of tissue responses they evoke is similarly wide.

The general characteristics of a virus

As a group, viruses constitute the smallest infectious agents known. The largest ones are just visible with the light microscope, but the majority can only be seen on electron microscopy, their diameters ranging from 20 to 300 nm (1 nm = 10^{-3} μm). Each true virus contains only a **single** nucleic acid as its genome, either DNA or RNA; the type of nucleic acid forms one of the bases for viral classification. The nucleic acid is covered by a symmetrically arranged protein shell which is known as the **capsid**. The capsid consists of clusters of polypeptides which form ultrastructurally recognizable units called **capsomeres**. The arrangement of the capsid falls into two distinct structural patterns. It may confer either an **icosahedral** (20-sided) appearance to the virus or a **helical** one. All viruses in which the nucleic acid is DNA are icosahedral (apart from the **poxviruses**); RNA viruses may be either icosahedral or helical. The mature infective virus particle is called a **virion**. In the case of some viruses this may refer to the nucleic acid genome and the capsid only, but in others these are surrounded by a glycoprotein **envelope**. Most of the DNA viruses have no envelope (with the exception of the **herpesviruses**); most RNA viruses are enveloped (with the exception of **picornaviruses** and **reoviruses**).

A true virus possesses several basic characteristics:

1. It contains one type of nucleic acid only.
2. Viral replication is controlled entirely by this nucleic acid.
3. Unlike bacteria, viruses cannot undergo binary fission.
4. Viruses lack the genetic information required to produce energy generating systems.
5. Viruses only replicate intracellularly and make use of the ribosomes of the host cell in the course of replication.

Viruses and the Target Cell

The **functional** implications of a viral infection derive from:

1. Changes directly produced by the virus in the host cell
2. The host tissue reactions to these changes
3. The responses of the immune system, both to the presence of the virus and to the cellular changes which it has produced

Integral to any understanding of these is some knowledge of how viruses enter a host cell and replicate within it. This can be regarded as an overlapping sequence of discrete steps which can be summarized as follows.

1. Virus attaches to cell surface membrane

Contact between the virus and its target cell occurs more or less randomly. However, **attachment** of the virion to the cell surface will not take place unless the surface membrane of the cell has a specific viral receptor site which is complementary to an attachment site on the surface of the virus. The necessity for such a specific affinity between the virion and its target is well demonstrated in the cases of **poliovirus** and the **influenza virus.**

For poliovirus to attach to a target cell, the latter must possess a specific lipoprotein receptor on its plasma membrane. This is present in primate cells but absent from those of rodents. The poliovirus virion will, therefore, attach to the former but not to the latter, and rodents cannot be infected by poliovirus.

Similarly the influenza virus attaches to cells because of the presence of a specific glycoprotein receptor (**N-acetylneuraminic acid; NANA**) on the cell surface. The receptor on the target cell is a binding site for a **haemagglutinin** (so-called because it can cause red cells to clump) carried on the envelope of the influenza virus. This receptor can be destroyed by treating cells in culture with bacterial neuraminidase (sialidase) and influenza virus will not attach to cells which have been treated in this way.

2. Virus penetrates the cell

Once attachment to the plasma membrane of the target cell has occurred, the virion becomes engulfed within the cell by a process akin to phagocytosis, the jargon term for which is **viropexis**. This is a temperature- and energy-dependent step and can be inhibited by treating the target cells with various metabolic poisons. The virus enters the cell within a membrane-bound vesicle. In the case of some enveloped viruses, the envelope fuses with the plasma membrane of the cell and the nucleocapsid is released directly into the host cytoplasm.

3. Viral nucleic acid is uncoated

The term uncoating means exposure of the viral nucleic acid. Sometimes this commences during the attachment stage. Commonly, however, it occurs within the host cell cytoplasm and lysosomal enzymes are thought to play some part in the process. In the case of a few viruses of the **reovirus** family, uncoating may never be completed.

From this point, the events in viral replication differ according to whether the nucleic acid genome is DNA or RNA.

DNA virus replication

The viral DNA is transcribed in two stages, giving rise to messenger RNA at two points in time which are characterized as **early** and **late** (Fig. 17.1). Early transcription from the viral DNA takes place in the nucleus and the mRNA produced reaches the cytoplasm and is then translated by the host ribosomes into **early proteins** required for the synthesis of **new viral DNA**, which again takes place in the host cell nucleus. **Late mRNA** is then transcribed. This leaves the nucleus and is translated in the cytoplasm into **late proteins**, which constitute the material from which the capsomeres are made. These proteins then enter the nucleus and the virions are assembled there before leaving the host cell. This last move is accomplished by a bursting open of the cell, with release of the new virions into the surrounding extracellular environment. All DNA viruses replicate in this way, with the exception of the poxviruses which do so within the host cell cytoplasm. The polymerases concerned in the transcription of viral DNA are derived from the host cell in most instances. The poxviruses, however, have their own DNA-dependent RNA polymerase.

RNA virus replication

With one exception, all classes of RNA viruses replicate within the cytoplasm of the host cell. **Orthomyxoviruses** (responsible for influenza), however, replicate within the host cell nucleus. Since normal cells do not copy RNA, the RNA viruses need to have their own RNA-dependent polymerase for replication to take place. The details of RNA replication vary depending on the nature of the viral RNA, and both new viral RNA and messenger RNA are produced from the original viral genome. After uncoating, the viral RNA may serve as its

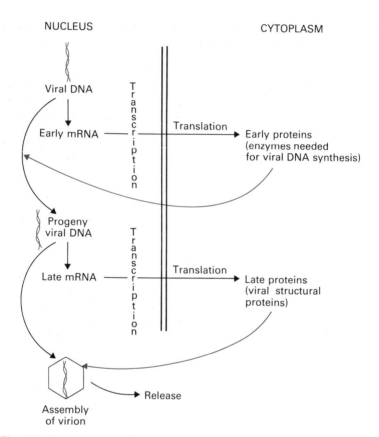

Fig. 17.1 Replication of a DNA virus.

own messenger RNA. This is then translated, resulting in the formation of an RNA polymerase, which in turn is necessary for the formation of a replicative, intermediate form of the viral RNA. This is double-stranded and contains one strand from the parent RNA and one which is complementary to it. At this time a series of **inhibitors** are formed which effectively switch off the normal synthetic processes of the host cell. From the double-stranded **'replicative'** RNA, single-stranded viral RNA molecules are formed. These may then function in three ways:

1. They may serve as templates for further viral RNA synthesis.
2. They may serve as mRNA for capsid protein synthesis.
3. They may themselves become encapsidated forming mature virions.

In one group of RNA viruses, the **retroviruses**, which are known to produce neoplasms in many animal species, the pattern of replication is different, since genetic information derived from the virus is inserted into the **host's genome** and this inserted segment must, of course, be DNA. The existence of this DNA means that **viral RNA must be copied into DNA.** For viral replication to occur, new mRNA must be transcribed from this newly formed DNA in order for new viral proteins to be synthesized. The formation of the DNA replica from the viral RNA is accomplished by a unique enzyme system known as **RNA-dependent DNA polymerase (reverse transcriptase).**

During all the events which follow penetration of the virions into the host cells, virus particles *cannot be detected* within the infected cells. This is known as the **eclipse phase.** Its length varies from virus to virus, ranging from minutes in the case of certain bacterial viruses (**bacteriophages**) to hours in the case of some animal viruses. Once the viruses have been assembled they are **released** from the infected cell. This may occur by bursting or lysis of the host cell or by budding from the host cell membrane. In the latter case the host cell is not destroyed. Where release occurs by budding, the virus is frequently enveloped. The viral glycoproteins which constitute the envelope are inserted into the plasma membrane of the host cell in the form of spikes. Beneath this there may be a matrix protein (M protein) which serves as an

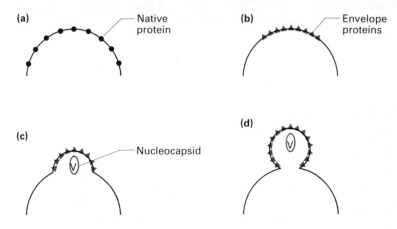

Fig. 17.2 Release of an RNA virus by budding from the cell surface. (a) Surface membrane of the host cell with 'native' proteins. (b) A segment of the host cell membrane expresses the virally coded envelope proteins. (c) The nucleocapsid adheres to the altered segment of the host cell surface membrane. (d) The altered segment of the cell surface membrane becomes wrapped round the nucleocapsid.

attachment point for the nucleocapsid. This altered segment of the host cell plasma membrane is wrapped round the nucleocapsid and the completed virion can then bud off from the cell in which replication has taken place (Fig. 17.2).

A Brief Classification of Viruses

Most known viruses can be separated into clearly defined groups on the basis of a number of criteria. These include:

1. The type and form of the nucleic acid genome
2. The size and morphology of the virus
3. The natural method of transmission from host to host
4. Susceptibility to a variety of chemical and physical agents
5. Viral preference for certain hosts, tissues and cells

DNA-containing viruses

Poxviruses

The viruses of the pox group are the largest and most complicated known. They are brick-shaped or elliptical and contain double-stranded DNA. The nucleocapsid is enveloped by a double membrane. Unlike most of the other DNA viruses, the poxviruses replicate solely within the cytoplasm of the host cell, where the site of viral replication may appear as an inclusion body (see p. 268). In man, these viruses cause smallpox (now eradicated), vaccinia, alastrim, and a curious mild disorder characterized by waxy nodules on the skin and trunk known as molluscum contagiosum.

A large number of poxviruses infect animals exclusively, but some cause disease both in animals and man.

Herpesviruses

Viruses of this group are medium-sized (the nucleocapsids measuring between 90 and 110 nm and the enveloped forms 150 and 200 nm in diameter) and contain double-stranded DNA. The capsid possesses icosahedral symmetry and is surrounded by a lipid-containing envelope.

These viruses are responsible for cold sores and genital blistering (herpes simplex virus), chickenpox and shingles (varicella zoster virus), infectious mononucleosis (Epstein–Barr virus) and intrauterine infections (cytomegalovirus). The Epstein–Barr virus probably also plays a role in the induction of Burkitt's lymphoma (see p. 460) and nasopharyngeal carcinoma (p. 461).

Herpesvirus infections show a marked tendency to become latent for long periods; once infection has occurred, the virus may remain latent within the infected individuals for the remainder of their lives.

Adenoviruses

Like the herpesviruses, the adenoviruses are also medium-sized (70 to 90 nm). They contain double-stranded DNA and are icosahedral. Most of the 252 capsomeres are hexons but 12 are pentons in which the cytotoxic potential of these viruses resides. From the pentons which form the corners of the virion, fine fibres project, each terminating in a knob-like structure. These terminal knobs are responsible for the agglutination of red blood cells and for adhesion to host cells. The nucleocapsid is not enveloped and the virus resists treatment with ether.

Adenoviruses can be divided into four main groups on the basis, inter alia, of the animal species whose red cells they agglutinate. They can be further subdivided into 33 subtypes on the basis of antigenic differences in hexon and fibre proteins. Of the subtypes which cause infections in man, many exhibit **latency** and may survive in lymphoid tissue such as the tonsil for many years. Clinically, they tend to affect mucous membranes and cause acute respiratory diseases characterized by fever, myalgia, nasopharyngeal inflammation, pharyngitis and conjunctivitis.

Papovaviruses

This family derives its name from its three members:

papilloma virus
polyoma virus
vacuolating virus in monkeys

These viruses are small (43 to 53 nm) and contain double-stranded DNA arranged in a circular pattern. In animals, papilloma viruses cause a variety of neoplasms; in humans they cause the common wart and may have a role in the pathogenesis of cervical neoplasia. Polyoma virus infections are also associated with **progressive multifocal encephalopathy,** a rare degenerative condition of the cerebral white matter seen in immunosuppressed patients, usually with malignant lymphomas (see p. 262).

Parvoviruses

As their name implies ('parvus' = small), these are very small viruses with a diameter of about 20 nm. They contain single-stranded DNA and their replication takes place in the nucleus of the infected cell. Parvovirus infection in man causes temporary erythroid aplasia, a common rash illness of childhood (erythema infectiosum), and may be involved in one variety of gastroenteritis occurring particularly in cold weather ('winter vomiting disease').

RNA-containing viruses

Picornaviruses

Picornaviruses ('pico' = small) are very small (20 to 30 nm), non-enveloped, icosahedral viruses. They contain single-stranded RNA and are resistant to treatment with ether. This family includes important human pathogens, including the viruses responsible for poliomyelitis and the common cold. The picornaviruses are divided into two genera: the **enteroviruses** and the **rhinoviruses.** Enteroviruses include:

1. Three types of poliovirus
2. Twenty-nine types of coxsackievirus
3. Thirty-two types of **ECHO** virus (enteric cytopathic human orphan virus). The term 'orphan' refers to the fact that for some time they were regarded as 'viruses in search of a disease'.

The enteroviruses cause a wide range of diseases in man. These include poliomyelitis, aseptic meningitis, myocarditis (chiefly in the newborn), myositis, herpangina, and upper respiratory tract infections.

Infection occurs via both the alimentary and the respiratory tracts, the former being much more important in the case of poliovirus infections. There is no natural animal host. This has interesting implications in respect of poliovirus, of which there are only three types. Vaccines have been prepared against all of these and it is quite possible that, following widespread immunization, the disease may be eliminated in a similar way to smallpox.

Most poliovirus infections are symptomless but the virus, which is cytocidal, may spread to involve the anterior horn cells with resulting paralysis. (The pathogenesis of full-blown poliovirus infections of this kind is shown in Fig. 17.15 on p. 272.)

Rhinoviruses, of which there are 113 types, cause the common cold.

Orthomyxoviruses

As defined currently, the orthomyxoviruses contain only those viruses which cause human influenza. They are medium-sized with a helically arranged capsid, contain single-stranded DNA and are enveloped. The lipid envelope is somewhat unusual in that it is studded with spike-like projections called peplomers. These are of two varieties, the first being a viral haemagglutinin which binds to the N-acetylneuraminic acid on the surface membrane of most cells, and the second being a neuraminidase. In morphological terms it is pleomorphic, some viruses being spherical in shape while others are filamentous.

The arrangement of the RNA is distinctly unusual. Instead of being a continuous thread, it exists in the form of eight segments, each of which represents a single gene. These eight gene segments code for 10 or 11 viral proteins, this being explained by the pattern of splicing of two of the mRNAs.

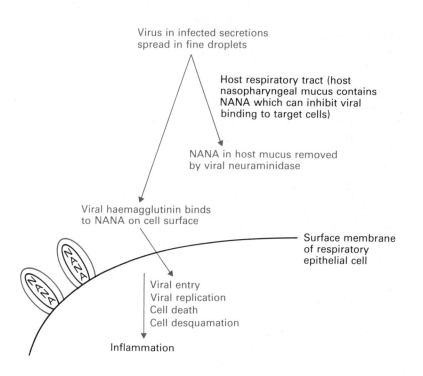

Virus in infected secretions
spread in fine droplets

Host respiratory tract (host
nasopharyngeal mucus contains
NANA which can inhibit viral
binding to target cells)

NANA in host mucus removed
by viral neuraminidase

Viral haemagglutinin binds
to NANA on cell surface

Surface membrane
of respiratory
epithelial cell

Viral entry
Viral replication
Cell death
Cell desquamation

Inflammation

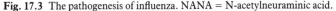

Fig. 17.3 The pathogenesis of influenza. NANA = N-acetylneuraminic acid.

The acute respiratory disease caused by the influenza virus in man can be fatal and may occur in very large scale local epidemics, usually every two to four years, or even on a world-wide basis (pandemics) every 10 to 20 years. A single influenza virus infection does not confer lifelong immunity to the disease. An important part of the reason for this curious epidemiological behaviour lies in the fact that the viral genome is continually changing. Minor changes in the haemagglutinins of a particular strain may occur, as a result of a series of point mutations, over a long period, this process being called **antigenic drift**. From time to time a much more fundamental change occurs in which multiple alterations in the antigenic make-up of the viral strain, probably as a result of recombination of genome segments, appear suddenly. This is known as **antigenic shift**. The appearances of new subtypes of influenza virus as a result of antigenic shift are likely to be associated with the occurrence of pandemic outbreaks.

The pathogenesis of influenza is shown in Fig. 17.3. Sporadic cases are usually fairly mild and self-limiting. Sometimes, especially in the elderly, severe pneumonia supervenes. This is most commonly due to a secondary bacterial infection, although in rare instances it is a primary viral pneumonia, in which intrapulmonary haemorrhage is a conspicuous feature.

Paramyxoviruses

These viruses were originally grouped with the orthomyxoviruses. They are roughly cubical in shape. They are somewhat larger than orthomyxoviruses, but share with them a number of characteristics such as the presence of haemagglutinins and neuraminidase (which, in contrast to what is seen in the influenza virus, coexist on the same 'spike' on the envelope).

Viruses of this group cause sore throats and croup (parainfluenza virus), measles, mumps, and infections of the lower respiratory tract (respiratory syncytial virus). In animals, paramyxoviruses cause Newcastle disease in birds, distemper in dogs and rinderpest in cattle. One of the interesting characteristics of viruses of this family is that they promote cell fusion with the formation of multinucleate cells (see p. 267). This feature has been used extensively in the production of hybrid cells, the virus employed for this purpose being Sendai virus (which causes parainfluenza in mice). The ability to promote cell fusion is conferred on the virus by its possession of a spike on the envelope which is quite distinct from the haemagglutinin, called the F glycoprotein. This glycoprotein is also necessary for penetration of the target cell to occur and strains which lack the F glycoprotein are not infective.

Rhabdoviruses

Viruses of this group have a rather curious shape, being flattened at one end and rounded at the other. The genome consists of single-stranded RNA and the nucleocapsid is enclosed in an envelope which bears spikes which are about 10 nm in length. This group includes the **rabies virus**, which causes one of the most serious of all viral infections. Many warm-blooded animals such as dogs, foxes, bats, skunks and jackals are reservoirs for rabies virus. Victims of the disease are infected by the bite of a rabid animal, the virus being present in the saliva. The rabies virus appears to have a special affinity for nervous tissue and travels slowly up the peripheral nerves to reach the central nervous system where it causes the encephalitis characteristic of the disease. In experimental rabies infections, where it is possible to examine specimens of peripheral nerves, viral particles have been seen in the axons on electron microscopy.

Arenaviruses

Arenaviruses derive their name from the Latin word '**harenaceus**' meaning 'sandy'. This term was coined because of the presence of electron-dense granules which can be seen within the virions on electron microscopy.

The natural hosts of arenaviruses appear to be rodents, which are often persistently infected. Man is infected more or less by accident on exposure to rodent excretions. The resulting infections include some of the most lethal viral disorders known: Lassa fever and Argentinian and Bolivian haemorrhagic fevers. The natural host of the Lassa fever virus is a West African rodent, the multimammate rat, which is persistently but apparently harmlessly infected.

Another example of arenavirus infection in animals discussed later in this chapter is the virus which causes **lymphocytic choriomeningitis** (LCM) in mice. The LCM virus is transmitted **vertically** (from mother to progeny) and exerts its damaging effect through the formation of soluble immune complexes which are filtered out in the glomerulus and cause a type III (Gell and Coombes) reaction at this site.

Coronaviruses

Viruses of this family include several which, in man, cause the common cold. They are medium-sized, rather pleomorphic viruses which have widely spaced club-shaped peplomers in their lipoprotein envelope; it is the arrangement of these 'clubs' which gives this virus its distinctive appearance and its name.

Togaviruses

Togaviruses are spherical, closely enveloped, RNA viruses which contain single-stranded RNA. They multiply within the cytoplasm of their target cells and mature by budding from cytoplasmic membranes. All the togaviruses, with the exception of rubella, belong to a larger grouping known as the **arborviruses** (*arthropod borne* viruses). Arthropods are not only the vectors for these viral infections, but are the primary natural **hosts** in which viral multiplication occurs before transmission to a secondary vertebrate host by insect bite. These vertebrates act as a **reservoir** for the viruses and are unaffected by the presence of the arboviruses. However, when man, an unnatural host, is infected, serious and often lethal disorders arise such as **yellow fever**, various encephalitides, and some of the haemorrhagic fevers (Fig. 17.4).

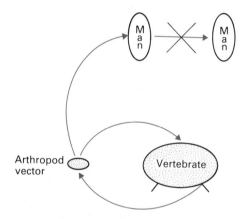

Fig. 17.4 Vector and vertebrate reservoirs for viral infections such as yellow fever.

In human infections, the virus in the saliva of the insect, in the course of biting, is injected into capillaries. Viral multiplication occurs in the first instance in the vascular endothelium and in the fixed phagocytic cells of the reticuloendothelial system. There is a short-lived viraemia and this may be followed by a variety of clinical developments, depending on the precise nature of the virus and its localization. In the haemorrhagic fevers, bleeding occurs from many sites and death may result from hypovolaemic shock. In yellow fever, the liver and kidneys are affected, leading to jaundice and impairment of renal function. There is massive necrosis in the mid-zones of the liver lobules and, as a consequence, a decrease in the synthesis of those clotting factors formed in the liver.

Rubella. Rubella virus is a member of the togavirus family, but is not transmitted via an insect vector and is classified as being in the genus **Rubivirus.** Infection by the rubella virus has no serious consequences unless it occurs in utero, especially in the first three months of pregnancy. When this happens there is a very high risk that the infants will be born with a wide range of congenital defects, most notably in the heart, ears (nerve deafness) and eyes (cataract). Many other organs may be affected, and hepatitis and pneumonia in the neonatal period are quite common. The risks are so serious that rubella occurring in the first three months of a pregnancy constitutes good grounds for termination of that pregnancy. In order to prevent intrauterine infections with the rubella virus, girls may be immunized with an attenuated viral vaccine in their early teens. Alternatively, the vaccines may be given to all children in an attempt to eliminate the infection altogether.

Reoviruses

The acronym 'reo' is derived from respiratory, enteric and orphan. This is because the initial sites of isolation were the respiratory and gastrointestinal tracts, and because no diseases were known to be

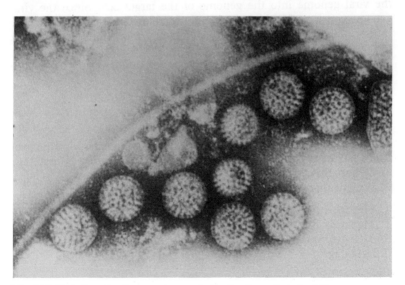

Fig. 17.5 Rotavirus. An electron micrograph showing the typical wheel-like appearance of this virus. This appearance is due to the presence of a double-layered capsid, the outer layer being smooth and the inner layer being symmetrically roughened on electron microscopy. (Photograph by courtesy of Professor J. Pattison.)

associated with this group of viruses (hence 'orphan'). Three genera are known, of which only two, **rotavirus** and **orbivirus**, cause disease in man. Orbivirus is an arborvirus and causes Colorado tick fever. Rotavirus has a curious double-layered capsid, the outer layer appearing smooth on electron microscopy and the inner layer symmetrically 'roughened'. This gives the virion a wheel-like appearance, hence the name (Latin 'rota' = a wheel) (Fig. 17.5).

Rotaviruses are an important cause of gastroenteritis, mainly in young children, and of a similar syndrome in a variety of young animals. Diagnosis of gastroenteritis caused by these viruses can be made by examining stool samples either by electron microscopy, since the highly characteristic virions are present in very large number in the faeces, or by immunological methods.

Oncornaviruses

These are oncogenic RNA viruses belonging to family Retroviridae and responsible for the production of a wide variety of neoplasms of connective, lymphoid and haemopoietic tissue in a number of different animal species. They are also capable of inducing malignant transformation in cultured cells. This involves the insertion of part of the viral genome into the genome of the target cell. Since the viral genome consists of RNA only, clearly some mechanism must exist for transcribing DNA from the viral RNA: this is accomplished through the action of a virally coded enzyme system known as **reverse transcriptase**. The activity of these viruses is discussed in a little more detail in Chapter 30.

Unclassified viruses

Some viruses do not fit conveniently into the groups described above. Amongst these are a group whose only unifying feature is that they cause **hepatitis.**
At present this group is regarded as having three members:

1. Hepatitis A
2. Hepatitis B
3. Hepatitis non-A non-B (this probably includes at least three or four different agents)

Hepatitis A

This is a small RNA virus, some of the features of which suggest a relationship with the picornaviruses. It is transmitted by the faecal–oral route and the disease has an incubation period of between two and six weeks. Hepatitis A affects chiefly children and young adults. Onset of symptoms is acute, with nausea, vomiting and anorexia being prominent. Jaundice usually appears within a few days and lasts for two to three weeks in most cases. Massive liver necrosis can occur but is very uncommon and complete recovery is the rule.

Hepatitis B

Hepatitis B virus has nothing in common with the A variety. It is a DNA-containing virus with a small nucleic acid genome (approximately 3200 base pairs) which is arranged as a circle of double-stranded DNA with a gap in one of the strands. The nucleic acid is contained within an icosahedral capsid; these two elements together constitute the **core.** The core is surrounded by a second shell of lipid and protein and the complete virion is termed the 'Dane particle' after Dr David Dane who first described it.

Three types of viral particle can be identified by electron microscopy in the sera of infected individuals (Fig. 17.6). The first of these, which is the infectious agent of hepatitis B, is the virion or Dane particle. The

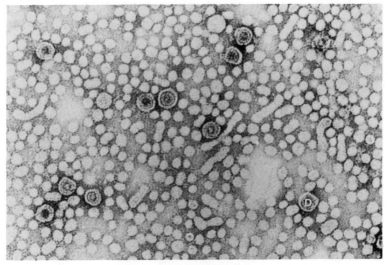

Fig. 17.6 Hepatitis B virus. This concentrated preparation shows the three morphological forms in which the virus may be seen in the serum of infected individuals: (1) the Dane particle or complete virion (D); (2) small spherical particles composed of the same lipid and protein which constitutes the outer shell of the complete virion; (3) long particles which represent aggregates of the spherical particles. (Photograph by courtesy of Professor J. Pattison.)

second, and most numerous, is a small spherical particle about half the size of the complete virion. This is composed of the same lipid and protein which constitutes the outer shell of the complete virion. Lastly, there are long filamentous particles (50 to 200 nm in length) which represent aggregates of the spherical particles. All these particles can be detected immunologically, and collectively constitute the surface antigen (**HBsAg**) (originally known as the Australia antigen). Other antigens have been identified which elicit an antibody response in infected individuals: the **c** or core antigen, which consists of capsid protein, and an **e** antigen, the presence of which in serum correlates with high infectivity.

The main route of transmission is via injection into the bloodstream or tissues. Since the virus can be shown to persist in blood for prolonged periods, both after clinically apparent and subclinical infections, this carrier state constitutes a potent reservoir for infection. Originally blood transfusion was thought to be the major risk factor in spreading hepatitis B. It is now known, however, that infections can occur in the course of transfers of much smaller amounts of blood or plasma, such as might occur with sharing of needles by heroin addicts, tattooing, etc. Male homosexuals also appear to have a high risk of contracting hepatitis B.

In the UK, the carrier rate is low (about 0.1%), but in other parts of the world, notably Asia and certain parts of Africa, it may reach very much higher levels (commonly 5 to 15%).

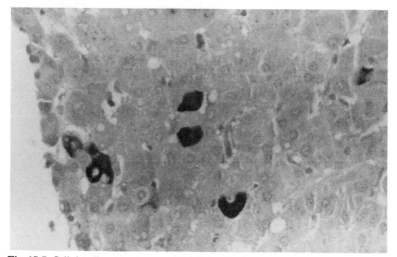

Fig. 17.7 Cells in a liver biopsy showing the presence of hepatitis B surface antigen. This section has been treated with an antibody prepared against the surface antigen of hepatitis B virus. Binding of the antibody to cells containing the antigen has been demonstrated by use of the immunoperoxidase method, in which cells containing antigen stain brown.

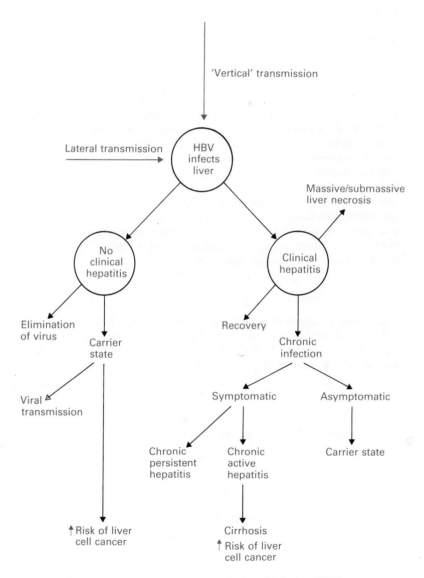

Fig. 17.8 Possible natural histories of infection with hepatitis B virus (HBV).

The incubation period is much longer than that of hepatitis A (seven weeks to six months) and, in general, the disease is more severe. Damage to the infected liver cells does not appear to be brought about by any direct action of the virus itself, but by cell-mediated immune mechanisms evoked by the presence of viral surface antigen expressed on the surface of the affected cell (Fig. 17.7). This is an example of a mechanism of viral elimination being responsible for the pathological and clinical features of a disease. It follows from this that if surface antigens are not so expressed, viral replication can continue within the liver cells with no associated liver cell damage to call attention to the presence of an HBV infection. Such persistent infections in the liver may, however, be associated with continuing liver damage; this state is known as **chronic active hepatitis.** This is thought to occur in about half the patients in whom there is persistent infection. If unchecked, the continuing liver cell necrosis leads to fibrosis and nodular regeneration with disorganization of the normal lobular architecture of the liver (**cirrhosis**). This, in its turn, can lead to chronic liver failure and portal hypertension (Fig. 17.8). There is a strong association between persistent hepatitis B infections and a high risk of liver cell cancer. This is discussed in Chapter 30.

Non-A non-B hepatitis

This group of agents is now thought to be responsible for the majority of cases of post-transfusion hepatitis and also some of the largest outbreaks of hepatitis in India and other parts of the Far East. They may also be associated with chronic hepatitis and cirrhosis. A possible non-A non-B viral particle has been identified by electron microscopy. It is serologically distinct from the other hepatitis viruses.

The Natural History of Viral Infections

Viral infections may be divided into two main groups:

1. Superficial infections, e.g. influenza and other viral infections of the respiratory tract
2. Infections associated with systemic spread, when viruses travel from the **portal of entry** to the **target organ**, producing the typical disease, e.g. poliomyelitis

Many of the effects of a viral infection will depend on the rate at which viral replication proceeds and whether the infected host cells are killed, either because of lysis or because of inhibition of their own synthetic processes by viral proteins.

Acute infections

Where a virus replicates actively within an infected cell and new viruses are released from such a cell, the infection is spoken of as being **productive**. This may lead to the patient experiencing an acute illness, often febrile, the clinical picture of which will be modified by the nature of the cells which are killed. For example, poliomyelitis is associated with necrosis of the anterior horn cells in the spinal column and therefore paralysis may develop. Within a few weeks either the virus is eliminated or the infected person dies. Not all acute infections, however, produce a clinically apparent disease. In many instances viral infections are subclinical and the only objective evidence that they have occurred is the presence of appropriate antibodies in the plasma.

Failure of viral elimination

Failure to eliminate the virus from the host may lead to a number of different situations. Such infections can be:

1. **Latent**, in which the virus is not normally detected. The infection persists in an occult, quiescent form with episodes of reactivation in the form of acute, self-limiting illnesses.
2. **Persistent** and **slow** infections, in which the infection persists and causes a prolonged disease which is slow to develop and often inexorable in its progress
3. **Oncogenic**, in which part of the viral genome is incorporated into the host genome, resulting in malignant transformation

Latent infections

True latency in relation to viral infections implies the persistence of virus in such small amounts that ordinary methods fail to detect its presence, though the virus will usually appear if the infected tissue is cultured and may be identified by using specially radioactively labelled viral probes.

Latent infections tend to occur especially with viruses of the herpes group. Amongst the commonest clinical expressions of this are the 'cold sores' or 'fever blisters' which affect many people at frequent intervals throughout their lives (Fig. 17.9). These are due to infections with the **herpes simplex virus**, which produces clusters of little vesicles, usually at the mucocutaneous junctions of the lips. The vesicles rupture, leading to painful ulcerations which heal with scarring. At various times, often in association with fever, sunburn, menstruation, etc., the vesicular lesions recur, always at the same site. Between these clinical episodes the virus can be recovered only with difficulty or often not at

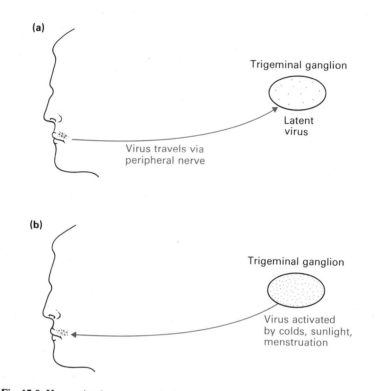

Fig. 17.9 Herpes simplex: an example of latency in viral infection. (a) Primary infection leading to latency. (b) Recurrent infection following activation of latent virus ('cold sore').

all. It remains latent within the cells of the trigeminal ganglion between attacks and is released from the cells of the ganglion when they are cultured. The trigeminal ganglion is believed to harbour the herpes virus in about 80% of adults.

Another virus of the herpes family, the varicella-zoster virus provides another common example of latency with occasional reactivation. The latter manifests as herpes zoster or shingles. This is characterized by a painful rash, usually limited to an area of skin or mucous membrane served by a single sensory ganglion. It occurs for the most part in individuals over 50 years of age and is only found in those who have had chicken pox (**varicella**) in the past. Zoster and varicella are two distinct manifestations of infection by a single virus. Varicella represents the primary infection, and zoster the reactivation of the virus which has lain latent in sensory ganglia since the attack of varicella, which may have occurred many years before. Zoster is infectious to those who have not had varicella; infection in such an individual leads to an attack of chicken pox, not to an attack of shingles.

Zoster seems to increase in frequency in relation to x-irradiation and a similar increase is seen in patients suffering from Hodgkin's disease. This suggests that the expression of infection and the appearance of clinical manifestations are controlled by the state of immunity of the host. However x-irradiation of mice does not seem to have this effect.

Persistent infections

These may be due to:

1. Well characterized viral agents such as measles or hepatitis virus
2. Agents of unknown nature

In this situation the virus is not eliminated from the host and goes on replicating inside infected cells, usually at a rate which does not cause any direct tissue damage. Very often the infected individual will **carry** the virus in blood or other tissue fluids; such a patient may be a dangerous source of infection to others. Roughly one-third of patients who have an acute episode of hepatitis due to hepatitis B virus (HBV) will become carriers, and there are many more with no history of a diagnosable episode of jaundice. It is estimated that there may be as many as 100 000 000 carriers of HBV in the world. It is obvious that there is a considerable risk of the virus being passed on through the medium of blood transfusion, etc., and screening of donors for this and, indeed, other carrier states is clearly important. Other types of viral infection in which this asymptomatic carrier state can develop include **cytomegalovirus** infection and infections with the **Epstein–Barr virus** (which causes infectious mononucleosis and is believed to be causally associated with certain neoplasms.

In some instances chronic asymptomatic infections may lead eventually to the appearance of serious, clinically apparent disease. An example of this is **lymphocytic choriomeningitis** (LCM) in the common household mouse. The virus (one of the **arenavirus** family) is vertically transmitted from generation to generation, the infection being acquired in utero. This infection appears to be associated with low zone tolerance in which T lymphocytes are tolerant but B lymphocytes are not. Low levels of antibody to viral antigens are produced over a long period and soluble immune complexes are produced which eventually cause the appearance of glomerulonephritis in old mice. The tolerance which develops is associated with the fact that the LCM infection occurs during the perinatal period. If mature, immunologically competent mice are infected with this virus, they develop a severe inflammation in the brain (**encephalitis**).

A rather different type of chronic infection is seen in a small number of patients as a result of infection with **measles virus**. The disease which follows the very long-continued localization of measles virus in the brain is known as **subacute sclerosing panencephalitis**. The peak incidence of this, happily, rare condition is during adolescent life. Affected patients present with increasing reduction of intellectual function, motor abnormalities and fits. An inexorable downward path is followed by death within a year of the appearance of symptoms. The patients' brains show degenerative features with loss of myelin and a mild increase in the supporting glial fibres. There is also evidence of an encephalitis in the form of a perivascular lymphocytic infiltrate. Cerebrospinal fluid contains high titres of measles antibody and viral antigen, and nucleocapsid material can be identified in cells within the brain as well as within lymph nodes. It has been suggested that the disorder is an expression of an aberrant T cell response to the presence of virus in the brain, but this is still a matter of debate.

Slow progressive infections

The term 'slow virus infection' was introduced to describe certain very slowly developing and chronic diseases in sheep, originally observed in Iceland, caused by members of the Lentivirus group — visna and maedi. It has now been extended to cover a number of curious disorders in which the only unifying feature is slowness of development.

Slow infections may be caused by conventional viruses. Subacute sclerosing panencephalitis, described above as a chronic infection, could just as well be regarded as a slow virus infection, since the onset of symptoms usually follows on a considerable period after the original measles infection.

Another slow viral infection in man is **progressive multifocal leucoencephalopathy** (PML), a rare disease of the brain leading to focal demyelination in many areas of the white matter. It is caused by infections with members of the **papovavirus** group and only occurs in patients who are immunosuppressed. Such immunosuppression may be seen in patients with neoplastic disease involving the lymphoid system, such as Hodgkin's disease, and also in those who are receiving cytotoxic chemotherapy in the course of treatment for malignant disease. The papovaviruses which have been isolated from the brains of affected individuals are widespread, at least in Europe and the USA, and papovavirus infections, in the general population, are usually acquired fairly early in life.

In animals, slow virus infections occur in three disorders:

1. Maedi produces a slowly progressive pneumonia in Icelandic sheep.
2. Visna produces a progressive demyelinating disease, also of sheep.

Both these diseases are caused by retroviruses and are transmissible with incubation periods of several years.

3. Aleutian mink disease is a slowly developing syndrome caused by chronic infection by a member of the **parvovirus** group. There is a humoral immune response but this does not succeed in eliminating the virus. Soluble immune complex formation is a prominent feature and most of the affected animals develop an immune complex mediated glomerulonephritis. Other evidence of a disturbance in the regulation of the immune response is present in the form of hypergammaglobulinaemia and antibodies directed against red cell antigens.

Slow infections in the nervous system which do not appear to be due to 'conventional viruses'. There is a group of slow, relentlessly progressive disorders of the central nervous system occurring both in man and animals, which, while being clearly **transmissible**, do not appear to be caused by agents which have the characteristics of true viruses. These disorders have been termed the **spongiform encephalopathies** because of the histological changes seen in the central nervous system. They include:

In man:
kuru
Creutzfeldt–Jakob syndrome
Gerstmann–Straussler syndrome

In animals:
scrapie
transmissible mink encephalopathy

The clinical and pathological features of all these disorders suggest that they are closely related. Kuru, scrapie and the Gerstmann–Sträussler syndrome all begin with difficulty in walking and loss of coordination, suggesting dysfunction of the cerebellum. In Creutzfeldt–Jakob disease, dementia is an early feature but usually develops late in kuru. In **none** is there any sign in the brain of an inflammatory response such as is seen in the encephalitides caused by true viruses, no antibodies are formed, and the cell count in the cerebrospinal fluid is unaffected.

The pathological changes are confined to the central nervous system. Proliferation of supporting cells, the astrocytes, is a constant feature. In the neurones there is a depletion of dendritic spines (which are believed to play a part in the transmission of nerve impulses) and numerous vacuoles give the brain a spongy appearance (hence the term 'spongiform encephalopathies').

Kuru. Kuru is a chronic disorder of the central nervous system found only among the Fore tribe in the highlands of New Guinea. It is characterized by cerebellar degeneration leading to ataxia, tremors and loss of coordination; death usually occurs within a year of the onset of symptoms. It was unknown in this area until about 1920, but by 1960 was said to be responsible for a high proportion of deaths among children and young adults, and a similarly high proportion of deaths among women. The predilection of the disease for these groups has been related to the practice of a modified form of cannibalism which was introduced into this area sometime between 1910 and 1920. This involved the eating of the remains of deceased relatives, the meal being accompanied by elaborate ceremonies. The brain was consumed by women and children only. With the advent of an Australian administration, this method of disposing of one's nearest and dearest was forbidden and kuru has now become much less common, with the average age of onset rising each year. There is, thus, every reason to believe that this strange disease will disappear. These epidemiological data and the demonstration in 1965 by Gadjusek (a recent Nobel laureate) that kuru could be transmitted to chimpanzees by intracerebral inoculation strongly suggest an infectious origin.

Creutzfeldt–Jakob disease. This is a very rare syndrome encountered in early middle age in which the patients complain of abnormal sensations in their limbs and develop spasticity and jerky movements. Mental changes appear early in the disease and lead to a profound dementia. The pathological changes seen in the brain are similar to those encountered in kuru and, as with kuru, the disease can be transmitted to chimpanzees (also to goats and cats) by intracerebral inoculation of brains from Creutzfeldt–Jakob patients, even if the brain tissue has undergone prolonged fixation.

Scrapie. Scrapie is a chronic disorder occurring in sheep which has been recognized since the eighteenth century. It is characterized clinically by incoordination of the hindquarters and a pruritus (itching) which leads to compulsive rubbing or scraping against fixed objects (hence the name 'scrapie'). Eventually paralysis and death supervene. Scrapie can be transmitted to sheep, goats and rodents by intracerebral inoculations of brain and spinal cord from affected animals.

Agents responsible for the spongiform encephalopathies. All these disorders have been shown to be transmissible by intracerebral inoculation of brain or cord. The infective agent, however, differs greatly from true viruses:

1. It is extremely small (molecular weight about 50 000).
2. It fails to elicit an antibody response in the disease situation.
3. No virus particles can be seen on electron microscopy.
4. The agent **resists** heat (90°C), ultraviolet light, formaldehyde, RNase, DNase, x-irradiation (unless in high dose), nucleases and zinc, despite the fact that all these agents damage **nucleic acids**. The resistance to ultraviolet light may be due to the close association of the infective particle with lipids of cell membranes. If chlorpromazine is added to the infective preparation, ultraviolet irradiation reduces infectivity. Chlorpromazine is known to penetrate lipid bilayers and to induce single-strand breaks in nucleic acid in the presence of ultraviolet light.

The agent of scrapie, which has been the most extensively studied, is inactivated by some proteases, phenol and sodium dodecyl sulphate, all agents which damage **protein**. Thus the pattern of agents which inactivate or fail to inactivate the infective agent suggests that it is proteinaceous in nature and does not contain any nucleic acid.

Studies of the scrapie agent, which can be concentrated from the hamster brain, confirm that its biological activity depends on the presence of a protein which can be isolated from the brain tissue. This infective agent has been termed a '**prion**' (proteinaceous infective particle). The bulk of the protein isolated from the brains of scrapie-infected animals appears to consist of a single molecule which has been given the name PrP (prion protein). PrP is a comparatively small molecule, less than half the size of haemoglobin. In infective material which has been concentrated, the PrP can be seen with the electron microscope to be aggregated in rod-shaped particles.

Thus far no nucleic acid has been detected in the prion by available methods. However, it is possible that a very small amount of nucleic acid might escape detection and the recent finding that ultraviolet irradiation can reduce infectivity in the presence of chlorpromazine suggests that this might be so.

The most important biological question relating to the prion is **how it replicates**. Some of the explanations which have been canvassed seem very implausible and do not conform with current thinking on molecular biology. One suggestion that merits consideration is that the prion is encoded by a gene in the **host genome** and that infection by prions might, in some way, activate this gene. The answer to this question may well be available in the not too distant future. Part of the amino acid sequence of PrP is now known and from this, DNA with a series of nucleotides complementary to the one which would encode the known part of the protein, has been prepared. This complementary DNA could be used as a probe to see whether a prion-encoding gene does exist within host cells or not.

It may seem a little strange to emphasize these rare disorders which may be of little importance in human medicine. However, the recognition of such unusual biological events, which appear to break the rules relating to viral infections, must lead eventually to an understanding of new areas of host–parasite interaction.

Transforming infections

Viruses can produce **malignant neoplasms** in a variety of animal species and may play a part in the induction of some human neoplasms. They can also induce transformation of cells (chiefly of connective tissue origin) in culture. Viral transformation of this type is discussed in Chapter 30.

The Effects of Viruses on Host Cells

The range of structural changes which can be produced by viral infections is extensive (Figs 17.10 and 17.11). They include:

1. **No change.** Cells in which the viral infection is of the **latent** variety show no structural abnormalities.
2. **Cell death.** Cell death is an extremely common outcome of viral infections and the type of cell affected may play a dominant role in

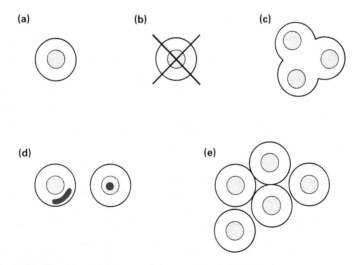

Fig. 17.10 The effects of viruses on their target cells. (a) No change (latency). (b) Cell death. (c) Cell fusion. (d) Formation of inclusion bodies. (e) Cell proliferation.

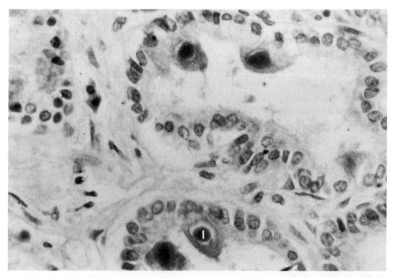

Fig. 17.11 Kidney from infant dying of cytomegalovirus (CMV) infection. Two of the renal tubules show marked enlargement of some of the epithelial lining cells. The nuclei of these cells contain large deeply eosinophilic inclusions (I) with a clear halo round them. This virus, a member of the herpes group, causes a wide range of effects which depend largely on the time of infection. Intrauterine infections may have a devastating effect on neonates. In adults, CMV infections are seldom serious other than in the immunosuppressed.

determining the clinical pattern of the disease, as for example in poliomyelitis. In cell culture systems, the morphology of the changes leading to cell death which are produced by different viruses may be so distinct one from another as to constitute a useful method for diagnosis. The cause of cell death in viral infections is not always obvious. On some occasions it may be due to cell lysis caused by the release of large numbers of newly formed virions. More often, however, cell death is caused by cessation of the normal synthetic activity of the target cell due to suppression by virus-specified proteins, not all of which are components of the virion.

3. **Alterations to cell surface membranes.** Some viruses, especially certain members of the paramyxovirus group, cause **fusion** to take place between infected and non-infected cells, with the formation of multinucleated giant cells. This is seen not uncommonly in the tissues of patients suffering from measles, the giant cells being found chiefly, but not exclusively, in lymphoid tissue. The highly characteristic mulberry-like giant cells are known as Warthin–Finkeldy cells and may be useful in the diagnosis of measles in tissue sections from patients who may have died from measles pneumonia.

4. The formation of inclusion bodies. In terms of the light microscope an inclusion body is a localized change in the staining properties of either the nucleus or the cytoplasm of cells which have been infected by certain viruses. They are rounded, sharply demarcated areas which usually show a marked affinity for acid dyes and are thus strongly eosinophilic in sections stained with haematoxylin and eosin.

Intracytoplasmic inclusions are found in cells infected by poxviruses, paramyxoviruses, reoviruses and one of the rhabdoviruses (rabies), in which pathognomonic inclusions are present in neurones within the brain and spinal cord (Negri bodies).

Intranuclear inclusions may be present in cells infected by herpesviruses and adenoviruses.

Inclusion bodies have been helpful from time to time in the diagnosis of certain viral infections. For example, if difficulty were experienced in distinguishing between a severe case of chickenpox (varicella) and smallpox, examination of cells scraped from a lesion would reveal intranuclear inclusions in the former and intracytoplasmic ones in the latter. These criteria for diagnosis have been largely superseded by electron microscopy.

Most inclusion bodies have been shown either by immunofluorescent or electron microscopic studies to be sites of viral synthesis within the cell. However, on some occasions, as in the case of herpesvirus infections, the inclusions do not consist of viral elements and may represent accumulations of by-products of viral replication.

5. Cell proliferation. Independent of any oncogenic effect, some viral infections can cause cells to proliferate. This is seen in a very common, self-limiting disorder, **infectious mononucleosis**, in which the patients, usually young adults, present with malaise, sore throat and enlarged lymph nodes. Infectious mononucleosis is caused by a herpesvirus, the **Epstein–Barr virus** of which the target cell is the B lymphocyte. B lymphocytes proliferate and develop new antigens on their cell surface membranes. These elicit a T cell reaction which brings the virus-induced B cell proliferation to an end.

Protective responses of host cells against viral infections

The interferons

Approximately 50 years ago the phenomenon of **viral interference** was first discovered. This term was coined to describe the situation in which a viral infection in an animal appeared, in some way, to protect against subsequent infections by another virus. In 1957, Isaacs and Lindenmann showed that cells infected with inactivated influenza virus released soluble compounds into the culture medium. These soluble compounds inhibited the replication of normal influenza virus within other cells. The blanket name '**interferon**' was applied to these substances, which are now known to be protein in nature.

At least three distinct types of interferon are known. These are:

alpha interferon (released chiefly from leucocytes)
beta interferon (released chiefly from fibroblasts)
gamma interferon (released by activated T lymphocytes)

Despite this tendency to identify certain interferons predominantly with certain cell types, it is likely that all cells can produce alpha and beta interferons when suitably stimulated.

The most important inducers of alpha and beta interferon release are viral infections, though the production can be triggered by rickettsiae, protozoa, bacterial endotoxins and even certain synthetic polynucleotides [poly I (polyriboinosinic acid) : poly C (polyribocytidilic acid)].

Interferons induced by viral infection are species specific (i.e. chick interferon will not protect rat or monkey cells against infection), but are not virus-specific. They appear between 12 and 48 hours after infection and shortly after they make their appearance, viral replication starts to decline.

The stimulus to interferon production in virus-infected cells appears to be foreign double-stranded RNA formed in the course of viral replication. How this induces the formation of the interferons is not known (Fig. 17.12).

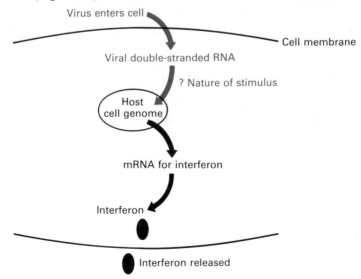

Fig. 17.12 Production of interferon in a cell infected by a virus.

Action of interferon. The reason that the protective effect of interferon is not limited to a single virus is that, unlike antibody, it does not interact directly with the virus. The interferon secreted by an infected cell diffuses from that cell and binds to a membrane receptor on the surface of neighbouring non-infected cells.

There is no inhibition of viral attachment or penetration of the cell to which the interferon has bound. The protective effect is mediated though blocking the translation of viral messenger RNA in the host cell polyribosomes. There are two ways in which this can be done. First, cells to which interferon has bound contain increased amounts of an adenine trinucleotide, which activates a ribonuclease which can destroy

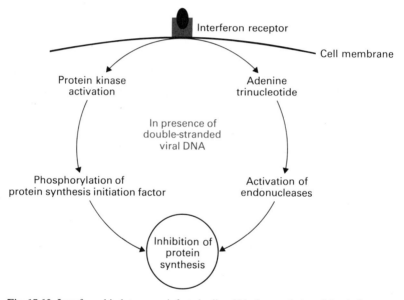

Fig. 17.13 Interferon binds to a non-infected cell and blocks translation of the viral messenger RNA.

certain messenger RNAs. Second, the bound interferon stimulates a protein kinase which phosphorylates the protein initiation factor and thus inhibits synthesis. In both these situations double-stranded RNA is required, so that the inhibition of translation only occurs in cells which are infected by a virus (Fig. 17.13).

Other effects of interferon. In addition to the protection of cells against viral infection outlined above, the interferons have other actions. At high dose levels interferons can inhibit cell proliferation and this has drawn attention to a possible role for them as **antitumour agents.**

Unfortunately, high doses of interferons are associated with a number of unpleasant side-effects such as nausea, loss of hair, fever, and depression of platelet and leucocyte production by the bone marrow. The interferons also have an effect on some immune functions, being associated with increased T cell and natural killer cell activity and decreased antibody formation.

Protective response of the immune system

The ways in which the elements of the immune system respond to viral infections has already been discussed in Chapter 10 and will not be repeated here.

Interaction between Virus and Host Species

The production of a viral illness involves several steps. The virus must have an appropriate route of access to the host and there must be a

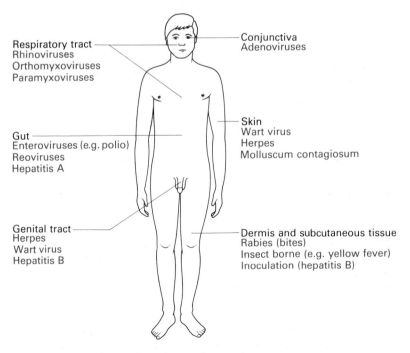

Respiratory tract
Rhinoviruses
Orthomyxoviruses
Paramyxoviruses

Conjunctiva
Adenoviruses

Gut
Enteroviruses (e.g. polio)
Reoviruses
Hepatitis A

Skin
Wart virus
Herpes
Molluscum contagiosum

Genital tract
Herpes
Wart virus
Hepatitis B

Dermis and subcutaneous tissue
Rabies (bites)
Insect borne (e.g. yellow fever)
Inoculation (hepatitis B)

Fig. 17.14 Portals of entry of some human viruses.

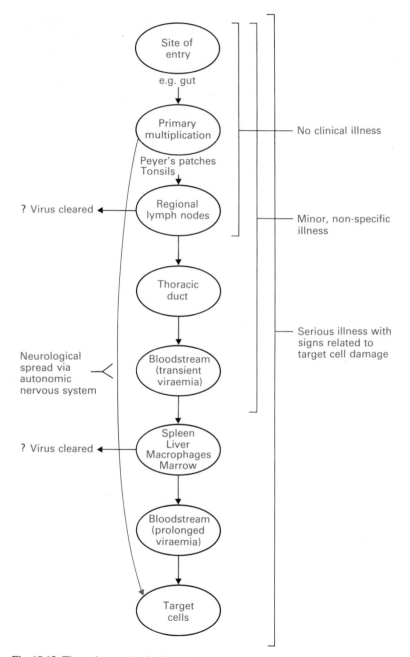

Fig. 17.15 The pathogenesis of a viral disease such as poliomyelitis.

mechanism or mechanisms for the virus to reach its ultimate target, for example the anterior horn cells in poliomyelitis. Routes of access to the host include the skin and subcutaneous tissues, the conjunctiva, the respiratory tract, and the genital and gastrointestinal tracts. These and the possible outcome of viral entry are shown in Figs. 17.14 and 17.15.

Chapter 18

The Pathological Bases of Ischaemia I: Atherosclerosis

Ischaemia is the term used to define a state in which the arterial perfusion of an organ or tissue is insufficient to cater for the metabolic needs of that tissue. The circumstances which modulate the appearance of ischaemia in any vascular bed and the effects which it produces will be considered in a later chapter.

It must be clear, however, that any pathological change causing either narrowing or blockage of an artery is likely to produce ischaemia in the tissue supplied by that vessel and distal to the point of narrowing or occlusion. In arteries, such narrowing is brought about by a widely prevalent disease of the wall of large elastic and muscular arteries known as **atherosclerosis**. The eventual occlusion of the arterial lumen is caused by **platelets**, first adhering to an abnormal vascular surface and later aggregating one with another to form a plug which is capable of blocking the artery. Such a plug, which can form within a few seconds, is known as a **thrombus**, a solid mass formed within the heart, arteries, veins and capillaries from the components of **streaming** blood. The process of thrombus formation is known as **thrombosis**. In arteries, thrombosis is a frequent complication of atherosclerosis. Indeed, many workers hold the view that platelet deposition on the artery wall is intimately involved in the process of atherogenesis. There are also very close associations between the processes of thrombosis and those involved in clotting of the blood.

In the Western World, the complications of atherosclerosis kill more people than any other single disease, including all the forms of cancer. More than 150 000 patients die each year in Britain alone from the effects of coronary artery narrowing and occlusion; roughly one person for each three minutes of the day. Put another way, rather more than one-quarter of all deaths occurring in this country are due to atherosclerosis.

What is atherosclerosis?

The term atherosclerosis is derived from two Greek words — '**sclerosis**' which means **hardness** and '**athere**', meaning a sort of gruel

274

or porridge. A commonly used synonym is **atheroma**, a term first used in connection with arterial lesions by Albrecht von Haller in 1755. 'Porridge-like hardness' seems a very odd combination. It owes its adoption to the fact that many atherosclerotic lesions, which consist essentially of localized thickenings in the arterial intima, contain soft, pultaceous material in their deeper portions. This material, which is very rich in lipids, can ooze out into the arterial lumen and be carried away in the bloodstream if the more superficial parts of the atherosclerotic lesions rupture.

Definition

Our understanding of the aetiology and pathogenesis of atherosclerosis is still far from complete and for this reason we are forced to define the disease in terms of its **morphology.** On this basis it has been defined as a widely prevalent disorder affecting large elastic and muscular arteries (such as the aorta, the coronary, carotid and cerebral arteries). It is characterized by the presence of focal thickenings of the innermost layers of such arteries (the tunica intima), these thickenings being composed partly of connective tissue and partly of tissue debris which is rich in lipid. Most of this lipid is derived from the plasma.

Connective Tissue Proliferation in Atherosclerosis

Intimal smooth muscle proliferation may be a reaction to injury

Atherosclerotic lesions owe much of their bulk, and hence their ability to encroach on vessel lumina, to proliferation of certain connective tissue elements in the arterial intima. The key to this process lies with the intimal **smooth muscle cell** which expresses, not only the contractile properties expected in a muscle cell, but also the ability to synthesize and secrete extracellular components of the artery wall such as collagen. In vivo the intimal smooth muscle cell can be induced to multiply in any situation where the lining endothelial cells are damaged and platelets adhere at the site of injury (Fig. 18.1). The trigger for such proliferation is the release of a low molecular weight basic protein known as **platelet-derived growth factor** (**PDGF**), which is stored in the alpha granule of the platelet (see p. 298). In vitro PDGF also acts as a mitogen for arterial smooth muscle cells in culture. No such effect is seen if platelets which have *no* alpha granules ('the grey platelet syndrome') are used. PDGF is also mitogenic for other types of connective tissue cell in culture, stimulating both DNA synthesis and cell division. It differs from other growth factors in also being

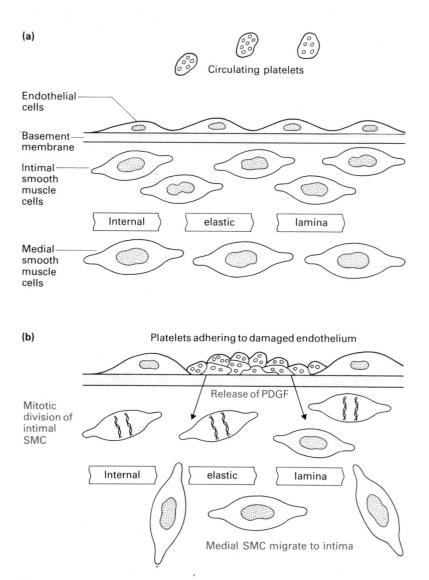

Fig. 18.1 Platelet interaction with smooth muscle cells (SMC) of the artery wall. (a) Normal endothelium. (b) Damaged endothelium. PDGF = platelet-derived growth factor.

chemotactic for fibroblasts, smooth muscle cells, macrophages and neutrophils, and thus may well play a part in the inflammatory reaction and its sequelae. The experimental models associated with such 'platelet-driven' smooth muscle proliferation are perhaps rather artificial and we do not know yet whether they have a counterpart in human atherogenesis.

Intimal smooth muscle proliferation may be akin to tumour growth

An alternative explanation for local smooth muscle proliferation in atherosclerotic plaques has been offered which implies that this process has more in common with what happens in tumour growth than with the events associated with repair. This suggestion stems in the first instance from the Lyon hypothesis, which states that in any normal, mammalian, female, eukaryotic cell, one of the X chromosomes is inactivated. This deletion is random and, thus, each female is, in a sense, a phenotypic mosaic with individual cells containing either an active maternal or active paternal X chromosome. In most instances this is of no significance, since both X chromosomes code identically. However, the enzyme glucose-6-phosphate dehydrogenase (G-6-PD) is a special case since it exists in at least two isoenzymic forms which are easily separable by electrophoresis. About one-third of the black females in the USA are heterozygous in respect of this enzyme and extracts of their tissue are usually found to contain **both** isoenzymes of G-6-PD. Samples of smooth muscle tumours of the uterus in these heterozygous females have been found to contain only **one** isoenzyme per tumour and this has led to the view that the cell population of each tumour is made up of the progeny of a **single** cell which has been induced to proliferate. Such a cell population is spoken of as being **monoclonal.**

Similarly it has been found that samples of atherosclerotic plaques from Negro females heterozygous in respect of G-6-PD usually contain only one isoenzyme, while samples of the macroscopically normal aorta contain both isoenzymes. The same interpretation has been given of these findings as of those relating to the smooth muscle tumours in the uterus: i.e. that the local proliferation of arterial smooth muscle cells is monoclonal in nature and cannot therefore be a repair process, as this would be characterized by a polyclonal cell response.

If atherosclerotic plaques do indeed have something of the nature of smooth muscle tumours in miniature, then one must ask what triggers these focal proliferations. One suggestion is that potentially mutagenic hydrocarbons derived from cigarette smoke may reach the arterial intima, having been carried there in association with lipoprotein fractions in the plasma. Samples of some aortas have been shown to contain mixed function oxidases which could transform premutagens into substances which are capable of binding covalently to DNA and thus able to trigger smooth muscle proliferation through some genomic alteration.

This view of the nature of the connective tissue response in atherogenesis is certainly novel and challenging, but should not be accepted uncritically. Not all plaques show a convincing degree of monotypism, and there may be explanations for such monotypism other than monoclonality.

The Lesions of Atherosclerosis

In any disease process where tissue changes occur, it is logical to examine the relationship between the morphology of the lesions and the pathogenesis by first describing the earliest lesions and then the sequence of changes that lead to the full-blown picture of the disease. This is something that, in terms of human atherosclerosis, we cannot do. There is controversy as to what constitutes the early lesion of atherosclerosis, no certainty that the common endpoint (the raised lesion or fibro-lipid plaque) may not be reached from different beginnings, and certainly no agreement that what many pathologists regard as the early lesions develop inevitably into mature atherosclerotic plaques. A histopathologist, for the most part, can view a lesion in humans at only one point in its natural history. What has gone before and what may follow can, at best, be only the result of a more or less skilled and imaginative reconstruction, a point which should be borne in mind when considering the morphology of the lesions that are regarded as being part of the spectrum of atherosclerosis.

The fatty streak

This lesion, which is regarded by many as being the precursor of mature atherosclerotic plaques, is found in large elastic and muscular arteries in all population groups from childhood onwards. In very young patients coming to necropsy the lesions occur chiefly in the region of the aortic valve ring and the ductus scar. With growth, the aortic arch and the posterior part of the thoracic aorta become involved and this is followed by the appearance of streaks in the abdominal aorta. In the coronary arteries, fatty streaks appear in the proximal parts of the vessels about the time of puberty. In these large arteries the fatty streak appears first as a minute round or oval yellowish patch, minimally, if at all, elevated above the surface of the surrounding intima. The tiny dot-like lesions become arranged in rows of differing lengths, roughly parallel to the streamlines of the flowing blood, and coalesce to form the characteristic streak. In humans the fatty streak has a fairly constant relation to the mouths of aortic branches. The streaks are concentrated in the **proximal** portions of the ostia of the branches, the actual flow divider being spared. These proximal areas are those in which the wall shear rates are lowest and in which the duration of contact between blood cells and the vessel wall is, for haemodynamic reasons, likely to be longest.

Histological appearances of the fatty streak

Light microscopic examination of these lesions requires the preparation of both frozen and paraffin sections of the material since all stainable fat is removed from the latter by dehydration in a graded series of alcohols. Frozen sections stained with fat-soluble dyes such as Oil-Red O show droplets of fat that, for the most part, are concentrated within smooth muscle cells and macrophages in the immediate subendothelial region. A small amount of lipid may be distributed in a finely divided form along the internal elastic lamina which separates the intima from the media. The number of macrophages in fatty streaks is small but they may play an important role in **removing** excess lipid from the arterial intima. Monocytes have been shown to penetrate the intima in lesion-prone areas of the aorta in pigs fed a diet high in fat and cholesterol, this penetration being noted before the appearance of fatty streaks. It has been suggested, therefore, that these monocytes are acting as a clearance system by endocytosing intra-arterial lipid and migrating back into the bloodstream with a cargo of lipid. If this is true, then the development of fatty streaks might be viewed, at least in part, as a failure on the part of the monocyte/macrophage system.

Is the fatty streak the precursor of the fibro-lipid plaque?

There is universal acceptance that the raised lesion or fibro-lipid plaque is the archetypal lesion of atherosclerosis. No such agreement exists in relation to the fatty streak; controversy still clouds the question of whether or not the streak lesion is the precursor of the mature plaque. Certainly the fatty streak seen so commonly in the aorta of young patients coming to necropsy does not appear to predict well for the development of atherosclerosis in the population group to which the patient had belonged. In addition, its topographical distribution differs from that of mature lesions, as does its fatty acid pattern. In the coronary arteries, however, the distribution of fatty streaks does mirror that of fibro-lipid plaques. Some workers have suggested that the term **fatty streak** is an umbrella for a number of different lesions, and that there is a subset, characterized by focal necrosis and an inflammatory cell infiltrate, which does predict for the subsequent development of mature, raised lesions. As in so many other areas of human pathology, the Scottish verdict of **not proven** is, for the moment, the most appropriate one.

The gelatinous lesion

In recent years increasing attention has been directed to the possibility that small blister-like elevations in the arterial intima are the precursors of fully developed plaques. These small lesions are translucent and have, thus, been termed **gelatinous elevations.** They are not easy to see on naked-eye examination and there are few data as to their frequency and distribution pattern. These little droplet-like lesions are either colourless or a very pale pink in colour. Their histological appearances are banal in the extreme, consisting essentially of separation of the connective tissue elements of the intima by oedema. On biochemical analysis, all the constituents of the intima which could be derived from the plasma are increased (there is twice as much albumin and about four times as much fibrinogen and lipoprotein as in the normal intima). As in the case of the fatty streak the relationship of this lesion to the subsequent development of atherosclerotic plaques remains unproven.

The fibro-lipid plaque

The raised lesion or fibro-lipid plaque is the characteristic lesion of atherosclerosis. Within given population groups its extent and severity predict well for the subsequent development of occlusive arterial disease. In the aorta, plaques are more frequent in the abdominal than in the thoracic portions of the vessel and often involve the mouths of the intercostal and lumbar arteries. Haemodynamic factors obviously play a part in the localization of lesions and in the modulation of their growth. For example, in the cervical portion of the carotid system, it is rare that lesions other than fatty streaks are found in the common carotid. However, once the point at which branching into internal and external carotids occurs has been passed, raised plaques, frequently subject to complications such as ulceration and thrombosis, are common.

Morphology of the fibro-lipid plaque

In contrast to the fatty streak, the fibro-lipid plaque is elevated considerably above the surface of the surrounding non-involved intima. The increase over normal intimal thickness may be so great that the intima may equal or even exceed the underlying media in thickness.

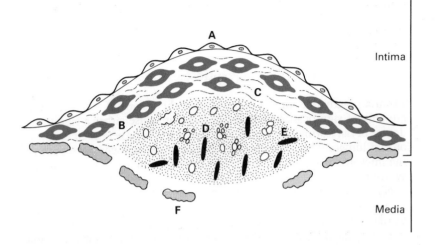

Fig. 18.2 The anatomy of a fibro-lipid atherosclerotic plaque. Medial thinning is usually present under the plaque. A = endothelium; B = intimal smooth muscle; C = collagen, elastin and glycosaminoglycans; D = lipid-rich tissue debris ('atheroma'); E = cholesterol crystals; F = internal elastic lamina (often shows focal damage).

The underlying media is often thinner than the media in adjacent non-involved areas of the artery, chiefly due to loss of smooth muscle cells between the elastic laminae. The weakening of the artery wall consequent on this effect on the media may lead to a localized dilatation of the vessel known as **aneurysm**. Such aneurysms may have significant effects on adjacent tissues as a result of pressure or may rupture, this being associated with catastrophic haemorrhage. In its characteristic form the lesion consists of a lipid-rich basal pool that is covered on its luminal aspect by a connective tissue 'cap' which varies in thickness from lesion to lesion (Fig. 18.2). In some, the proliferated connective tissue that constitutes the cap is the predominant element; this gives the luminal aspect of the plaque an opaque, white, 'pearly' appearance. When such a lesion is cut into, the yellow, lipid-rich 'atheromatous' base may be inconspicuous or even absent. In other lesions, the basal accumulations of lipid and tissue debris may be of massive proportions, and are separated from the artery lumen only by a thin, easily ruptured sheet of fibrous or fibromuscular tissue. All gradations between these two extremes may be seen, and various complicating factors such as ulceration, thrombosis, intraplaque haemorrhage and calcification are often superimposed on the basic plaque pattern. The end result may be a marked degree of morphological heterogeneity within the plaque population in any given vessel.

The Effects of Atherosclerotic Lesions

From a pragmatic, clinical point of view the lesions of atherosclerosis are only of significance in so far as they can cause either a significant degree of narrowing of the artery lumen or a total or near total blockage of that lumen. The ischaemia that results from such encroachment on the integrity of vessel lumina can be expressed in a number of clinical syndromes.

Narrowing of the arterial lumen may be caused by a gradual increase in plaque bulk, this being due either to connective tissue proliferation mediated by smooth muscle cell hyperplasia, an increase in the amount of accumulated lipid, or both of these acting in concert. A considerable degree of lumen reduction (perhaps as much as 70%) is required before perfusion of the tissue begins to suffer to any significant degree.

Of equal or perhaps more importance are the acute **occlusive** events which occur, usually against a background of severe stenosing atherosclerosis. The most frequent site for this is the coronary artery tree, in which acute occlusion may have lethal or crippling effects.

Coronary artery thrombosis

The most important event in the natural history of an atherosclerotic plaque is **thrombosis.** In large calibre vessels such as the aorta, the consequences of such thrombosis are not necessarily severe or even clinically apparent, but in smaller vessels such as the coronary arteries, the occurrence of large-scale thrombosis is often catastrophic.

In the coronary arteries, the key event which precedes the formation of occlusive thrombi appears to be splitting of the connective tissue cap with consequent exposure of the underlying subendothelial tissues to the passing stream of blood. Blood flows rapidly into the soft atheromatous pool at the base of the plaque and very rapid aggregation of platelets takes place, often with the formation of a 'dumb-bell' shaped thrombus, masses of aggregated platelets being present both within the plaque and within the vessel lumen (Fig. 18.3). Such splitting of plaques is unlikely to take place in the absence of a significant degree of softening of the plaque base, and the cause of this softening remains one of the most significant, unsolved problems in the natural history of atherosclerosis.

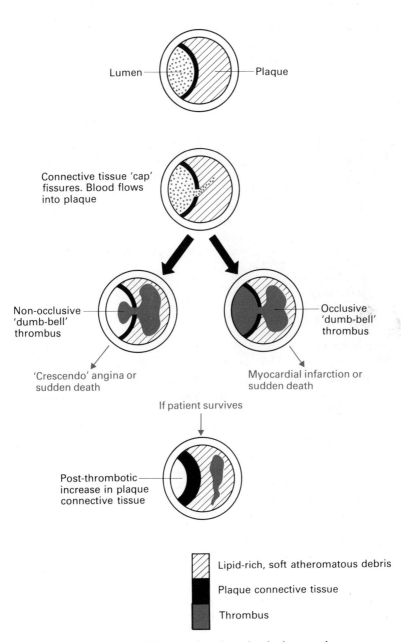

Fig. 18.3 The consequences of fissuring of an atherosclerotic plaque, such as may occur in the coronary arteries.

Risk Factors in Relation to Atherosclerosis

Any variable that is associated with a significant increase in the chance of developing either a specific disease or a specific lesion can be regarded as a **risk factor.** The risk factor concept is an important one for the prevention of disease rather than its cure. If such primary prevention is to be brought about, the identification of potentially reversible risk factors must be of great importance. However, it must be borne in mind that not all the factors that have been found to be associated with the prevalence of a given disorder have a direct causal relationship and thus the removal or reversal of such a factor may not materially affect the frequency and severity of the disease.

Many risk factors have been canvassed as playing a role in the development of occlusive arterial disease and hence, by implication, in the development of atherosclerosis. Apart from such inescapable variables as age, sex and race, which are discussed briefly below, the most important of these appear to be:

hyperlipidaemia
hypertension
cigarette smoking
diabetes mellitus

Age

Of all these variables, age has the strongest and most constant association with atherosclerosis. The different arterial areas are, however, affected at different rates. Lesions appear in the aorta in the first decade of life, in the coronary arteries in the second, and in the cerebral vessels in the third. It would be useful to know whether the fact that the lesions are closely age-related is due to some intrinsic ageing process or whether it is simply a reflection of the time during which other factors can exert their effect. It seems likely that the second of these possibilities is true since population groups exist whose lifespan is not significantly different from the human species in general and in whom ageing is not accompanied by clinical manifestations of atherosclerosis.

Sex

There is no doubt that clinical events related to atherosclerosis are far commoner in males than in females during the middle decades of life. With increasing age this difference diminishes but never disappears. These clinical differences are, to a considerable extent, mirrored by differences in the prevalence and severity of arterial lesions as seen at necropsy. It is obviously tempting to describe these differences in terms of a role for sex hormones. In experimental atherogenesis, the use of oestrogens as a modulating factor has given conflicting results. Since such studies have, for the most part, been performed in small animals not known for their propensity to develop atherosclerosis spontaneously, it is difficult to know how much significance to attach to these results. In human males the use of oestrogens in a large scale secondary prevention study has not proved encouraging. Some sex differences appear to exist in lipid metabolism and merit further exploration. In females taking oral contraceptives, the effect on plasma lipids depends on the type of compound: high doses of oestrogen increase the plasma concentrations of high density lipoproteins, while the reverse is true of progesterone and its analogues.

Race

The prevalence of atherosclerosis-related clinical disease is strikingly influenced by geography. These differences correspond roughly to the distribution of various racial groups and are also mirrored in the prevalence and severity of atherosclerotic lesions. Within individual racial groups, quite steep gradients exist in the extent and severity of coronary artery atherosclerosis; these large intra-group variations suggest that membership of one or other racial group does not per se confer relative immunity from or increased susceptibility to atherosclerosis. This view gains strength from considering the experience of immigrant groups. They appear to acquire a risk for the development of atherosclerosis-related disease much closer to that of their host population than to that of the community from which they came.

Lipid metabolism and atherosclerosis

A vast amount of literature exists relating to the association between lipid metabolism, atherosclerosis and occlusive arterial disease. Despite the complexity of this subject, this association can be expressed in a number of simple propositions:

1. Atherosclerotic lesions contain far more lipid than adjacent, non-involved areas of the intima. Most of this lipid, in mature plaques, is derived from the plasma.
2. Increasing the plasma concentrations of certain lipid classes in a variety of animal species by dietary and/or pharmacological means leads to the appearance of focal intimal lesions which have some features in common with human atherosclerosis.
3. In populations in which the prevalence of atherosclerosis-related

diseases and of raised fibro-lipid plaques is high, plasma concentrations of certain lipids (notably cholesterol in the form of low density lipoproteins) are also high. Where the prevalence of such lesions is low, the reverse is true.

Plasma concentrations of two **lipid transport proteins** — low density lipoprotein and high density lipoprotein — are related to the probability of coronary heart disease and hence, by implication, to atherogenesis. There is a strong positive association between the risk of coronary heart disease and high levels of low density lipoprotein (LDL). In contrast, there is a strong **inverse** relationship between high plasma concentrations of high density lipoprotein (HDL) and coronary heart disease risk.

LDL concentrations are affected by both genetic and environmental factors

Genetic factors. It has been suggested that some 30% of the variance in plasma cholesterol concentrations (which correlate closely with LDL concentrations) in a given population may be due to genetic determinants. This excludes a number of diseases in which single mutant genes with powerful effects can cause elevated levels of LDL, low levels of LDL, or absence of LDL. In familial hyperlipidaemia type IIa (see p. 10), the increase in LDL concentration in the plasma is due to a reduction in the function of cell surface receptors for low density lipoprotein. These receptors are responsible for at least 30% and possibly much more of the catabolism of this lipid transport protein. This variety of hyperlipidaemia is transmitted in an autosomal recessive manner. Homozygotes are relatively rare and most of them die from coronary heart disease by the time they reach their early 20s. The incidence of the heterozygous form of familial type IIa hyperlipidaemia is about 2 per 1000 in most communities.

Much more common is **familial combined hyperlipidaemia**, in which a familial clustering of different forms of hyperlipoproteinaemia is found. The primary defect here may be excess secretion of one of the carrier proteins (apoprotein B) leading to an overproduction of LDL and very low density lipoprotein (VLDL). Coronary heart disease is strongly associated with this disorder.

Environmental factors. The most important environmental factor regulating lipoprotein concentrations is diet. The intake of fat and the type of fat consumed are the most powerful dietary factors though dietary cholesterol, fibre, protein and carbohydrate all affect plasma lipids. There is a strong correlation between plasma cholesterol concentrations and the intake of saturated fatty acids. However, a substantial part of the differences in LDL concentrations that exist between members of the same population group cannot be explained on the basis of dietary differences.

An additional factor which has to be taken into account is the large individual differences in the **response** of plasma cholesterol to dietary intake. In humans and in several animal species, a wide variation in response to a high intake of cholesterol has been found. Both in vivo and ex vivo studies suggest that this variation is due to differences in the degree of suppression of endogenous cholesterol synthesis and hence in the degree of down-regulation of HMG CoA reductase (see p. 11).

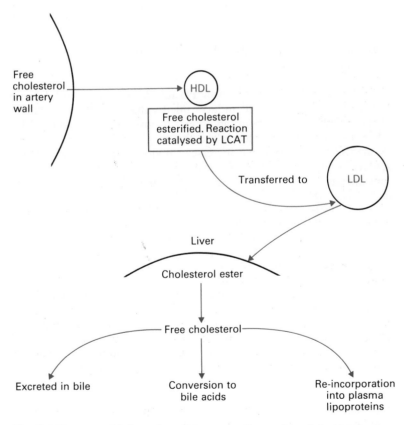

Fig. 18.4 Transport of cholesterol out of the artery wall: a possible role for high density lipoprotein (HDL). LDL = low density lipoprotein; LCAT = lecithin–cholesterol acyltransferase.

High density lipoproteins (HDL)

High plasma concentrations of HDL are inversely related to the risk of subsequently developing coronary heart disease. Similarly, low concentrations constitute an efficient predictor for coronary heart disease. The question which arises from this is whether HDL has some protective role and can partially inhibit the development of atherosclerosis or whether it functions merely as a predictor. Animals with high plasma concentrations of HDL are resistant to atherosclerosis, and in humans there is a strong inverse relationship between coronary artery narrowing (seen on angiography) and a subfraction of HDL.

It has been suggested that HDL may take up free cholesterol from extrahepatic tissues (Fig. 18.4). The free cholesterol is then esterified, transferred to LDL and returned to the liver, where the cholesterol esters are hydrolysed. The free cholesterol so formed in the liver enters a pool of free cholesterol which is available for removal in bile, conversion into bile acids which can also be removed, or re-incorporated into lipoprotein.

Determinants of HDL concentration. Plasma concentrations of HDL are increased by agents that induce microsomal enzymes, including phenobarbitone, phenytoin and certain insecticides. Alcohol also produces a rise in HDL levels and this may well be due to the same mechanism. Any factor that increases adipose tissue lipoprotein lipase activity, such as insulin or physical exercise, tends to increase HDL concentrations. HDL levels tend to be low in obese people and increase following weight reduction.

Genetic factors also play a part in regulating the plasma levels of this lipid fraction and are believed to be of more importance here than in determining LDL concentrations. Interestingly enough, in this respect, a familial syndrome has been recognized in which HDL levels are very high and this is associated with longevity.

Hypertension

It is quite clear, from a number of studies, that high blood pressure is associated with an increased risk of death from coronary and cerebral artery disease. While this does not necessarily indicate that hypertension also increases the degree of atherosclerosis, careful necropsy studies show that this is in fact the case. There are significant differences in respect of raised atherosclerotic lesions between hypertensive and non-hypertensive cases at all ages, in both sexes and in both the aorta and coronary arteries.

High blood pressure may affect the development of atherosclerosis in a number of ways. However, no convincing evidence exists to persuade us that factors other than the raised pressure itself are responsible. In patients with coarctation (congenital segmental narrowing) of the aorta, atherosclerosis develops in the high pressure area proximal to the stenosis but not distal to it where the pressure is normal. A fascinating experiment of nature which reinforces this view is a rare congenital anomaly in which the left coronary artery originates from the pulmonary artery and is thus perfused at low pressure. In patients with this abnormality who survived to middle age, atherosclerosis was present in the right coronary artery but not in the left.

Cigarette smoking

Cigarette smoking is strongly correlated with a high risk of occlusive arterial disease affecting both the coronary arteries and the arteries of the lower limb. British data show that the risk of dying from coronary heart disease in men aged between 45 and 54 is **trebled** if they smoke more than 15 cigarettes per day. The risk seems to be related to the number of cigarettes smoked rather than to the duration of the habit. The increase in risk diminishes fairly rapidly in those who give up smoking. This suggests that smoking may have an effect over and above an increase in atherosclerosis, though post-mortem studies have shown that the extent and severity of atherosclerosis is greater in smokers than in non-smokers.

Many possibilities have been canvassed in the search for mechanisms to account for any effects of cigarette smoking on the arterial wall. These include a possible direct effect of nicotine, high carbon monoxide levels in the blood, the action of free radicals, and possible hypersensitivity to glycoprotein antigens in tobacco. At this time it is impossible to say whether one, more, all or none of these plays a role.

Diabetes mellitus

In over-privileged Western communities there is no doubt that diabetes is a powerful additional risk factor for atherosclerosis-related clinical disease. For diabetes to operate in this way, a certain background level of atherosclerosis appears to be necessary, since in those parts of the world where atherosclerosis is not a serious problem, diabetes does not produce any significant effect on the frequency of the major clinical syndromes associated with atherosclerosis. The question of whether diabetes increases the severity of artery wall disease is not easy to answer. Ideally one would need to compare two groups coming to necropsy who were alike in every way other than in respect of the presence or absence of diabetes. Such data as do exist suggest that there is a real difference between diabetics and non-diabetics in respect of raised atherosclerotic lesions in both the aorta and coronary arteries.

The Pathogenesis of Atherosclerosis

At the beginning of this chapter atherosclerosis was defined in morphological terms. It may now be appropriate to look at this condition in terms of the processes involved in atherogenesis, even though our knowledge of these is still incomplete. The key processes in atherogenesis are:

1. Proliferation of smooth muscle cells within the arterial intima and the synthesis and secretion by them of extracellular connective tissue elements such as collagen, elastin and the glycoproteins and glycosaminoglycans of the intimal matrix.

2. The accumulation of lipid, both intra- and extracellularly. In the raised lesion most of this lipid, which consists predominantly of esterified and free cholesterol in a ratio of 3:1, can be shown to be derived from the plasma and to enter the artery wall as intact lipoprotein. The entry of excess amounts of such lipoprotein forms the basis of what is known as the **infiltrative** theory of atherogenesis. The supporters of this view hold that lipoprotein entry and accumulation is the primary event in atherogenesis and that the connective tissue proliferation represents a reaction to the presence of excess lipid.

3. Once the two processes mentioned above are well developed, a variety of other events can occur. These include the death of intimal smooth muscle cells, dystrophic calcification, and necrosis and softening at the plaque base. As previously stated, this last circumstance is a major contributor to splitting of the connective tissue cap of the plaque and consequent thrombosis.

It is possible to regard atherogenesis as being, in the broadest sense, **a reaction to injury** associated with exposure of the subendothelial cell population to a variety of growth factors. It is equally possible to regard it as a **paraneoplastic** process triggered by the activation, within the intima, of potential mutagens as outlined in the monoclonal hypothesis. The evidence relating to these has been outlined briefly on p. 277. Irrespective of which of these views one favours, it is highly probable that atherosclerosis is initiated and probably modulated either by changes in some of the many functions of the endothelial cells or by actual loss of endothelium.

The endothelial cell and atherogenesis

In a happy phrase, the endothelium has been described as 'the guardian of the smooth muscle cells of the intima'. While it is certainly this, endothelium has a range of activities which extends far beyond that of a selective permeability barrier. Endothelial cells can produce and metabolize a large number of substances which may have important roles both in relation to thrombosis and to blood clotting.

Changes in permeability

Atherosclerotic lesions contain plasma-derived macromolecules in much larger amounts than are found in the normal intima. This suggests that atherogenesis involves an increase in the permeability of the endothelium. Even in normal arteries, permeability is not uniform within a single vessel, and those areas which normally show the greatest permeability are those in which atherosclerosis occurs preferentially. On electron microscopy these areas also show evidence of endothelial damage and some thinning of the surface glycocalyx. It is not known with certainty whether those factors thought to increase the degree of atherosclerosis also increase the permeability of the endothelium, though the results of some morphological studies of the aortic intima following the exposure of rats and rabbits to cigarette smoke would support this view.

Endothelial cell loss

There is no lack of evidence to show that injury of the endothelium aggravates experimental atherosclerosis or, conversely, that some models of atherosclerosis are associated with changes in endothelial cells. If these results are to be extrapolated to the human situation, a need exists for a model in which it can be shown clearly that endothelial changes precede the atherosclerotic lesions. One model which meets these demands, at least in part, is the White Carneau pigeon. Virtually all these birds develop atherosclerosis in both the aorta and the coronary arteries. In some instances, focal loss of endothelial cells and adhesion of platelets (which presumably release PDGF) to the exposed subendothelial surface have been seen to antedate the appearance of atherosclerotic plaques.

Apart from hyperlipidaemia and cigarette smoking, endothelial alterations can also be brought about by immune mechanisms and by certain viral infections in a variety of animals. Infection of chickens with the virus of Marek's disease leads to the development of atherosclerotic lesions in a significant proportion of the affected birds. The induction of hypercholesterolaemia does not materially affect these lesions. Transformation of endothelial cells in culture by exposing them to mutagens can also alter their functions very significantly: cloned bovine endothelial cells showed morphological changes and failed to express factor VIII of the clotting system following exposure to the mutagen 2-chloroacetaldehyde.

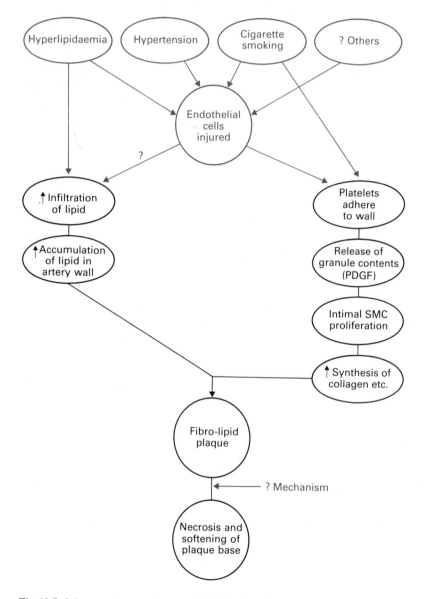

Fig. 18.5 Atherogenesis: a reaction to multiple injurious factors? PDGF = platelet-derived growth factor; SMC = smooth muscle cell.

How relevant any of these experimental data are to human atherosclerosis is still unknown. What seems certain is that it is necessary to interpret the concept of endothelial injury in a broader sense than has been done hitherto and to extend the definition of injury (as we do in other situations) to circumstances in which cell function may be altered without evidence of cell death. A speculative scheme of how the factors discussed in this chapter may interact to produce atherosclerotic lesions is shown in Fig. 18.5, but it must be emphasized that our knowledge is far from complete and that the scheme represents informed speculation and not revealed truth.

Chapter 19

The Pathological Bases of Ischaemia II: Thrombosis

A **thrombus** is a **solid mass or plug formed within the heart, arteries, veins or capillaries from the components of the streaming blood.** It is a matter for regret that many speak of thrombosis as being more or less synonymous with clotting of blood, as it is important that the fundamental differences between the two processes should be appreciated (Fig. 19.1). In **clotting** the initiation of a cascade system within the blood leads to the generation of thrombin and thus to the

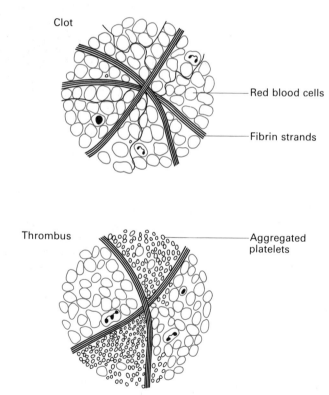

Fig. 19.1 Clot and thrombus.

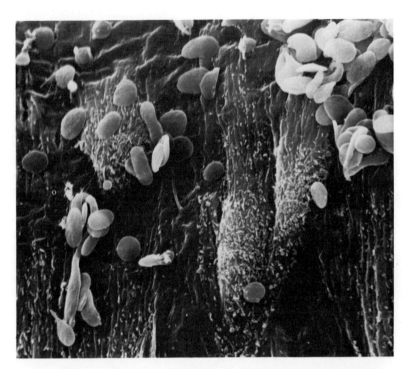

Fig. 19.2 Platelets adhering to the intimal surface of an artery. Scanning electron micrograph of rat aorta following exposure of the animal to cigarette smoke. Numerous platelets can be seen to be adhering to the endothelial surface. Many of these are still disc-shaped and have not undergone the release reaction; others have clearly been activated and have undergone a shape change.

conversion of the soluble plasma protein fibrinogen to the insoluble fibrin polymer. **Thrombosis**, on the other hand, is characterized by a series of events involving the blood **platelets**. These cells **adhere** to sites of endothelial cell loss or areas where the endothelial cells are otherwise abnormal and, in the course of undergoing a shape change, **release a number of very potent factors**, which lead to the **aggregation** of further platelets at the site of the initial adhesion, to the local formation of fibrin, to changes in vessel permeability and to a stimulatory effect on the connective tissue cells in the underlying vessel wall (Fig. 19.2).

Platelets and Haemostasis

The fact that thrombosis and clotting are different processes should not obscure the fact that both contribute to haemostasis. It has been known for many years that **normal platelets in normal numbers are essential if bleeding from a damaged blood vessel is to be brought under control**; the formation of a haemostatic plug and the formation of an arterial thrombus are essentially similar. Both are composed largely of platelet aggregates which adhere at sites of injury to the endothelial surface. Strands of fibrin around the platelets serve to stabilize the platelet mass. Thus a significant decline in the number of circulating platelets (thrombocytopenia) or some intrinsic abnormality either in the platelets or in the endothelial cell (e.g. von Willebrand's disease) may be associated with abnormal bleeding.

The primary event in the interaction between the platelet and the vessel wall is **adhesion**. If this adhesion does not take place then an abnormal bleeding tendency may show itself. The two most commonly encountered failures of platelet adhesion are **von Willebrand's disease** and the **Bernard–Soulier syndrome**. In the first of these there is a lack of a large multimeric protein, the factor VIII related antigen (or von Willebrand factor) which appears to be essential if platelets are to adhere to a damaged intimal surface. The Bernard–Soulier syndrome is due to the absence of a receptor in the glycoprotein outer coat of the platelet (GPIb), which thus renders the platelet 'deaf' to the signals which normally start the adhesion process.

The anatomy of the platelet

Of all the cells in the circulating blood, the platelets are the most sensitive to a wide range of chemical and physical agents. For instance,

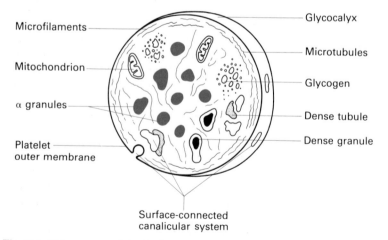

Fig. 19.3 Microanatomy of the platelet.

minute amounts of catecholamines, which cause little or no response in neutrophils, monocytes, lymphocytes or red cells, can trigger irreversible changes in the platelet. Understanding platelet physiology and pathology is made easier if we have some knowledge of the structure of the platelet; since it is so small, only ultrastructural studies are capable of providing this essential information.

The platelet circulates in the blood in the form of a flat disc. If such a disc is cut in the equatorial plane, **four major zones** can be seen on examination with the electron microscope (Fig. 19.3). These are:

1. The **peripheral** zone
2. The **sol–gel** zone
3. The **organelle** zone
4. The **membrane** zone

The peripheral zone

This consists of the surface membranes and structures closely associated with the surface. There is an **exterior coat** or **glycocalyx**, which is rich in glycoproteins. This houses the receptors for the signals which trigger platelet activation and the substrates for adhesion and aggregation reactions. Several different glycoproteins have been identified and some of these clearly serve important roles in relation to platelet/platelet and platelet/vessel wall reactions. Platelets from patients with **thrombasthenia** lack glycoproteins IIb and IIIa and fail to adhere or aggregate both in vitro and in vivo. In Bernard–Soulier syndrome, platelets aggregate normally but fail to adhere to damaged blood vessels in vivo, or to bovine fibrinogen or the antibiotic ristocetin in vitro. This indicates that the glycoprotein Ib, which is absent from these platelets, is the receptor for the von Willebrand factor.

The middle layer of the peripheral zone is made up of a typical unit membrane rich in asymmetrically distributed phospholipids, which are essential for reacting with coagulant proteins. During platelet aggregation, a substance essential for accelerating the clotting process is derived from the lipid-rich unit membrane. This is known as **platelet factor 3.**

The third component of the peripheral zone is the area which lies just deep to the unit membrane. It contains a system of filaments, which appear to be similar to microfilaments. They may contribute to maintenance of the normal discoid shape of the unstimulated platelet and also interact with other elements of the platelet's contractile system.

An important element of the peripheral zone is the open canalicular system. This is a series of invaginations of the cell surface which ramify deeply within the platelet and thus markedly increase its surface area in a manner analogous with the structure of a sponge. Its functions are closely interrelated with those of the membrane system, but structurally it shares the same features as other portions of the cell surface membrane.

The sol–gel zone

Early studies with the phase-contrast microscope suggested that the formed elements within platelets float in a fluid suspension. It is now known, as a result of ultrastructural studies, that fibres of various types are present in the cell matrix and that changes in the state of polymerization and movement of these fibres are intimately related to maintenance of the discoid form and to internal contraction. At least three systems of fibres are present within the matrix:

the submembrane fibres mentioned above
microtubules
microfilaments

The **microtubules** are arranged as a circumferential band near the peripheral zone, which suggests that their role is to contribute to the support of the discoid shape of the unstimulated platelet. Agents such as colchicine, which interfere with the assembly of microtubules (see p. 48), dissolve platelet microtubules and cause loss of the discoid shape.

Microfilaments exist in a dynamic balance of sol–gel transformation and, like microfilaments in other cells, appear to consist of actin and myosin.

The organelle zone

Like many other cells, platelets contain mitochondria, lysosomes and peroxisomes. There are, in addition, two other types of intracytoplasmic organelle which are peculiar to the platelet. The first of these is known as the **alpha granule**. Its contents, which are released after activation, consist of:

platelet-derived growth factor
platelet factor 4
beta-thromboglobulin
factor V
factor VIII related antigen
albumin
fibrinogen
thrombospondin

fibronectin
antiplasmin
alpha-1-antitrypsin
alpha-2-macroglobulin
permeability factor
chemotactic factor
glycosaminoglycans

A rare defect (the grey platelet syndrome) is characterized by the absence of alpha granules. These platelets lack all the proteins listed above. None of these is essential for platelet aggregation so long as the plasma concentration of fibrinogen is adequate. The only abnormalities noted are a somewhat prolonged bleeding time and easy bruising.

The other granule peculiar to the platelet is the so-called **dense body**, which, as its name suggests, is much more electron-dense than the alpha granule. Its contents, also released following activation of the platelet, consist of:

adenosine diphosphate (which causes platelets to aggregate)
adenosine triphosphate
calcium and/or magnesium
5-hydroxytryptamine (serotonin)

Dense bodies may be absent from platelets in a number of rare inherited syndromes, including the Hermansky–Pudlak syndrome and the Wiskott–Aldrich syndrome. The lack of releasable adenosine diphosphate (ADP) has its main effect on **aggregation**, but the bleeding problems in these patients are generally not severe since aggregation can be induced via other pathways.

The membrane zone

Two elements make up this part of the platelet structure. The first of these, which has been referred to earlier, is the so-called **surface-connected open canalicular system**. This is a series of invaginations of the surface membrane which tunnel through the cytoplasm of the platelet in a serpentine manner. These channels remain open whether the platelet is inactive and discoid in shape, or activated, contracted and changed in shape. This suggests that the canaliculi serve not only as a means for increasing the surface area of the platelet susceptible to chemical signals, but also as a series of conduits for secretions produced by platelets in the course of the **release** phase of activation.

In addition to these channels, there is an additional membrane-related system of tubules known as the **dense tubular system**. These tubules are made up of smooth endoplasmic reticulum derived from the parent megakaryocyte. In some areas within the cell the membranes of the dense tubular system and those of the open canalicular system are closely apposed in a manner similar to the relationship between sarcotubules and transverse tubules in muscle cells.

The role of these membrane systems can be appreciated most easily if one looks upon the platelet as being in some respects rather like a muscle cell, in that both cells contract on stimulation. The contraction of platelet actomyosin, as in other situations, is modulated by calcium flux. In the platelet calcium is sequestered in the dense tubular system when the cell has not been activated. Signals reach the platelet interior via the open canalicular system and the connections between this and the dense tubular system lead to the extrusion of calcium from the dense tubular system into the cytoplasm. This is followed by contraction of actomyosin and a change in the shape of the platelet. When the platelet is not activated by a chemical signal, the cytoplasmic calcium is maintained at low levels by the operation of a calcium pump which transports cytoplasmic calcium into the dense tubular system, and which appears to be essential for maintaining the platelet in its resting, discoid form. If there is a rise in intracellular cAMP, the activity of the calcium pump is enhanced. It is not without interest that chemical agents which appear to inhibit platelet activity, such as the anti-aggregatory prostaglandins E_1, D_2 and I_2, act by stimulating the platelet adenylate cyclase to produce a rise in intracellular cAMP. In addition to a role in modulating contractile functions, the dense tubular system also appears to be the site of prostaglandin synthesis within the platelet.

Mechanisms of platelet activation

Adhesion

During the formation of a haemostatic plug or arterial thrombosis, platelets react with exposed subendothelial tissue components. They then change from the normal disc shape, becoming more rounded, and put out pseudopodia. Alternatively, if polymerizing fibrin is present, they may adhere to the fibrin strands and undergo a similar shape change, this probably being brought about by the local accumulations of thrombin, which is responsible for the conversion of fibrinogen to fibrin. How collagen influences platelet behaviour is not clear. There does not appear to be a specific collagen receptor on the platelet surface, and it is possible that several sites on the platelet membrane are cross-linked by the collagen fibril.

The release phase

Once platelets have adhered to collagen fibrils their shape changes and the contents of the intracellular granules are discharged. Some of the compounds released at this point are believed to be deeply involved in the next phase, **aggregation**, when platelets stick to one another to form a clump. Many substances can cause platelets to aggregate (at least in vitro) and most of these also induce granules within the platelets to release their contents. The compounds likely to be operating in real life as opposed to the laboratory include ADP, which can be released from activated platelets, damaged red cells or injured cells of the vessel wall, or formed from ATP, which is also released from platelets. Another powerful aggregator of platelets is thrombin, which can exert its effect via a number of different pathways. In addition, an important group of both pro- and anti-aggregatory compounds can be released from activated platelets as a result of metabolic pathways which have **arachidonic acid**, derived from the platelet surface membrane, as their starting point.

Products of arachidonic acid metabolism in the platelet. In platelets that adhere to collagen or are acted upon by thrombin or some other agent capable of inducing the release reaction, two phospholipases, C and A_2, are activated. Phospholipase A_2 releases arachidonic acid from platelet membrane phospholipids, while phospholipase C frees the arachidonate from phosphatidyl inositol (aided by mono- and diglyceride lipases) (Fig. 19.4). The arachidonate is converted via the cyclo-oxygenase pathway to the prostaglandin endoperoxides, prostaglandins G_2 and H_2. These are then converted to thromboxane A_2 under the influence of thromboxane synthetase. Other products formed in platelets from the prostaglandin endoperoxides include prostaglandins D_2 and E_2. Prostaglandin D_2 is a powerful inhibitor of platelet aggregation because of its ability to stimulate adenylate cyclase. Thromboxane A_2 and its endoperoxide precursors are all platelet-aggregating agents and also cause contraction of vascular smooth muscle.

Just as certain prostaglandins are powerful agents for inducing aggregation of platelets, so the most potent inhibitors of aggregation are those prostaglandins which stimulate the adenylate cyclase system and thus produce an increase in the cAMP content in the platelet. One of these, prostaglandin I_2, is produced by stimulated endothelial cells. Its effects are directly opposite to those of thromboxane A_2 and it is the most powerful inhibitor of platelet aggregation known. Prostaglandin I_2 formed locally may affect the extent of platelet accumulation at that site, though it seems unlikely that it can act as a circulating hormone.

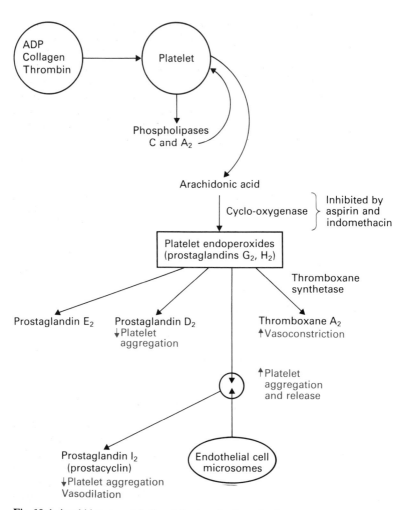

Fig. 19.4 Arachidonate metabolism following platelet activation.

Platelet factor 3 and surface glycoprotein receptors

As stated earlier, when platelets undergo the release reaction, a phospholipoprotein called platelet factor 3 becomes available on their surface. This accelerates the generation of thrombin by taking part in two steps of the intrinsic clotting pathway: the interaction of factors VIIIa and IXa to form factor Xa from factor X, and the interaction of factors Xa and Va to form thrombin from prothrombin.

Shape change in the platelet is also associated with a rearrangement of two glycoprotein receptors on the surface. These form a complex with calcium and this complex acts as a receptor for fibrinogen. The fibrinogen then reacts with this receptor and forms bridges between adjacent platelets. This is an important mechanism in aggregation. If these glycoproteins are missing from the surface (as in thrombasthenia), the platelets will not aggregate, though they can respond to stimuli by discharging their granule contents. Similarly, in severe afibrinogenaemia, effective platelet aggregation does not occur.

Factors Promoting Thrombosis

The very complexity of the interrelating processes involved in platelet adhesion, release and aggregation which have been described above suggests that a number of different circumstances may influence platelet/vessel wall behaviour. In the 1860s, when thrombosis was recognized (but not the existence of the platelet), Rudolf Virchow suggested that the factors likely to promote thrombus formation fell naturally into **three** major groups:

1. Changes in the intimal surface of the vessel
2. Changes in the pattern of blood flow
3. Changes in the constituents of the blood

These are known as **Virchow's triad.**

Changes in the pattern of blood flow

The important changes in blood flow pattern which are believed to increase the risk of thrombus formation are, first, changes in the **speed** of normal laminar flow and, second, actual **loss of the normal laminar pattern** and its replacement by a **turbulent pattern.** Slowing of the speed of blood flow without loss of the normal laminar pattern appears to be of particular significance in relation to the formation of thrombi in **veins**, while, in the **heart** and **arteries**, turbulence plays a more important haemodynamic role.

A reduction in the speed of blood flow may be either a general or a local phenomenon. The first of these may occur in patients with severe congestive cardiac failure, in whom the circulation time can be reduced significantly. Local slowing tends to occur particularly in the veins of the leg under a number of different circumstances, of which the most important are:

prolonged dependence of the limb
reduced muscle pumping activity
proximal occlusion of the venous drainage

These circumstances are most likely to arise in a patient immobilized in bed, especially after surgery. So far as the development of venous thrombosis is concerned, hospital is a very high risk area. Dissection of the deep veins of the calf has shown the presence of thrombi in more than 30% of medical patients coming to necropsy and about 60% of surgical patients. The clinical diagnosis of such thrombi is difficult; only a small minority are correctly diagnosed during life by the presence of some swelling and tenderness in the affected calf and by pain in the calf being elicited on dorsiflexion of the foot (Homan's sign). Rational prevention related to minimizing changes in the pattern of blood flow, which is likely to be much more useful than treatment of an established thrombus, should include routine physiotherapy with exercises emphasizing calf and thigh muscle contraction, early postoperative ambulation, and avoidance of prolonged dependency of lower limbs.

Stasis of blood can also occur in the heart and large vessels such as the aorta if either the cardiac chambers or a segment of a major artery are abnormally dilated. This is found in aortic and other arterial **aneurysms**, in the dilated chambers of the heart in a disorder of heart muscle known as **congestive cardiomyopathy**, and in the dilated atria of patients with mitral valve disease, especially if there is associated atrial fibrillation. A situation rather similar to this occurs in patients in whom a large segment of the left ventricular wall has been rendered severely ischaemic following coronary artery occlusion (**myocardial infarction**). The dead heart muscle is replaced by scar tissue which is non-contractile and this can lead to local disturbances of flow during ventricular systole and the formation of thrombi over the area of lost cardiac muscle.

Turbulent flow is of particular importance in relation to areas where arteries branch and to narrowed segments of arteries, chiefly due to atherosclerosis. The haemodynamics at points of branching are such that platelets tend to collect on the outer walls of branches. This has been demonstrated by introducing extracorporeal shunts, made either of glass or plastic, into the arterial system of animals, and then studying the sites at which platelets preferentially accumulate. In such a model system, the wall surface is uniform and thus the effect of flow can be studied in isolation.

Changes in the vessel wall surface

Changes in the surface of the vessel wall are recognized to be of major importance in the pathogenesis of arterial thrombi. The most important of these changes is **atherosclerosis**, the lesions of which are described in Chapter 18. However, injury (using the word in its broadest sense), inflammation or neoplasms may also be associated with damage to the vessel wall. Of all the structural elements of the vessel wall, the one most likely to be implicated in thrombus formation is the endothelial cell. In any situation where there is actual loss of endothelial cells with exposure of the subendothelial collagen, platelet adhesion is the inevitable sequel. This certainly happens in complicated atherosclerotic plaques when splitting of the connective tissue 'cap' of the plaque occurs. Endothelial cell desquamation can also take place in the rare inherited metabolic disorder homocystinuria, and it has been claimed that endothelial cells can be identified in significant numbers in the blood following smoking.

One of the dogmas of vascular pathology is that platelets do not adhere to intact endothelium. However, in some experimental models, such adhesion has been seen. This has followed infusions of the enzyme neuraminidase, which alters the proteoglycans in the luminal glycocalyx of the endothelial cell, and has also been noted in animals exposed to fresh cigarette smoke. A reduction in the amount of prostaglandin I_2 (prostacyclin) produced by aortic rings from rats exposed to fresh cigarette smoke has also been reported. These data, scanty as they are, suggest that certain factors may alter the structure and function of endothelium in such a way as to promote platelet/vessel wall interactions, without it being necessary for focal necrosis of endothelium to take place.

Trauma to the endothelium of a sufficient degree to cause thrombosis can occur under a number of circumstances. At a rather extreme level, thrombosis can occur after burning or freezing (e.g. capillary thrombosis in 'frostbite'). Mechanical trauma to endothelium occurs in association with the presence of indwelling cannulas. Another type of much less easily provable endothelial trauma has been suggested as being one of the factors involved in the production of postoperative venous thrombi in the lower limb. During anaesthesia there is loss of the normal muscle tone, and the dead weight of the limb and the hard surface of the operating table might be sufficient to cause trauma to the venous endothelium. There is no direct evidence for such trauma at the moment, though surgery certainly appears to be a very potent thrombogenic stimulus as far as the veins are concerned.

Chemical trauma certainly exists and thrombosis may follow infusion of certain compounds into veins. This fact is made use of in certain treatments of both varicose veins and haemorrhoids, where sclerosing chemicals are injected into the affected veins with the deliberate intention of causing thrombosis.

Inflammation

Thrombi occur frequently in situations where the vascular channels are involved in an inflammatory process. This may occur in the heart valves in patients with either rheumatic or infective endocarditis. Arteries involved in an immune complex mediated inflammatory reaction such as occurs in **polyarteritis nodosa** or **temporal arteritis** are often thrombosed; both veins and capillaries passing through an inflamed area may also be affected in the same way.

Neoplastic involvement

The invasion of small venules by malignant cells is often accompanied by thrombosis and there is evidence to suggest that fibrin formed in relation to the tumour cells in the course of this process may enhance their chances of survival and, hence, of multiplying.

Changes in the constituents of the blood

Platelets

It seems obvious that platelet function should be considered in relation to the three main constituents of their behaviour: adhesion, release and aggregation. In addition, their concentration within the blood should be determined, since it is known that a low platelet count is associated with abnormal bleeding and a high one with an increased tendency towards thrombosis.

In the laboratory it is common practice to measure the aggregatability of platelets to a given stimulus. ADP, collagen or thrombin are added to a suspension of platelets in a cuvette and the turbidimetric changes resulting from aggregation measured. Platelet adhesiveness can also be measured: the suspension of platelets (of known concentration) is passed at a constant rate across glass beads and the drop in platelet numbers occurring as a result of this passage is determined. The release reaction can be monitored by measuring changes in concentration of two products derived from the alpha granules — platelet factor 4 (an anti-heparin factor) and beta-thromboglobulin. If sufficient care is taken in the sampling of the blood, a rise in the concentration of these compounds is prima facie evidence of thrombosis having taken place. However, the half-lives of both platelet factor 4 and beta-thromboglobulin in plasma are very short and thus the timing of the sampling is critical.

Risk factors for clinically evident thrombotic events and platelet function

Prostaglandins

The results of epidemiological studies among the Eskimos of north-west Greenland suggest that alterations in the plasma concentrations of certain lipids may influence the balance between thromboxane

A_2 and prostaglandin I_2. The incidence of ischaemic heart disease in this Eskimo community is very low. They have low levels of cholesterol and low density lipoprotein in the blood and correspondingly high levels of high density lipoprotein. This plasma lipid pattern is not genetic in origin but appears to be brought about by the diet. In addition, platelet aggregatability is lower than in age- and sex-matched Danes and the bleeding time is prolonged. One of the outstanding features of the Eskimo diet is a high intake of eicosapentaenoic acid (EPA) (which is present in fish), and Eskimos have high plasma concentrations of this fatty acid and low concentrations of arachidonic acid. Eicosapentaenoic acid is a starting point for the synthesis of prostaglandin I_3, which is anti-aggregatory, but the thromboxane derived from EPA is said not to be pro-aggregatory. Diets rich in cod-liver oil, which contains large amounts of EPA, have been shown to reduce the tendency to thrombosis in extracorporeal shunts inserted into rat aortas.

Platelet aggregation and plasma lipid patterns

Other evidence that the pattern and concentrations of plasma lipids may influence platelet behaviour is derived from patients with type IIa hyperlipidaemia. Their platelets are many times more sensitive to doses of aggregating agents such as collagen, ADP or thrombin than are those of normal subjects, though the lipid composition of the platelets themselves differs little, if at all. However, platelets from patients with hyperlipidaemia convert more arachidonic acid to thromboxane A_2 than do those from normal subjects.

In rabbits, feeding a diet high in saturated fat results in an increase in aggregatability of platelets in response to a standard dose of thrombin. This change takes place before any increase in the cholesterol concentration in the artery wall can be demonstrated. Similar data have been obtained from human studies.

Cigarette smoking and platelet function

There is a strong positive correlation between heavy smoking of cigarettes and the risk of one of the major clinical manifestations of occlusive arterial disease. Cigarette smoking could operate as a risk factor in a number of ways and, clearly, the possibility of an effect on platelet behaviour is an area which requires investigation. Acute smoking experiments have yielded conflicting data on platelet aggregatability, but some studies suggest that smoking may have an effect on the adhesion of platelets to the underlying arterial wall.

The Evolution of Venous Thrombi

The process of thrombus formation in a non-inflamed vein is usually termed **phlebothrombosis.** When thrombosis occurs in a vein which is inflamed, it is spoken of as **thrombophlebitis.** This is most commonly seen in superficial veins.

The site of initiation of the process is usually the valve pocket. If these areas are examined in sections of thrombosed veins, small clumps of platelets can be seen adhering to the luminal surface. It is a moot point whether this is preceded by damage to the endothelium in this area. Thus far no positive evidence that such damage occurs has been presented, but the technical problems in carrying out such a study are daunting and it is, perhaps, too early to write off endothelial injury as

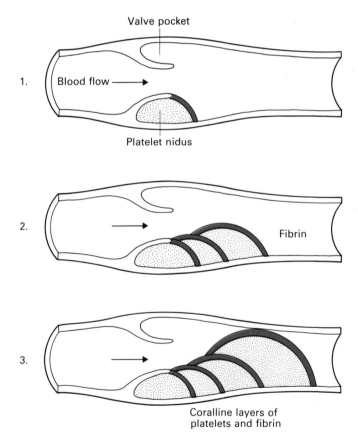

Fig. 19.5 The evolution of a venous thrombus.

being an important starting point for the process of venous thrombosis. Some workers have noted the presence of leucocytes rather than platelets in these valve pockets and it is possible that these cells could bring about changes in the endothelium. Once platelets are aggregated, clotting factors are activated locally and fibrin strands stabilize the platelet aggregate and help to anchor it to the underlying vein wall. A second phase then begins in which a further batch of platelets are laid down over the initial aggregate. At this stage of the development of the thrombus, the platelets can be seen to have aggregated in the form of laminae which project from the surface of the initial aggregate and lie across the stream of blood. As a result of the forces exerted by the streaming blood, these platelet laminae are bent in the direction of flow and form a somewhat coralline structure (Fig. 19.5). Between the platelet laminae are large numbers of red cells, some fibrin strands and a moderate number of leucocytes. The laminar arrangement of the platelets coupled with shortening of the fibrin strands between the laminae gives rise to a curious 'rippled' appearance when the thrombi are viewed from above. The appearances are reminiscent of what one

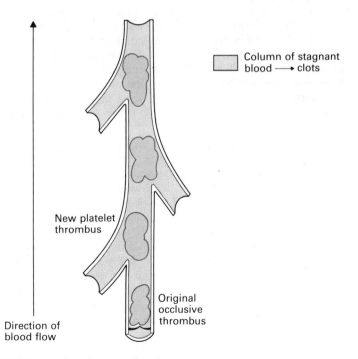

Fig. 19.6 Propagation of a venous thrombus.

sees when a wind has blown across a beach and produced rippling of the sand. In both instances the 'ripples' lie concave to the direction of the force; in the case of the platelet laminae this force having been the bloodstream. These elevated ridges on the surface of thrombi are known as **lines of Zahn** in commemoration of the pathologist who first described them. They are clearly visible with the naked eye, but may be seen best with the aid of a hand lens. The more rapid the streaming of the blood in the segment of vessel where thrombosis has occurred, the more prominent are the lines of Zahn. They are most easily seen, therefore, in large arteries such as the aorta.

At this stage the process may come to an end. The thrombus will then become covered by new endothelial cells and be incorporated into the structure of the underlying vessel wall. However, if the deposition of platelets and fibrin continues, a third phase ensues. As the coralline mass of platelets admixed with clotted blood continues to grow, the stream of blood through the affected segment slows still further and occlusion may ultimately occur. This phase is predominantly mediated by activation of the coagulation pathways rather than by platelet adhesion and aggregation.

Once a segment of vein is occluded in this way, the flow of blood cephalad to the occlusion stops. Thus a stagnant column of blood exists between the point of occlusion and the point cephalad to it where the next venous tributary enters (Fig. 19.6). This stagnant column of blood coagulates and forms what is termed a 'consecutive clot' in continuity with the original thrombus. This is the first step in a process known as **propagation** of the thrombus. This process may occur in two basic patterns:

1. As mentioned above, consecutive clot forms between the original occlusion and the tributary immediately cephalad to it. At this point, blood enters from the tributary and passes across the surface of the clot. Platelets then adhere to the fibrin meshwork and aggregation follows with the formation of another small platelet thrombus. If this too grows enough to occlude the lumen, propagation may occur again and another segment of vein may fill with fresh clot. In effect, a long segment of the venous drainage of the limb can become occluded in a series of 'jumps' or episodes of clotting, each of which is triggered by the adhesion of platelets. The mixed mass of platelet thrombi and consecutive clot is anchored to the underlying vein wall only at those sites where there has been adhesion of platelets.
2. If the venous return from the limb as a whole is slowed down, propagation by the formation of consecutive clot may occur on a massive scale. Cephalad to the original, occlusive platelet/fibrin thrombus, a long cord of clotted blood may form which fills the vein

lumen and which is anchored only at its origin. With the eventual shortening of fibrin strands that takes place more or less inevitably after the formation of any clot, this mass of clotted blood comes to lie quite loosely within the lumen except at the point where the original thrombus is attached. If the thrombus becomes dislodged from its attachment point, then the whole mass is carried away in the systemic venous circulation until impaction takes place within the pulmonary arteries (pulmonary embolism).

The Natural History of Thrombi

Some thrombi may undergo lysis through the action of plasmin and 'like some insubstantial pageant faded, leave not a wrack behind'. From the pragmatic point of view this is clearly the most desirable outcome, especially in relation to occlusive thrombosis within the arterial tree. It is not without interest that plasminogen activator, which converts plasminogen to the active form plasmin, is present in greater concentrations within venous intima than within arterial intima.

Thrombi may become detached from the underlying vascular wall, be it vein, artery or heart. When this occurs, the detached portion of thrombus travels at high speed in the systemic venous circulation (if its origin is a vein) or within the systemic arterial circulation (if the site of origin was an artery or the heart). At some point a vessel will be reached whose calibre is less than the diameter of the thrombotic material and impaction occurs. This **embolization** can have serious structural and functional consequences which will be discussed in Chapter 20.

If the thrombus persists, the processes of organization, as described in Chapter 8, are triggered. Much will depend on whether the thrombus is occlusive or whether it lies in a plaque-like fashion on the surface of the vessel wall without seriously impeding the flow of blood. This latter case is known as a **mural thrombus.**

The organization of occlusive thrombi

If a segment of a vessel remains plugged by thrombus, new capillary vessels of granulation tissue type grow out from the vasa vasorum in the adventitia, across the media, into and across the intima and, ultimately, into the thrombus itself. At the same time, the removal of thrombotic material, largely through the action of macrophages, is proceeding. Eventually, at the worst, the occlusive thrombus may be replaced by a solid plug of collagenous tissue and all chance of re-establishing flow is lost (Fig. 19.7).

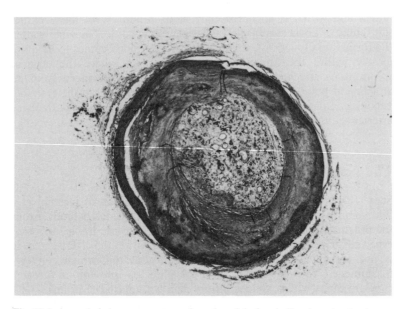

Fig. 19.7 An occluded coronary artery where the original occluding thrombus has been replaced, through the process of organization, by vascular granulation tissue.

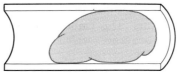

Segment of artery occluded by recent thrombus

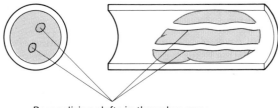

Recanalizing clefts in thrombus may re-establish some degree of flow

Fig. 19.8 Recanalization of an occlusive thrombus.

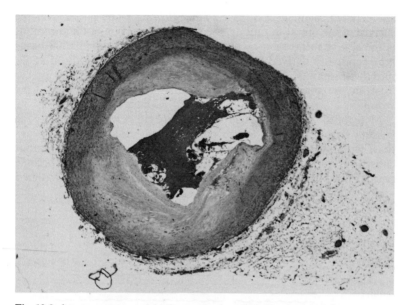

Fig. 19.9 A coronary artery originally completely occluded by thrombus. In some areas the thrombus has retracted from the underlying vessel wall, thus re-establishing some flow through the previously blocked segment.

Fortunately, however, the picture is not by any means always so gloomy. Quite early on after the formation of an occlusive thrombus, clefts may appear within the thrombotic material. These clefts often lie in the long axis of the occluded segment and hence, by implication, in the same axis as the blood flow. Not infrequently they link up with one another to form new channels which pass through the occluding plug of thrombus/granulation tissue from one patent segment of the vessel to another (Figs 19.8 and 19.9). Within a few days the clefts become lined by flattened cells of mesenchymal origin which ultimately differentiate into endothelial cells. Occasionally some of the mesenchymal stem cells close to the new vascular channels differentiate into smooth muscle and arrange themselves round the clefts in a concentric fashion. The whole process by which a greater or lesser degree of blood flow is re-established through the occluded segment of vessel is known as **recanalization.**

The organization of mural thrombi

In this situation the pattern of organization is different because the pathophysiological circumstances differ so much from what obtains in an occluded segment of a vessel. Since flowing blood passes over the surface of the mural thrombus, the superficial portion of the thrombus is the seat of infiltration by oxygenated plasma and granulation tissue type capillaries derived from the vasa grow only very slowly, if at all, into the thrombus. The lack of this feature may be mediated, in part at least, by the normal intramural tension within the affected part of the vessel.

Many of the platelets disaggregate and are either washed away by the passing stream of blood or are phagocytosed. In arteries this means that, within a short time, the major part of the remaining thrombus consists of a spongy mass of polymerized fibrin which tends to become packed down onto the surface of the underlying vessel wall. Within a

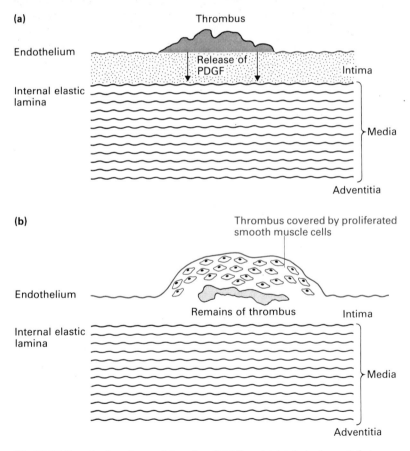

Fig. 19.10 Organization of a mural thrombus. PDGF = platelet-derived growth factor.

few days the surface of the thrombus becomes partly covered by a layer of flattened cells. Originally it was thought that these were new endothelial cells but there is some evidence to suggest that the cells making up the early neo-intima are smooth muscle cells.

As in other situations where organization is taking place, the mass of fibrin and platelets becomes vascularized. An unusual feature, however, is the fact that the new vascular channels, which can be seen within a few days of the thrombus being formed, are derived from the main lumen of the vessel and grow down into the thrombus rather than upwards across the media from the vasa vasorum.

The picture is further complicated by the interaction of platelet-derived growth factor with smooth muscle cells in the underlying vessel wall. The major part of the proliferation of smooth muscle cells which ensues after the formation of a mural thrombus appears to take place on the lumenal aspect of the thrombus, so that the thrombus eventually lies deep within the thick new intima (Fig. 19.10). The possibility that this process may play a part in the growth of atherosclerotic plaques is discussed in Chapter 18.

Chapter 20

The Pathological Bases of Ischaemia III: Embolism

An **embolus** is an abnormal mass of material, either solid or gaseous, which is transported in the bloodstream from one part of the circulation to another and which finally **impacts** in the lumen of vessels which are of too small a calibre to allow the embolus to pass. Emboli may consist of:

thrombus
mixed thrombus and blood clot
air
nitrogen
fat
small pieces of bone marrow
debris from the base of atherosclerotic plaques
groups of tumour cells (embolization constitutes an important means of tumour spread)

Most major emboli are derived from thrombus

Roughly 99% of emboli are derived from thrombus or from thrombus mixed with blood clot such as is found in the veins of the lower limb.

When the origin of the embolus is a venous thrombus, the end result must be impaction in the pulmonary arterial tree. This is one of the commonest forms of embolization in man and also one of the most dangerous. Some 600 000 cases of pulmonary embolization occur each year in the United States, the number of patients dying ranging from 20 000 to 50 000 annually. In unselected necropsies, pulmonary emboli can be identified with the naked eye in about 10% of cases. If the necropsy sample is a more selective one (patients who have had orthopaedic operations on the lower limb, patients with severe burns or with fractures), the frequency with which emboli can be identified rises steeply. The pathophysiological effects of pulmonary embolization depend on the interaction between two factors:

1. The **size** of the embolus and hence the degree of mechanical obstruction which it causes
2. The presence or absence of **congestion** in the pulmonary circulation at the time of impaction

316

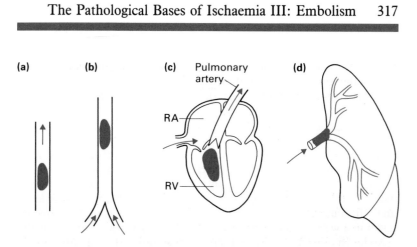

Fig. 20.1 Pulmonary embolism. (a) A thrombus becomes detached from the leg vein wall, forming an embolus. (b) The embolus travels up the inferior vena cava. (c) It enters the right side of the heart. RA = right atrium; RV = right ventricle. (d) Impaction occurs in the pulmonary artery or one of its branches, depending on the size of the embolus.

Massive pulmonary emboli (Fig. 20.1)

The logical correlate of massive pulmonary embolization is that the embolus has been derived from thrombus **occluding a long segment of the venous drainage of the lower limb.** In effect this means that the thrombotic process has involved the iliofemoral part of the venous system. Even then it must be remembered that the calibre of the main pulmonary arteries exceeds that of the iliac or femoral veins, and in order for blocking of one of the major pulmonary vessels to occur, the length of mixed thrombus and clot must be loosely bundled together to form a mass of the appropriate dimensions. Massive pulmonary embolism usually presents extremely suddenly. Often the symptoms appear when the patient is straining, for example at stool. Affected patients may die suddenly or complain of chest pain and experience shortness of breath. The signs of circulatory collapse are usually present. It is humiliating to have to confess that the mechanisms involved in the production of the dramatic clinical picture are still not well understood. It has been suggested that the sudden blockage to the flow of blood through one of the main pulmonary arteries is responsible, though, if this is the case, it is hard to see why patients can withstand ligation of the main pulmonary artery in the course of surgical removal of a lung without any obvious circulatory problems. Other explanations which have been suggested are:

1. A vagal reflex inducing spasm of the coronary and pulmonary arteries

2. A reflex which produces marked peripheral vasodilatation
3. A reflex producing cardiac arrest
4. A massive release of prostaglandins which can provoke vasospasm

Small pulmonary emboli

Small emboli are usually clinically 'silent' and are often multiple. Retraction of the thrombotic material from the wall of the vessel in which they are impacted frequently takes place, and the combination of such retraction with the organization described in Chapter 19 may leave small fibrous tissue cords, criss-crossing the lumen of the affected vessel in a web or band-like fashion, as the only marker of the embolic episode. In other cases the emboli retract so much that the thrombotic mass becomes packed down onto the vessel wall in the same way as occurs with a mural thrombus. These emboli then become covered by new endothelium and are incorporated into the vessel wall, this process of incorporation being accompanied by the proliferation of smooth muscle cells and the formation of a thicker than normal intimal layer. If this sequence of events is repeated many times, the increased thickness of the intima in the pulmonary arterial bed leads to a decrease in the compliance of the vessels and ultimately to a rise in pulmonary artery pressure (pulmonary hypertension).

Under certain circumstances, pulmonary emboli of **moderate size** (i.e. large enough to block secondary or tertiary branches of the pulmonary arteries) may reduce the perfusion of a segment of lung tissue sufficiently to produce a localized area of necrosis. Such areas of necrosis secondary to ischaemia are known as infarcts; these are discussed in Chapter 21.

Systemic emboli

Most thrombotic, systemic emboli are derived from the left side of the heart. The thrombi may arise in the atrial appendages (this being particularly likely to occur in patients with atrial fibrillation). Intraventricular thrombi may occur as a consequence of transmural myocardial infarction (see p. 331) or in congestive cardiomyopathy, a muscle disorder in which the myocardium is flabby and the ventricles are dilated. There is a marked decrease in the systolic ejection fraction and thus a volume overload on the ventricular muscle. In life, the presence of these thrombi can be detected by echocardiography. Thrombi affecting the heart valves and of a size sufficient to give rise to significant emboli are usually related to the presence of **infective endocarditis**, a disorder produced by the combination of haemodynamically induced endocardial injury and bacteraemia. The infected thrombi, or **vegetations** as they are often called, may be bulky and friable. Portions of the vegetations can break off readily and travel in the systemic arterial circulation until they impact. This may, of course, occur in a very large number of places, but the brain, lower limbs, spleen and kidneys are favoured sites. When an infected thrombus impacts, it may set up a localized inflammatory reaction leading to partial destruction of the wall of the vessel in which impaction has taken place. This leads to a dilatation of the affected arterial segment, and rupture followed by haemorrhage may occur. Such a lesion is termed a **mycotic aneurysm**, a misleading term since fungi have nothing to do with the pathogenesis ('mycos' = mushroom).

Small **platelet thrombi** occur quite commonly in relation to atherosclerotic plaques at the point in the neck where the common carotid artery divides. Emboli derived from these platelet masses lodge in the cerebral circulation, often in small vessels, where they may give rise to permanent or transient neurological deficiencies.

Gaseous emboli

Air may be introduced into the systemic circulation under a number of circumstances. These include:

1. Operations on the head and neck where a large vein is opened inadvertently
2. Mismanagement of blood transfusions where positive pressure is being used to speed up the flow of blood
3. During haemodialysis for renal failure
4. Following insufflation of air into the fallopian tubes in the course of investigation of sterility
5. Interference with the placental site during criminal abortion

The air enters the right side of the heart where, in the right ventricle, it is whipped up into a frothy mass. This mass can block the flow of blood through the pulmonary arteries. The clinical picture that develops closely mimics that of massive pulmonary embolization by thrombus derived from the leg veins. In some cases the froth may gain access to the systemic arterial circulation and impact there. The most frequent site for this is the brain, but cases have also been reported of embolization of vessels supplying the spinal cord, with patients being investigated for sterility becoming quadriplegic following tubal insufflation. As little as 40 ml of air can have serious clinical results and 100 ml can be fatal, though there have been rare cases in which 200 ml have been tolerated. If air embolism is suspected as the cause of death, it is necessary to place the heart and pulmonary arteries under water when they are opened, in order to detect the escape of the air bubbles from the blocked vessels.

Nitrogen embolization occurs in decompression sickness, which is also known as 'caisson disease'. It is found in persons whose occupation causes them to work at very high pressures and who may then be returned too quickly to normal atmospheric pressure (deep sea divers, tunnellers, etc.).

At high pressures, inert gases, of which nitrogen is the most important, are dissolved in the plasma and in interstitial tissue, especially adipose tissue. If the persons at risk return too quickly to normal atmospheric pressure, the gas comes out of solution and small bubbles are formed within the interstitial tissues and blood, platelets often being associated with gas bubbles in the latter situation. These bubbles may coalesce to form quite large masses and the clinical features are produced either by emboli in the circulating blood or by the presence of bubbles in the interstitial tissues, especially in tendons, joints and ligaments. When this happens the patient complains of excruciating pain (the syndrome being known as '**the bends**'). The central nervous system may be affected and the sudden onset of respiratory distress has also been described. The symptoms may be relieved by placing the patient in a compression chamber and forcing the gases back into solution. Once this has been done, slow and careful decompression should avoid a recurrence. Occasionally the presence of nitrogen emboli in the systemic circulation is followed by ischaemic damage to the ends of long bones, this being associated with secondary damage to the articular cartilages and joints.

Fat emboli

Fat embolism is relatively common under certain circumstances, but significant clinical consequences are, happily, quite rare. It has been most frequently associated with fractures of long bones, with severe burns, and with severe and extensive soft tissue trauma, but may also be found in patients with hyperlipidaemias and following ischaemic bone marrow necrosis in patients with sickle cell disease. The fact that the syndrome can occur in the absence of trauma suggests a multifactorial pathogenesis.

In patients with fractures, especially multiple fractures, fat globules are thought to enter veins at the fracture site which have been torn at the time of injury. These globules are then carried in the systemic venous circulation to the lungs, where they may impact in small vessels and cause the sudden onset of respiratory distress some 24 to 72 hours following injury. In such patients it may be possible to identify droplets of fat in the sputum by staining sputum smears with fat soluble dyes such as Oil-Red O. Despite the fact that the fat is said to enter the venous circulation, some patients present with predominant involvement of the central nervous system. They may become agitated at first and then lapse into coma; a high proportion of such patients die. At autopsy, if they have survived the onset of unconsciousness for a day or two, the brain shows oedema and **very many tiny haemorrhages.** These occur in both the grey and the white matter but are more easily seen in the latter site. Frozen sections of brain stained with fat soluble dyes show the presence of fat globules within the lumina of cerebral capillaries.

As mentioned above, fat emboli occur more frequently than does the **fat embolization syndrome.** When autopsies were carried out on Korean war battle casualties dying within four weeks of having been injured, evidence of fat embolization was found in 90% of cases. However, in only 1% could any part of the clinical picture in these patients be attributed to the fat emboli.

The **pathogenesis** of fat embolism is a more complex matter than was previously thought. While one could accept the old simple hypothesis that it was due to the entry of fat into traumatized veins in patients with multiple fractures, this cannot account for those cases which occur in the absence of trauma. Other mechanisms that have been suggested include the possibility that under certain circumstances, particularly when there is a rise in endogenous catecholamine levels, chylomicrons much larger than usual are formed due to some instability of the normal emulsion which chylomicrons and plasma represent.

Bone marrow emboli

Bone marrow emboli are not infrequently found on histological examination of post-mortem samples of lung tissue from patients who have had episodes of cardiac arrest due to ventricular fibrillation and in whom the attempts at resuscitation have included external cardiac massage. In middle-aged and elderly people, in whom the costal cartilages have long since become ossified, repeated pressure on the rib cage usually results in the fracture of several ribs and it is from these sites that the bone marrow is squeezed into the veins. What the clinical effects, if any, of such emboli are is simply unknown.

Emboli derived from atheromatous debris

Atheromatous emboli obviously occur only in the systemic arterial tree. They are derived from plaques which ulcerate and in which there is a massive basally situated pool of lipid and tissue debris, as described in Chapter 18. The emboli are usually found incidentally on histological examination of tissue and can be easily recognized since they consist of a mixture of thrombotic material and lipid-rich debris in which highly characteristic, cigar- or torpedo-shaped cholesterol crystals are present.

Chapter 21

Ischaemia and Infarction

Ischaemia may be defined as **the state existing when an organ or tissue has its arterial perfusion lowered relative to its metabolic needs.** This definition is often broadened to include the functional changes which are produced by such a diminution of perfusion. An **infarct** is a **morphological** entity: a large, localized area of tissue necrosis which is brought about by **ischaemia.**

Ischaemia is most often caused by some local interference with the perfusion of the organ or tissue concerned. On some occasions, however, the ischaemic state may be generalized. This occurs only rarely and is associated with a fall in cardiac output. While acute reductions in cardiac output are by no means uncommon, they are not often expressed in the form of ischaemic changes in individual tissues. Rarely, gangrene of the extremities may be seen following either extensive myocardial infarction or the sudden onset of a ventricular arrhythmia, both of which may be associated with a severe drop in cardiac output. Disorders of cardiac rhythm, including pathological changes in the conducting system, are not uncommon causes of cerebral ischaemia. An obvious and important example of this is **complete heart block** in which sudden periods of unconsciousness (Stokes–Adams attacks) occur. If adequate perfusion of the brain is not restored within three to four minutes, irreparable damage to the neurones occurs.

Local Causes of Ischaemia

The most important of the pathological bases of ischaemia — atherosclerosis, thrombosis and embolism — have been described in Chapters 18 to 20. In addition, arterial perfusion may be interfered with by spasm of the smooth muscle in the vessel wall or by pressure on the vessel from without. However, it is worth remembering that interruption of arterial blood flow is not the only way in which ischaemia may be produced; pathological changes affecting veins and capillaries can also lead to underperfusion of tissues.

Ischaemia due to venous occlusion

The pathogenesis of ischaemia due to venous occlusion is outlined in Fig. 21.1. It should be obvious from this that ischaemia on such a basis

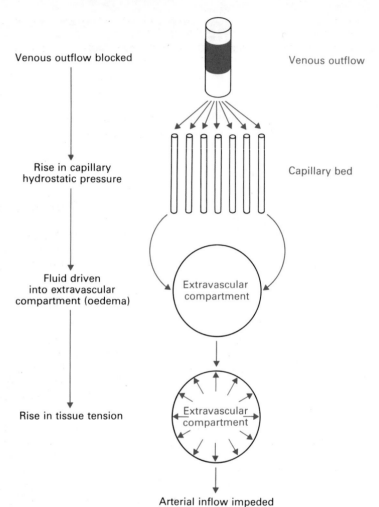

Fig. 21.1 Pathogenesis of ischaemia due to venous occlusion.

is likely to occur only in certain anatomical situations where it is not possible for the blood to bypass the obstruction via collateral drainage channels, and that, because of the local interruption to venous return, the affected tissues are likely to be **intensely congested** and possibly even **haemorrhagic.** The circumstances under which **venous infarction** is likely to occur include:

1. Extensive mesenteric venous thrombosis, leading to infarction of the small intestine

2. So-called strangulation of hernias, where entrapment occurs leading
to oedema and pressure on the draining veins
3. Cavernous sinus thrombosis, which may lead in turn to thrombosis
of the retinal vein and, ultimately, to blindness
4. Thrombosis of the superior longitudinal sinus within the dura. This
can occur in severely dehydrated children and leads to patchy
haemorrhagic necrosis in the cerebral cortex
5. A very rare variant of thrombosis in the iliofemoral system, which
may be followed by gangrenous changes in the lower limb

Ischaemia due to capillary obstruction

This can occur as a consequence of physical damage to the capillaries,
as in 'frostbite'. Capillaries may be occluded rarely by parasites, as in
cerebral malaria, by abnormal red cells in sickle cell disease or in certain
autoimmune haemolytic anaemias, by fibrin where disseminated
intravascular coagulation has occurred, by antigen/antibody complexes,
by fat or gas emboli, or by external pressure, such as is seen in 'bed
sores'.

Arterial obstruction

Obstruction of arterial inflow may be followed by a spectrum of
functional and/or structural changes which range from no effect to
extensive tissue necrosis. If neither functional nor structural changes
can be observed, we can infer that the collateral arterial supply to the
target area is good and that no significant reduction in perfusion has
occurred.

Functional disturbances are usually noted when the collateral supply
is only good enough to maintain adequate perfusion so long as the
metabolic demands of the tissue are at a basal level. If these demands
are increased, as for example in the heart or the muscle of the lower
limb during exercise, then a state of ischaemia will be produced and the
patient will experience either substernal pain (**angina pectoris**) or a
cramp-like pain in the calf (**intermittent claudication**). Cessation of
activity leads, in most instances, to disappearance of the pain.

The eventual changes in the function of an organ or tissue which has
been rendered ischaemic may result either from loss of cells or from
abnormal or deficient behaviour on the part of surviving cells. In
ischaemic myocardium there is a marked tendency for electrical
disturbances to occur and these frequently give rise to fatal arrhythmias
such as ventricular fibrillation. Indeed, at least half the patients who die
in the course of their first clinically apparent episode of myocardial
ischaemia, die in this way. Similarly the presence of ischaemic sensory
nerve bundles may lead to qualitative abnormalities in the sensory

patterns interpreted within the central nervous system, and it has been suggested that this mechanism may underlie the phenomenon of persistent pain in patients with limb ischaemia.

If the degree of ischaemia is greater than has been described above, then structural damage to cells and tissues will occur. This may take the form of patchy loss of parenchymal cells, such as is seen in the myocardium of patients with a long history of angina pectoris, or of massive necrosis. In either event, if the patient survives the ischaemic episode, the lost tissue is replaced, except in the case of the brain, by fibrous tissue in a manner identical with that occurring in repair (see Chapter 8). The degree of post-ischaemic necrosis is proportional to the degree of ischaemia, which, in turn, depends on the balance between the needs of an individual tissue and the degree to which arterial perfusion is compromised. When the ischaemia is slow in onset and chronic in nature, a characteristic feature is the tendency for cell death to affect either individual cells or small groups of cells. Initially these may show the changes of intracellular oedema (see p. 17) or fatty change, but eventually they die and are replaced by small foci of fibrous tissue. When such chronic ischaemia occurs in the heart it gives the muscle a curious flecked appearance because of the 'drop out' of small numbers of cells and their replacement by collagen fibres. In chronic lower limb ischaemia, the dermal papillae of the skin become flattened and both the epidermis and the dermis are thinned. Skin appendages such as hair follicles, sweat glands and sebaceous glands may also disappear. As a result of these changes, the skin appears shiny, hairless and dry.

The degree of ischaemia

The degree of ischaemia is determined by a number of interacting variables (Fig. 21.2). These include:

    the metabolic needs of the underperfused tissue
    the speed of onset of arterial occlusion
    the completeness or otherwise of the arterial blocking
    the anatomy of the local blood supply
    the state of patency of the collateral blood supply

The metabolic needs of the underperfused tissue. Tissues vary in their capacity to withstand a reduction in their arterial perfusion. The brain is the most sensitive in this respect, and deprivation of oxygen for more than three to four minutes will cause irreversible damage to the nerve cells. The myocardium is also very susceptible to damage following underperfusion. It is doubly unfortunate that both brain and heart

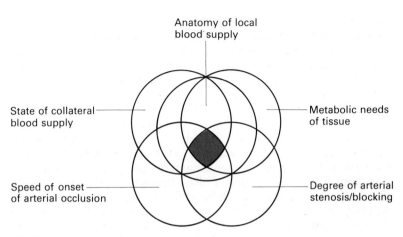

Fig. 21.2 Factors influencing the degree of ischaemia.

have, on the whole, rather poor collateral blood supplies and that neither heart muscle cells nor neurones are able to regenerate.

The speed of onset of arterial occlusion. If arterial occlusion takes place very rapidly as, for example, when an atherosclerotic coronary artery plaque ruptures, the effects of this are more severe than with slow narrowing of the same segment of artery, since there is little or no time for collateral vessels to open.

The completeness of the arterial blocking. Other things being equal, complete occlusion of an arterial lumen causes more extensive damage to the affected area than does severe stenosis. It must be equally obvious that the more proximally the occlusion is situated in a given arterial tree, the greater will be the area of tissue affected by ischaemia.

The anatomy of the local blood supply. Some organs or tissues have no collateral blood supply and the arteries which perfuse such parts are known as 'end-arteries'. The retina is an example of such a tissue. It is supplied by a single vessel, the central retinal artery, which only branches once it has reached the retina. If occlusion of the central retinal artery occurs and is not rapidly relieved, irreparable ischaemic damage will be produced within the retina. The smaller arteries within the cerebral cortex also function as end-arteries. In contrast, some tissues, such as the lung, have a **double** arterial supply. Occlusion of one part of this blood supply need not lead to necrosis of the underperfused area since the supply from the other source may be sufficient to maintain tissue viability.

Patency of the collateral blood supply. A good collateral supply, in the anatomical sense, can only compensate for blockage in the main arterial tree if the collateral vessels themselves are neither stenosed by atherosclerotic plaques nor in spasm.

Infarction

An **infarct** can be defined as **a fairly large area of tissue necrosis** (usually coagulative in type) **which results from ischaemia.** Blood may seep into the ischaemic area for some time, partly as a result of back flow from venules and escape of blood through the walls of vessels in the local microcirculation which have been damaged in the course of the ischaemic process. Thus many infarcts contain a good deal of blood in the early stages of their natural history. In spongy tissue such as the lung, the escape of red blood cells and fibrin is a conspicuous feature and the ischaemic lung tissue becomes firmer than normal. At necropsy, infarcts of this type can be appreciated as wedge-shaped lumps on the pleural aspect of the lung. When the lung is cut into, the infarcted area tends to bulge and to stand proud of the surrounding normal lung. This outpouring or 'stuffing' of blood into the devitalized areas is merely an epiphenomenon and is not the core event in infarction. Failure of pathologists to appreciate this led to the introduction of the archaic and essentially unhelpful term '**infarct**', which is derived from the Latin verb 'infarcire' meaning 'to stuff'.

With the passage of time the dying cells often swell. This tends to squeeze blood out of the interstitial tissue in the infarcted area and the infarct becomes much paler. In the heart, for example, it takes 24 to 36 hours for this process to become complete. The pallor is a useful marker for the macroscopic diagnosis of infarction at necropsy. However, because this pallor takes a considerable time to develop, it may be difficult to make such a necropsy diagnosis in the early stages of the natural history of a myocardial infarct. The application of enzyme histochemical methods to this problem can be of great assistance in arriving at an accurate diagnosis on macroscopic examination of the heart (see p. 331), but even these techniques fail to identify necrotic muscle tissue unless the patient has survived for six to nine hours after the cutting off of the blood supply to an area of the myocardium. The division of infarcts into '**pale**' and '**red**' varieties is pointless. Many infarcts start off as red and become pale as the blood is squeezed out of the infarcted area by swelling of the dying cells. Cerebral infarcts are usually pale ab initio (unless they are embolic in origin) and infarcts in the spongy lung tissue remain red and undergo repair while still at that stage.

The dead parenchymal cells in the infarcted area undergo autolysis and the diapedesed red cells haemolyse. At the same time a brisk inflammatory reaction occurs at the margins of the infarct and first neutrophils and then macrophages infiltrate the necrotic tissue. Breakdown products of haemoglobin — haematoidin (bile pigment) and haemosiderin (aggregated molecules of ferritin) — may be seen in relation to the infarcted area and are ingested by macrophages. At this stage, usually about one week after the cutting off of the arterial supply, an infarct in a solid organ is generally firm in consistency and a dull yellow in colour, with a red zone of hyperaemia at the margins.

The presence of large numbers of macrophages corresponds with what is seen in the **demolition** phase of an inflammatory reaction, and is of equal importance in the context of infarction. In some tissues, for example the **heart**, dead parenchymal cells are removed rapidly and there is an equally rapid replacement of these cells, first by granulation tissue and then by scar tissue. In other situations, such as the **kidney**, the infarcted area persists, sometimes for months, before being replaced by scar tissue. Histological examination of such an area shows the 'ghost outlines' of the architectural elements of the tissue, the tubules and glomeruli, although the constituent parenchymal cells are clearly dead. A slow but progressive ingrowth of connective tissue occurs even in these cases and, eventually, the infarct becomes converted to a fibrous scar in which calcium salts may be deposited (dystrophic calcification).

The sequence of events described above may be interrupted, at any time, by the death of the patient.

Infarction in Specific Sites

The central nervous system

The generalizations made above relating to the development of infarcts do not apply to the brain. Here the processes involved after part of the brain has been rendered ischaemic are somewhat different. The type of necrosis is typically liquefactive rather than coagulative and this may, in the long term, lead to the formation of a cavity. Histologically, the early stages of the development of a cerebral infarct are characterized by a transient neutrophil response which is followed by a period of intense phagocytic activity by the **microglial cells**. These cells, which, in their resting phase, are normally small, cluster in the infarcted area and phagocytose the lipid which is liberated from degenerate myelin. The cytoplasm of the microglia, therefore, increases in bulk very markedly and appears foamy or granular in appearance. (Classically these swollen microglia are referred to as **compound granular corpuscles**). Reactive astrocytes now gather at the margins of the infarcted area and synthesize new glial fibres, which eventually replace part or all of the infarcted tissue.

The heart

Cardiac ischaemia is the single most important cause of death in Western communities. Approximately 150 000 adults in the United Kingdom die every year from ischaemic heart disease (about 25% of all deaths). A decrease in the arterial perfusion of the myocardium may express itself in a number of ways, and it is important to realize that, while all occur against the background of myocardial ischaemia, the different clinical pictures may be brought about by different pathogenetic mechanisms. The patients may:

1. Complain of angina on effort
2. Die suddenly
3. Develop acute myocardial necrosis (infarction) of different patterns and with different underlying pathogenetic processes
4. Develop failure of muscle pumping activity

Angina pectoris

At autopsy on patients dying **with** rather than **from** angina pectoris, the myocardium may show no macroscopic abnormalities. In some instances there will have been ischaemic necrosis of small groups of heart muscle cells; the marker of this having taken place is the presence of small flecks of fibrous tissue in the muscle wall of the left ventricle. The coronary arteries invariably show the presence of stenosing atherosclerotic lesions which may affect one or more of the major coronary artery branches.

Sudden death

Sudden death may be defined as death occurring from myocardial ischaemia within one hour of the onset of acute symptoms. In practice many of these deaths occur within a few minutes. Sudden death is a major part of the overall problem of ischaemic heart disease, since at least 50% of the deaths due to a first attack of ischaemia occur in this way and without the patient having the benefit of medical attention. Death is due to the onset of severe ventricular arrhythmias, most notably ventricular fibrillation, these being associated with loss of cardiac output. Of the patients who collapse with such severe arrhythmias and who are resuscitated, only 16% develop a Q wave on electrocardiography (suggestive of myocardial necrosis involving most of the left ventricular wall thickness) and 45% show elevations in the plasma concentrations of enzymes derived from heart muscle. Thus a majority of these living patients show no clinical or biochemical evidence of their arrhythmia being associated with acute myocardial necrosis. Post-mortem examination of patients dying suddenly in this way reveals evidence of acute, though not necessarily occlusive thrombosis in a majority. The prevalence of **occlusive thrombi** is lower than in patients dying with myocardial infarction. Narrowing of coronary artery lumina by 80% or more is very frequent in these patients.

Acute myocardial necrosis

Acute myocardial necrosis occurs in two distinct patterns, although, from time to time, a combination of these may be seen. It is useful to be able to distinguish between these patterns since the pathogenesis of each differs considerably. Before being able to distinguish between the **patterns** of acute myocardial necrosis, it is necessary to be able to identify irreversibly damaged heart muscle. If the heart is examined some 18 to 36 hours after the onset of severe underperfusion there is no problem. The ischaemic heart muscle shows all the features of coagulative necrosis; macroscopically the necrotic area is a dull, yellowish, 'wash-leather'-like colour with a hyperaemic zone at the periphery. However, if the patient dies at an earlier stage of the natural history of myocardial necrosis, recognition of ischaemic damage is much more difficult. So long as the patient has survived six to nine hours after the onset of the acute ischaemia, the difficulty can be overcome by using a simple histochemical technique. This depends on the fact (see p. 19) that a cell which is irreversibly damaged loses its intracellular content of water-soluble enzymes. The presence of respiratory enzymes, such as succinic dehydrogenase, in normal heart muscle can be shown by immersing a slice of unfixed heart muscle in a solution of the dye nitroblue tetrazolium. This is a yellow dye which acts as a hydrogen acceptor. In the presence of a cell with a normal content of dehydrogenase, the yellow dye turns a bluish-purple colour and is deposited on the tissue at the site where the reaction has taken place. Where a cell has been irreversibly damaged and has lost its intracellular dehydrogenases, no such colour reaction takes place. Thus, viable and non-viable muscle can be distinguished from each other with relative ease.

Regional myocardial infarction. The commonest pattern of acute ischaemic necrosis in the myocardium is so-called regional infarction

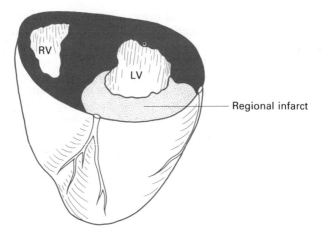

Fig. 21.3 Regional myocardial infarction with a large area of coagulative necrosis (more than 50% of the left ventricle thickness). The infarct is in the territory of the anterior descending branch of the left coronary artery. Occlusive thrombosis is found in about 95% of such cases. RV = right ventricle; LV = left ventricle.

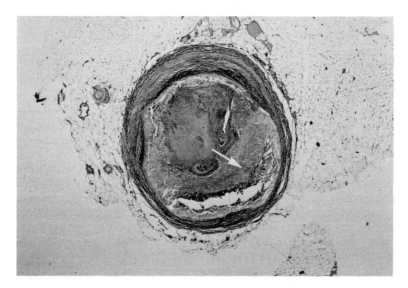

Fig. 21.4 Acute occlusive coronary artery thrombosis occurring in relation to a split in the thin connective tissue cap of an atherosclerotic plaque (arrow). Such fissuring of plaque with the formation of both intra-plaque and intra-luminal thrombi is the most frequent antecedent of acute occlusion in the coronary artery tree.

(Fig. 21.3). This occurs as a large single area of coagulative necrosis, measuring at least 3 cm along one of its axes and usually involving more than 50% of the thickness of the ventricular wall. In more than 90% of cases this pattern of necrosis is associated with occlusive thrombosis in the coronary artery segment supplying the affected area of muscle, and the majority of these thrombi occur in relation to breaks in the connective tissue caps of underlying atherosclerotic plaques (Fig. 21.4).

Subendocardial necrosis. Subendocardial necrosis in its pure form is much less commonly seen than regional infarction at necropsy. Here the ischaemic necrosis is confined to the **inner half** of the left ventricular myocardium, a very thin layer of viable muscle immediately beneath the endocardium always being present (Fig. 21.5). This type of

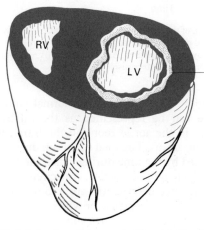

Subendocardial necrosis

Fig. 21.5 Subendocardial necrosis. The global involvement of the left ventricle wall suggests a generalized fall in perfusion. Occlusive thrombosis is found in about 15% of such cases. RV = right ventricle; LV = left ventricle.

necrosis may be segmental or can extend to involve the whole circumference of the left ventricle. Occlusive thrombi in the coronary arteries are found in only about 15% of cases, though severe stenosing atherosclerosis is widespread within the coronary artery tree.

Subendocardial ischaemic necrosis is the morphological expression of a **generalized lowering** of myocardial perfusion. It can occur in the absence of coronary artery disease in such situations as severe aortic stenosis or incompetence. Its pathogenesis can be understood most easily if one recalls two facts. These are (a) that perfusion of the myocardium takes place during **diastole**, and (b) that the wall tension in the left ventricular myocardium is greater in the subendocardial zone

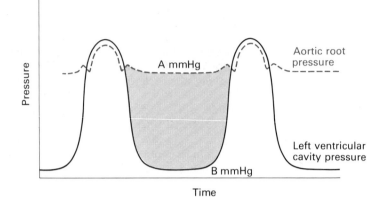

Fig. 21.6 Factors controlling perfusion of the subendocardial zone of the left ventricular wall. Perfusion 'drive' = A mmHg − B mmHg. Total diastolic perfusion = (A − B) × length of diastole, and is represented by the shaded area. Any decrease in (A − B) or in the length of diastole may lead to subendocardial necrosis.

than in the subepicardial region. In a person with normal coronary arteries, the **perfusion drive** can be represented as the difference between the diastolic pressure in the aortic root and the intra-cavity pressure in the left ventricle (Fig. 21.6). The total perfusion during any single cardiac cycle is determined by the time during which the drive is allowed to act and, hence, by the length of diastole. Any circumstances which lessens the pressure difference between the aortic root pressure and the intra-cavity pressure in the left ventricle or which shortens the diastolic interval may reduce myocardial perfusion sufficiently to produce ischaemic necrosis.

Complications of myocardial infarction. Each stage of the natural history of myocardial infarction may hold dangers for the patient (Fig. 21.7).

In the early stages the chief danger is the possible development of ventricular fibrillation leading to asystole and sudden death. As the coagulative necrosis develops and the dead muscle elicits a brisk acute inflammatory response, focal softening of necrotic muscle may occur. This can lead to rupture of the left ventricle, either of the free wall into the pericardial cavity, death being due to the rapid accumulation of blood within the pericardial sac (**cardiac tamponade**), or of the septum, with the production of a defect in the interventricular septum. Similar softening can affect the papillary muscles; if rupture of one or more of these occurs, the patient will develop a torrential regurgitant jet through the mitral valve. A somewhat less dramatic development of

Development of
arrhythmogenic
focus ↓

'Sudden death'

Infarct development

Very large area
of infarction
with acute
'pump failure'

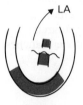

Rupture of
necrotic
papillary
muscle ↓

Acute severe
mitral
regurgitation

Rupture through infarct
(of free wall→haemopericardium;
of septum ──→ventricular septal
defect)

Mural thrombosis
over infarct

↓

May lead to
systemic emboli

Extensive
post-ischaemic
fibrosis
↓
Chronic 'pump
failure'

Post-ischaemic papillary
muscle atrophy

↓

Mitral regurgitation

Stretching of
scar tissue

↓

Ventricular
aneurysm

Fig. 21.7 Possible consequences of myocardial infarction.

mitral valve incompetence which is not uncommonly seen may occur simply as a result of ischaemic necrosis and scarring of papillary muscles.

The abnormal haemodynamics that can occur within the left ventricular cavity following infarction may lead to the formation of mural thrombi. Portions of these can break off and embolize the systemic circulation.

Healing of the infarcted muscle can also be associated with circumstances unfavourable to the patient. If there has been extensive loss of cardiac muscle in the process of infarction, correspondingly large amounts of fibrous tissue are formed during healing. This collagenous tissue lacks the power of recoil possessed by muscle and due to the normal rise of intra-cavity pressure during ventricular systole becomes gradually stretched and thinned. This may lead to a local dilatation or **ventricular aneurysm**, which can be a severe haemodynamic disadvantage to the patient. Extensive fibrosis following infarction of the anterior wall of the left ventricle may involve both bundle branches and lead to complete heart block.

The lung

Fewer than 10% of pulmonary emboli cause infarction in the lung, a figure which emphasizes the importance of the state of the pulmonary circulation at the time when embolization occurs. In young people, whose cardiac status is good, infarction is rare. This relative sparing is thought to be due, at least in part, to the double blood supply of the lung from the pulmonary and bronchial arteries.

Any rise in pressure in the pulmonary veins, as occurs in mitral stenosis or left ventricular failure, markedly increases the chances of infarction occurring if medium-sized branches of the pulmonary arteries become occluded. The vast majority of infarcts are due to emboli derived from thrombi in the leg veins; about 10% are, however, derived from thrombi formed in the right side of the heart.

Pulmonary infarcts are generally described as being wedge-shaped, with the base of the wedge situated towards the pleural aspect of the lung. In their early stages they are deep red in colour. At necropsy these infarcts are often more easily felt than seen. A fibrinous pleural reaction over the infarcted area is common and there may, on occasions, be small haemorrhagic effusions in the pleural cavity. Organization of pulmonary infarcts usually proceeds rapidly, perhaps because of the vascular network in the surrounding lung tissue. The infarcts are converted into inconspicuous scars, which tend to be concealed by the surrounding lung tissue, which often shows compensatory overdistension.

The liver

True infarcts in the liver are rare, presumably because spontaneous occlusion of the hepatic artery is correspondingly rare and because, like the lung, the liver has a double blood supply. However, accidental ligation of the hepatic artery in the course of surgery may produce true infarcts in the liver. Patchy hepatic infarction may also occur if hepatic artery branches within the liver are involved in immune complex mediated diseases such as polyarteritis nodosa.

The intestine

The commonest causes of intestinal ischaemia are mechanical: hernial strangulation, volvulus (twisting of a segment of intestine) and

(a)

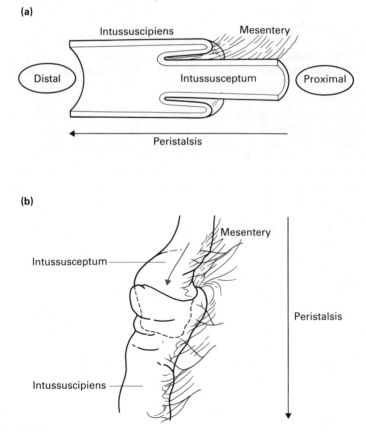

Fig. 21.8 Intussusception.

intussusception. In the latter, excessive peristaltic contraction drives the affected segment of bowel forward, so that the segment of bowel immediately distal lies in a sleeve-like manner over it (Fig. 21.8). Some of the mesentery is included in that portion of bowel which is pushed forward and the resulting local oedema leads to local ischaemia. Apart from such mechanical disasters, intestinal ischaemia can result from thrombotic or embolic occlusion of the mesenteric arteries or even from extensive mesenteric venous thrombosis (see p. 324). In this last instance the interference with venous drainage leads to a very marked degree of congestion affecting the mucosal and submucosal vessels and the patient may pass fresh blood per rectum. When the degree of intestinal ischaemia is sufficient to cause infarction, the bowel wall feels stiffer than normal and is a dark plum colour. The serosal surface is the site of a fibrinous inflammatory response, so that instead of the normal shiny appearance of the serosa, it is dull and slightly roughened. The necrotic bowel wall becomes colonized quite rapidly by the saprophytic organisms in the lumen and thus may show the features of true gangrene. Factors which may contribute to the death of such patients include intestinal paralysis (ileus) with loss of fluid and electrolytes into the gut lumen, haemorrhage, perforation, which causes generalized peritonitis, and bacteraemic shock.

Ischaemia of the gut need not lead in all cases to such a dramatic conclusion. It is now well recognized that periods of lowered arterial perfusion, affecting particularly the region of the splenic flexure, may lead to localized mucosal ulceration. Healing of these ulcers is accompanied by a very considerable degree of scar tissue formation, which may lead to localized narrowing of the gut lumen in the affected areas. During the healing phase these post-ischaemic ulcers show the presence of a broad band of granulation tissue extending into the submucosa and containing many macrophages laden with iron derived from broken-down red blood cells (haemosiderin).

Chapter 22

Abnormal Accumulations of Fluid and Disturbances of Blood Distribution

Among the most important requirements for good health is that there should be a normal quantitative relationship between intra- and extravascular fluid. A disturbance in this relationship can produce life-threatening situations in certain anatomical situations, notably the lung and the brain. Closely associated may be alterations in the distribution of blood in various tissue beds leading, for one reason or another, to local increases in the amount of blood present in a given organ or tissue.

Oedema

Oedema, in the context of the circulatory system, may be defined as an abnormal accumulation of fluid in the extracellular space. (This, therefore, excludes the increases in cytoplasmic sodium and water considered in the section on cell injury.) From a simple clinical point of view, the recognition of oedema depends on the identification of excess fluid within the interstitial tissues.

Total body water is of the order of 49 litres. Of this, the intracellular component accounts for about 35 litres and this varies very little. The intravascular compartment contains about 3 litres, and a further 11 litres are present in the extravascular compartment. The maintenance of a relatively constant relationship between intra- and extravascular water depends on a number of factors.

Those which tend to cause fluid to **leave the vascular compartment** include:

1. **Intravascular hydrostatic pressure**. An increase in hydrostatic pressure within the vascular compartment may produce profound changes in fluid distribution. For instance, severe mitral stenosis will lead to a chronic rise in the pulmonary venous pressure and hence to a rise in pulmonary capillary pressure. If such a patient takes severe exercise, the resulting increase in pulmonary artery pressure may be

sufficient on its own account to overcome all other relevant homeostatic mechanisms and fluid will pass from the pulmonary alveolar capillaries first into the alveolar walls and then into the air spaces themselves.
2. The **colloid osmotic pressure in the extravascular compartment.** If this is increased more fluid tends to leave the microvasculature.

Those factors which, under normal circumstances tend to **keep fluid within the vascular compartment** are:

1. The **osmotic pressure of the plasma proteins,** of which albumin, with its relatively low molecular weight and its high concentration relative to other plasma proteins, is the most important. A fall in the plasma concentration of albumin, due either to reduced synthesis, as in chronic liver disease, or to excessive loss, as in certain forms of kidney disease, may be associated with quite severe oedema.
2. The **selective permeability function of endothelium.** Normally albumin does not leave the vascular compartment in significant amounts. Should the permeability barrier function of the capillary wall become impaired, there will be a decline in the plasma concentration of albumin and a corresponding increase in the protein content of the fluid in the interstitial tissues.
3. The **tissue tension** in the interstitial tissue tends to limit the egress of fluid from the microvasculature. Normally this is low (less than 1 kPa).

All these physical factors can be summed up in the following mathematical expression:

$$\mathbf{J_v} = \mathbf{k}[(\mathbf{P_c} - \mathbf{P_i}) - \mathbf{II_c} - \mathbf{II_i})]$$

where $\mathbf{J_v}$ is the local rate of fluid flux along the length of a capillary; $\mathbf{k}$ is the capillary hydraulic permeability; $\mathbf{P_c}$ is the capillary hydraulic pressure; $\mathbf{P_i}$ is the hydraulic pressure in the interstitial fluid; $\mathbf{II_c}$ is capillary plasma colloid osmotic pressure, and $\mathbf{II_i}$ is the colloid osmotic pressure in the interstitial fluid.

Under normal circumstances there is a **nett loss** of fluid from the vascular compartment to the interstitial tissue but no oedema develops. This is because the excess fluid enters the lymphatic channels and drains away from the site where it might otherwise accumulate, eventually returning to the blood via the thoracic duct. Should the normal flow of lymph be obstructed, oedema fluid will collect.

Oedema may be either **local** or **systemic.** The characteristics of the oedema fluid depend on the mechanisms predominantly involved in its formation (Table 22.1). If the collection of fluid in the interstitial tissues is associated with an increase in **vascular permeability** then the fluid will contain large amounts of macromolecular proteins including fibrinogen and is termed an **exudate.** If the mechanisms involved are

Table 22.1 The characteristics of exudates and transudates.

Characteristic	Exudate	Transudate
Total protein	High	Low (1g/100ml)
Protein pattern	As in plasma	Albumin only
Fibrinogen	+ + (and clots)	Nil
Specific gravity	1.020	1.012
Cells	+ +	Few mesothelial cells

predominantly **hydrostatic** then the protein content of the oedema fluid will be low; such fluid is spoken of as being a **transudate**.

In practical terms the three most important factors which must be considered in the common forms of oedema are:

raised intracapillary pressure
low plasma oncotic pressure
retention of salt and water

The coexistence of any two of these is likely to be associated with oedema of considerable severity.

Systemic oedema

Cardiac oedema

Although the systemic oedema caused by congestive cardiac failure has been recognized for many centuries, the mechanisms involved are by no means simple or easy to understand. There is not only a redistribution but a general retention of fluid, this being shown by an increase in body weight of the patient. The distribution of the excess fluid is largely determined by gravity. When the patient is ambulant, the legs are first involved and swelling of the ankles at the end of the day is often the first sign reported. When the patient is confined to bed, the oedema appears in the sacral or, less commonly, in the genital regions. The oedematous areas pit readily on finger pressure. It would be tempting to ascribe this oedema purely to failure of the pumping function of the ventricles leading to an increase in venous pressure and a consequent increase in capillary hydrostatic pressure with the formation of a transudate. However, this would be not only a gross oversimplification, but also incorrect, though this mechanism does make some contribution to the development of cardiac oedema.

Doubt as to a significant role for back pressure in cardiac oedema arises from three observations:

1. There is an increased **blood volume** in heart failure, and this increase may occur before there is any rise in central venous pressure.

2. Oedema itself frequently occurs before there is any rise in central venous pressure.

3. The degree of oedema is not proportional to the height of the central venous pressure.

The most important mechanism in causing the oedema of cardiac failure is excess retention of sodium and water by the renal tubules. Failure of the heart as a pump leads initially to a fall in mean capillary pressure. This will in turn lead to a reduction in renal perfusion, which is aggravated by vasoconstriction mediated by the sympathetic nervous system. This relative renal ischaemia causes an increase in the production of renin and thus of angiotensin I. The rise in angiotensin causes an increased release of aldosterone from the zona glomerulosa of the adrenal cortex and retention of sodium and water (Fig. 22.1). At first, such retention of sodium and water has a good effect since it allows the mean filling pressure in the circulation to be increased. The

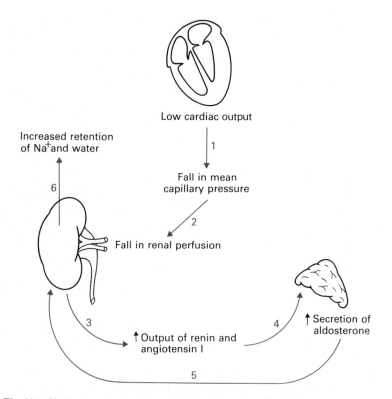

Fig. 22.1 Mechanisms involved in causing the oedema of cardiac failure.

increased filling of the heart stretches the heart muscle fibres and thus leads, in terms of Starling's law, to increased force of contraction. In due time, however, any advantage arising from sodium and water retention is lost.

Once cardiac filling pressure and hence stretching of muscle fibres exceeds a certain point, there is no further increase in cardiac output; indeed there is a decline in the work output of the cardiac muscle. Excess accumulation of fluid in the lung (pulmonary oedema) may ensue and this may interfere with gas exchange in the alveoli.

Renal oedema

Oedema related to renal disorders occurs under two different sets of circumstances.

Oedema associated with acute glomerulonephritis. Oedema is often a presenting feature in this disease, though it is usually not severe. The face and eyelids are affected predominantly, though on some occasions the ankles and genitalia may be involved as well. There is no entirely satisfactory explanation either for the cause of the oedema or for its distribution. However, it is likely that the control of sodium excretion in the urine is multifactorial and that states of sodium retention may exist in which there is no associated disturbance of plasma volume. Although in most examples of systemic oedema the kidney behaves as if it were responding to a low plasma volume stimulus, there are other factors such as intrarenal vascular resistance, renal nervous activity, circulating catecholamines, plasma levels of aldosterone, and intrarenal hormones such as prostaglandins or kinins which may all influence renal tubular handling of sodium. It has been suggested that the primary mechanism responsible for **nephritic oedema** is a fall in glomerular filtration rate, tubular reabsorption of sodium remaining more or less normal. The resulting increase in extracellular fluid volume would normally be followed by a brisk natriuresis but this response appears to be blunted in acute glomerulonephritis. The oedema fluid in acute glomerulonephritis has the characteristics of a transudate, indicating that no significant change has occurred in the permeability of the microcirculation.

Oedema associated with the nephrotic syndrome. The nephrotic syndrome encompasses a group of features which most notably includes heavy proteinuria (in excess of the ability of the liver to synthesize albumin) leading to hypoalbuminaemia and a resulting decrease in plasma oncotic pressure. While this loss of plasma protein certainly plays a part in the genesis of the systemic oedema encountered in this syndrome, other mechanisms also operate, including excess retention of sodium by the renal tubules. This is partly due to increased aldosterone production by the adrenal cortex, but some workers believe that non-systemic intrarenal mechanisms related to sodium reabsorption are of greater importance.

Nutritional oedema

Oedema is a well recognized feature of prolonged starvation. There is no correlation between the degree of oedema and the concentrations within the blood of albumin and other plasma proteins; indeed, oedema associated with starvation may be seen in the presence of normal concentrations of plasma protein. It has been suggested that the explanation for this variety of oedema lies in the loss of subcutaneous adipose tissue. This leads to a subcutaneous connective tissue of much looser texture than normal and an associated decline in the tissue tension within it. Bed rest is usually followed by a brisk diuresis and consequent lessening of the degree of oedema. An important and, regrettably, common variant of nutritional oedema occurs in **kwashior-kor**, which results from protein undernutrition in young children among economically deprived communities in Africa, Asia and Central and South America. These children, who fail to grow normally, are anaemic and have grossly fatty livers. They often exhibit a curious combination of oedema, mucocutaneous ulceration (the skin of the inner thighs often looks as if it has been scalded), and depigmentation of the hair. Adequate nutrition in terms of the protein content of the diet can produce a complete return to normal.

Oedema due to chronic liver disease

In so far as oedema is concerned, its chief expression in the context of chronic liver disease is the accumulation of fluid within the peritoneal cavity. This is known as **ascites**. Significant amounts of ascitic fluid are unlikely to accumulate in the absence of **obstruction to hepatic venous outflow**. The hepatic sinusoids are extremely permeable to protein, and hepatic lymph has a very high protein content. Plasma oncotic pressure is, therefore, unlikely to be a powerful determinant in maintaining normal relationships between intravascular and extravascular fluid in the liver, and the direction of fluid movement across the sinusoidal walls will be determined very largely by changes in sinusoidal hydrostatic pressure. With the development of portal hypertension, the 'holding capacity' of the splanchnic vasculature in terms of blood volume increases and the non-splanchnic or non-portal component of the plasma volume decreases. This results in the renal tubule being stimulated to retain sodium and water and, thus, in an increased total plasma volume. It is not clear whether the ascitic fluid accumulates purely because of an increase in hepatic lymph flow of a degree which results in the capacity of the thoracic duct to drain it away being exceeded, or whether sodium retention and expansion of the plasma volume are equally important. In this connection it is interesting to note that when ascitic fluid is drained in experimental situations it does not reaccumulate rapidly if the animal is kept on a sodium-free diet. Patients with chronic liver disease often have a decreased plasma concentration of albumin. As already noted, this can make no significant contribution to the passage of fluid from the intrahepatic sinusoids, which are very permeable to protein. However, this does not apply to the splanchnic capillaries and hypoalbuminaemia may well have a significant role in relation to fluid leakage from these vessels. It has also been suggested that in chronic liver disease related to prolonged excess alcohol intake, basement membrane-like material may be deposited in the walls of the sinusoids, making them relatively impermeable to protein. In these circumstances hypoalbuminaemia could make a contribution to the leakage of fluid from the sinusoids.

Pulmonary oedema

The blood pressure in the pulmonary circulation is about 2–3 kPa (15–23 mmHg) systolic and about 1–1.5 kPa (7.5–11 mmHg) diastolic. The pulmonary capillary pressure varies from 0.5–1.5 kPa (4–11 mmHg), being highest at the lung bases and lowest at the apices. In this connection it is not without interest that pulmonary oedema is usually most severe at the lung bases. The interstitial fluid pressure is negative owing to the elastic recoil of the lung tissue. The negative intrathoracic pressure is about −1 kPa (−7.5 mmHg) in forced inspiration and about −0.5 kPa (−4 mmHg) in forced expiration. Both these forces tend to drive fluid out of the capillaries into the interstitial tissue and thence into the alveoli, but under normal circumstances the plasma oncotic pressure within the alveolar capillaries is more than adequate to overcome these effects.

Causes of pulmonary oedema. In clinical practice the commonest causes of pulmonary oedema are left ventricular failure and 'tight' mitral stenosis. In both these situations the rise in pulmonary capillary pressure consequent on increases in pulmonary vein pressure plays an important role in the escape of fluid from the alveolar capillaries to the interstitial tissue. However, this is by no means the whole story, as anyone who has seen the swift relief conferred by an injection of morphine in the severe dyspnoea of acute pulmonary oedema will readily appreciate.

Especially in the acute variant of pulmonary oedema, which often occurs during sleep or in any event while the patient is lying down, there is an important sympathetic reflex component. Characteristically, such a patient shows an increase in heart rate and blood pressure, sweats profusely and has dilated pupils. This syndrome can be mimicked by giving adrenalin and can be aborted by quite small doses of drugs which block the sympathetic ganglia. It is believed that overaction of the sympathetic nervous system may cause systemic peripheral vasoconstriction with displacement of blood from the systemic to the pulmonary circulation.

The view that neurogenic factors can play a considerable part in the pathogenesis of heart disease-related pulmonary oedema is strengthened by the finding that severe pulmonary oedema may be induced in small animals by injecting protein solutions into the cerebral ventricles. This finding has some application in clinical medicine since patients with **head injuries** or suffering from **subarachnoid haemorrhage** sometimes develop severe pulmonary oedema.

Once a significant degree of pulmonary oedema has been established, there are local circumstances in the pulmonary vascular bed which tend to aggravate the situation. These are, first, the fact that the endothelial cells of the alveolar capillaries are oxygenated directly from the alveolar air rather than from the pulmonary vein blood, and, second, that plasma oncotic pressure is an extremely important mechanism in keeping the alveoli free from oedema fluid. The presence of a significant degree of oedema can lead to defective oxygenation of the alveolar endothelium and hence to some decline in its efficiency as a permeability barrier. The consequent loss of protein from the capillaries results in a lowering of the intra-capillary oncotic pressure and this tends to make the oedema worse. Such changes in the permeability of the pulmonary capillaries constitute the chief mechanism for the development of pulmonary oedema in the absence of heart disease. This is seen in a variety of circumstances, such as after exposure to irritating gases, in various inflammatory diseases affecting the lung, in patients or in domestic animals after having been transferred from sea level to very high altitudes, and in renal failure, and is known as the acute respiratory distress syndrome of adults.

Local oedema

Local oedema may occur as a result of three types of pathological disturbance. Firstly, a **local increase** in the **hydrostatic pressure within the microcirculation** may be operating. This can occur in pregnancy, in patients with occlusive venous thrombosis, and in those with varicose veins where the valves are incompetent. Secondly, **increased local vascular permeability** can result in local oedema, as in acute inflammation and type I hypersensitivity reactions such as urticaria and angioneurotic oedema. Lastly, the maintenance of the interstitial fluid volume within narrow limits requires normal lymphatic drainage, and any obstruction to the normal flow of lymph as a result of surgery or inflammation may cause quite severe local oedema. For example, some patients who undergo radical surgery for the removal of carcinoma of the breast and have the axillary tissue dissected and removed develop severe and intractable oedema of the arm on the side of the operation. The inflammatory disease classically associated with lymphatic obstruction is infestation by the nematode worm *Wuchereria bancrofti* (filariasis). In its adult form the worm inhabits the lymphatics in the groin. While it is alive the presence of the parasite produces little disability, but when it dies there is a brisk local inflammatory reaction which leads, eventually, to lymphatic obstruction. The resulting oedema of the lower limbs and the genitalia is severe and chronic — so severe that the condition is sometimes spoken of as **elephantiasis**. Sometimes lymphoedema may develop as a result of congenital malformations in the lymphatic drainage; an autosomal dominant variety of this is known as Milroy's disease.

Hyperaemia and Congestion

These two terms, which are used more or less as synonyms, mean that there is a **greater amount of blood than normal** in a given organ or tissue. Clearly there can be only two mechanisms for this: an **increased inflow** or a **diminished outflow** of blood.

Increased inflow of blood must be achieved by arteriolar dilatation and is known as **active** hyperaemia. It is seen in areas involved in acute inflammation, after exposure to excess heat, in flushing, and at the margins of areas of ischaemic necrosis.

Diminished outflow is essentially an obstructive phenomenon. The obstruction may be functional rather than structural. An example of this is to be found in some patients with chronic bronchitis in whom the resultant hypoxia causes reflex constriction of the pulmonary arterioles. This leads to a rise in pulmonary artery pressure and hence, in due time, to a rise in central venous pressure and congestion of various organs. Because of the basically obstructive nature of the phenomenon, congestion of this type is generally spoken of as **passive**. As in the case of oedema, passive congestion can be generalized or local.

Generalized venous congestion

In its acute form, generalized venous congestion may be seen in many patients who die suddenly from a variety of causes; it represents the sudden accumulation of blood behind a failing ventricle with resulting engorgement of the affected organs or tissues. However, in clinical practice, generalized venous congestion is most often manifest in its chronic form, the basic cause being, once again, a failing ventricle. The mechanisms involved in the accumulation of blood are covered earlier in the discussion relating to cardiac oedema (see p. 341). It results partly from the rise in pressure in the pulmonary and systemic veins, and partly (in so far as the pulmonary circulation is concerned) from the shift of blood from the systemic to the pulmonary circulation as a result of peripheral vasoconstriction.

This sequence of events can take place under a number of different sets of circumstances. These include:

1. Primary 'pump' failure. This may be due either to loss of heart muscle (following ischaemia or inflammation) or to some primary heart muscle disorder (cardiomyopathy).
2. Obstruction to normal outflow from the left ventricle. This may be due either to a **functional** cause (e.g. a rise in peripheral resistance, such as occurs in hypertension) or to a **structural** one (e.g. one of the variants of aortic valve stenosis).
3. Incompetence of either the aortic or mitral valve
4. Obstruction to ventricular inflow. This is seen classically in pure mitral stenosis where, despite the absence of cardiac failure, there is a rise in pulmonary venous pressure.

In all the forms of heart disease mentioned above, venous congestion is first evident in the pulmonary vascular bed, though in time systemic venous congestion also occurs.

Generalized venous congestion also occurs in a variety of pulmonary disorders associated with a rise in pulmonary artery pressure. This leads to a compensatory increase in the muscle mass of the right ventricle (work hypertrophy). In time the right ventricle may be unable to maintain a normal output in the face of the pulmonary hypertension and when this happens there is a rise in systemic venous pressure, and congestion in organs such as the liver and spleen. This form of cardiac failure is known as **cor pulmonale** and may be the result of disorders affecting the bronchioles and alveoli, thoracic movements, or the pulmonary vasculature.

Morphology and pathophysiology of cor pulmonale

The characteristic change seen in cor pulmonale is right ventricular hypertrophy secondary to pulmonary hypertension. The pulmonary circulation is a low pressure system where an increase in cardiac output (as with exercise) produces no increase in pulmonary artery pressure until the flow has increased to three times the normal. Once this level has been exceeded, there is a fairly steep, linear rise in pressure in proportion to the increase in flow. This ability of the pulmonary arterial bed to accept increased blood flow of a very considerable degree without a concomitant rise in pressure has important clinical implications. More than 50% of the pulmonary vascular bed must be destroyed or obstructed before pulmonary hypertension will be present at rest. Of course, any decrease in the pulmonary vascular bed will mean that smaller rises in cardiac output are required to raise the pulmonary artery pressure, and the more severe the reduction in capacity of the pulmonary circulation, the less the rise in cardiac output will need to be. Pulmonary hypertension, however, is quite common in the absence of destruction of part of the pulmonary vasculature. It arises due to pulmonary vasoconstriction which occurs in the pulmonary arterioles as a response to hypoxia. This is frequently seen in diseases associated with chronic obstruction to air flow, such as chronic bronchitis.

Morphological changes of chronic venous congestion

Generally speaking, chronically congested organs are swollen, darker in colour and firmer in consistency than normal.

The lung. On histological examination, marked engorgement of the alveolar capillaries is seen, each capillary being stuffed with blood. This distension of the capillaries gives the alveolar septa a beaded appearance. Quite often small intra-alveolar haemorrhages are seen due to rupture of the overdistended capillaries. This may be so marked a feature (especially in patients with severe pulmonary venous hypertension, as in mitral stenosis) that the patient coughs up blood-stained sputum (**haemoptysis**). The red blood cells break down and the iron-containing moiety of haemoglobin becomes converted to a yellow-brown crystalline pigment known as haemosiderin. This pigment is engulfed by alveolar macrophages, which then become known as **siderophages** or 'heart failure cells'. With the passage of time the congested alveolar septa become thicker than normal. In the early stages of chronic pulmonary venous congestion this is largely due to the presence of oedema fluid within the interstitial tissue of the septa. Later, fibrosis occurs within the septa and the lung tissue becomes much firmer than normal. The combination of a significant degree of iron pigmentation and interstitial fibrosis in long-standing pulmonary congestion is known as **brown induration**.

The liver. The structural changes seen in the chronically congested liver of a patient suffering from cardiac failure result from a combination of two processes. These are, firstly, a rise in pressure in the hepatic veins, central veins and sinusoids, and, secondly, poor perfusion of that part of the hepatic lobule which is furthest from its arterial supply.

As a result of the hepatic vein congestion, the central veins become distended and crammed with red blood cells. This overdistension may extend to involve the sinusoids in the central part of the lobule. The combination of high intra-sinusoidal pressure in the central part of the lobule and the poor oxygenation of the cells in this area leads to a decrease in the size of the liver cells and, eventually, to their disappearance (**atrophy**). In the centrilobular and midzonal areas the liver cells show evidence of hypoxia in the form of fatty change. Macroscopically, the combination of central congestion and paren-chymal fatty change leads to a characteristic mottled appearance which is known as '**nutmeg liver**'. In essence, this consists of an exaggeration of the normal lobular pattern, with the central veins and the sinusoids round them appearing as dark red spots. Surrounding this is a zone of pale yellow tissue which represents that part of the hepatic lobule in which fatty change is present. In examples of very severe and long-standing hepatic venous congestion, the reticulin strands along which the cords of liver cells are arranged collapse onto one another and the central zones of the lobules become fibrosed. This stage of the process is sometimes termed '**cardiac cirrhosis**', but the use of this term should be avoided since neither the pathological events nor the morphological alterations satisfy the criteria of a true cirrhosis (continuing liver cell loss, active formation of new fibrous septa, and parenchymal regeneration).

The spleen. The congested spleen is moderately enlarged (up to 250 g) and is of firmer consistency than normal. The cut surface is smooth and firm and the red pulp is a dark, purplish colour. Histologically, the presence of congestion is shown by the distension of the sinusoids, which are packed with red blood cells. There is some increase in the amount of reticulin in the walls of the sinusoids and also in the connective tissue in the trabecula.

Local venous congestion

This results from obstruction to the flow of venous blood from any part of an organ or tissue. It is usually due either to thrombosis in the local venous drainage or to pressure on veins from without as, for example, if a large tumour mass is present. The consequences will depend largely on the speed with which the obstruction to venous return develops and the effectiveness of any collateral draining systems.

Acute venous obstruction

If venous obstruction is acute, the presence of an effective collateral drainage system is vital if local oedema and, in some instances, haemorrhage are to be avoided. For example, if large veins in relation to the brain become obstructed, their tributaries will become severely engorged and, since collateral draining systems are absent, haemorrhages from the swollen tributary veins are not uncommon. A similar sequence of events may occur when a hernia becomes impacted. The venous drainage from a segment of the intestine may be obstructed completely; the bowel wall then becomes engorged with blood and may become necrotic.

When local venous obstruction is chronic, the collateral veins usually become markedly distended and may, under certain circumstances, rupture. This is seen in **portal hypertension**, which may occur as a result of disturbances in hepatic lobular architecture brought about by the processes involved in cirrhosis, as a result of pathological changes in the portal tracts, or as a result of obstruction to the portal vein itself. The rise in portal vein blood pressure leads to distension of the short gastric veins and of the anastomotic veins at the lower end of the oesophagus; this confers a risk of serious haemorrhage.

Chapter 23

Pigmentation and Heterotopic Calcification

Pigmentation

The pigments which may accumulate in excess amounts within the tissues or which may occur in abnormally small amounts can be separated into an endogenous group and an exogenous group.

Endogenous pigments are those which are produced within the body; there are three main types of such pigments:

1. Melanin
2. Pigments derived from haemoglobin
3. Pigments associated with fats

Melanin

Melanin constitutes the colouring matter of the hair, skin and eyes. It is also normally present in the leptomeninges, the nerve cells in the substantia nigra and the adrenal medulla. Limited pigmentation due to melanin may also occur in the juxtacutaneous mucous membranes of the vulva and mouth. Melanin-producing cells may also be found in small numbers in the ovary, gastrointestinal tract and urinary bladder.

Identification in tissues

As anyone who has moles and freckles will know, melanin usually produces a yellow-brown colour in the tissues where it is deposited. If present in very large amounts the local area of tissue may appear black.

On histological examination the melanin appears as brown intracellular granules. It possesses the ability to reduce solutions of ammoniacal silver with the consequent deposition of black granules of silver on the melanin granules. Substances which can do this are spoken of as '**argentaffin**'. Where pigmentation is very heavy the melanin can be removed from the tissue sections by bleaching them with oxidizing agents such as hydrogen peroxide.

Site of production

Melanin is produced by a specialized cell, the **melanocyte**, which can be seen in the greatest numbers in the basal layer of the epidermis. It is of neural crest origin and migrates to its various permanent homes during embryonic life. The average number of skin melanocytes is $1500/mm^2$, the number varying from $2000/mm^2$ in the forehead and cheeks to $800/mm^2$ in the skin of the abdomen. The number of melanocytes in the skin is constant (relatively) regardless of race. The darker skin of blacks, for example, is due to increased activity of the melanocytes.

Melanin is synthesized in small membrane-bound bodies known as melanosomes which are to be found in the Golgi apparatus. The melanin granules are transferred from the melanocytes to the neighbouring epidermal cells. At the point of contact between the dendritic process of the melanocyte and the plasma membrane of the epidermal cell, there is considerable excitation of the latter and clumps of pigment are taken into the epidermal cell and come to lie in a perinuclear position.

Formation

The basic starting point for the synthesis of melanin is the amino acid tyrosine (Fig. 23.1).

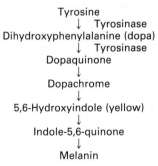

Fig. 23.1 The synthesis of melanin.

The most important functional aspect of the melanocyte is the presence of tyrosinase. Absence of this enzyme results in complete inability to synthesize melanin. The resulting syndrome is albinism (absence of pigmentation in skin, hair and conjunctiva). All normal melanocytes contain tyrosinase but not all are actively engaged in producing melanin. For this reason it is sometimes necessary to employ special means for the identification of melanocytes. This may be done by incubating the tissue sections in a solution of either dopa or tyrosine. If tyrosinase is present within the cells, melanin will be produced.

Clearly the intensity of skin colouring depends not only on the number of melanin-producing cells present in any site but also on their activity. This appears to be related to certain hormones of the pituitary and, to a lesser extent, the gonads. The pituitary secretes a hormone — **melanocyte-stimulating hormone (MSH)**, which shares part of its amino acid sequence with adrenocorticotrophic hormone (ACTH). In Addison's disease, where there is destruction of adrenal tissue due to either autoimmune processes or tuberculosis, there is loss of normal feedback mechanisms due to the fall in adrenal activity. Additional MSH is secreted by the pituitary; skin and mucosal pigmentation is thus a common feature of the disease.

Abnormalities in melanin pigmentation

Generalized hyperpigmentation. There are a number of diseases in which hyperpigmentation occurs:

1. Addison's disease
2. Acromegaly
3. Large doses of oestrogens given for treatment of prostatic cancer. These sometimes cause generalized hyperpigmentation. In addition, the effects of oestrogen may be the reason for the hyperpigmentation which sometimes occurs in chronic liver disease, in which it is alleged there is inadequate detoxication of oestrogen. In pregnancy, the nipples and genitalia become darker and there is sometimes a blotchy hyperpigmentation in the butterfly area of the face. This is known as chloasma.
4. Chronic arsenical poisoning
5. Haemochromatosis
6. Chlorpromazine. A curious violet-grey pigmentation occasionally develops after treatment with this drug; it may affect the eyes and those parts of the skin exposed to sunlight.

Focal hyperpigmentation. This may occur in a number of situations:

1. **Freckles** are an example of focal hyperpigmentation and are probably genetically determined.
2. **Café au lait spots** are large hyperpigmented macules. Unlike the common freckles, these show an increase in the number of melanocytes. They are found in two rare systemic conditions: firstly, neurofibromatosis, which is a condition characterized by the presence of multiple tumours derived from the fibrous element of the nerve sheath, and secondly, Albright's syndrome, which consists of a triad of

polyostotic fibrous dysplasia, hyperpigmentation, and sexual and skeletal precocity.

3. The **Peutz–Jeghers syndrome** is a rare syndrome inherited as an autosomal dominant. It has two main characteristics: a curious focal hyperpigmentation involving the lips and the circumoral skin, and multiple polyps in the gastrointestinal tract, which may cause acute or subacute intestinal obstruction.

4. **Lentiginosis** is the presence of multiple hyperpigmented spots characterized by an increase in the number of melanocytes. This has been reported to be associated with hypertrophic cardiomyopathy in a few cases.

5. Focal hyperpigmentation can result from exposure to ionizing radiation, ultraviolet light, heat (erythema ab igne) and chronic irritation (as in itchy dermatoses).

6. Tumours arising from melanocytes are most commonly seen in the skin but may occur at any of the sites in which melanocytes have been described. Most of these are benign — the 'moles' of various kinds — but a small proportion are malignant (mostly ab initio). These are termed 'malignant melanomas'. Other skin tumours may accumulate melanin and this may cause some concern as to their nature. This type of pigmentation is common in seborrhoeic warts and basal cell carcinoma.

Hypopigmentation. **Albinism**, as already mentioned, is due to a deficiency of tyrosinase. In classic cases the skin is very white, the hair pale, the irides transparent and the pupils pink. Such extreme cases are fortunately rare among humans. These patients tend to suffer from the skin tumours believed to be associated with exposure to sunlight, thus emphasizing the importance of melanin as a protective agent.

Focal hypopigmentation (**vitiligo**) is very common and is characterized by the presence of well-demarcated areas of depigmentation. Histological examination shows either paucity or absence of melanocytes.

Pigments derived from haemoglobin

In this section we shall restrict our consideration to the iron-containing pigments.

Excess iron, which may be either localized or systemic, is initially stored in the form of ferritin. This is a micellar structure about 5.4 nm in diameter which consists of a ferric core surrounded by a shell of protein subunits. Ferritin cannot be seen under the light microscope and does not give positive reactions with the staining methods commonly employed for the recognition of iron. It may, however, be seen fairly easily with the electron microscope.

With further increases in intracellular iron accumulation, the ferritin molecules aggregate to produce a coarse crystalline yellow-brown pigment which is very easily seen on light microscopy. This pigment is known as **haemosiderin**. These crystals are about 36% iron and can be identified with certainty by applying the Prussian blue method. This involves treating either tissues or tissue sections with a mixture of hydrochloric acid and potassium ferrocyanide. The iron in the tissues is present in a trivalent form and a blue precipitate of ferric ferrocyanide is produced. This method is both easy and sensitive.

Localized deposition of haemosiderin

Localized deposition of haemosiderin always implies that there has been haemorrhage at the site of the pigmentation. Haemosiderin pigmentation is therefore frequently seen in relation to bruises, organizing haematomas, fracture sites and haemorrhage infarcts as well as certain tumour-like lesions such as sclerosing haemangioma in the dermis and pigmented villonodular synovitis in the large joints.

The cells of the renal tubules can convert haemoglobin to haemosiderin and haemosiderinuria may sometimes follow haemoglobinuria.

One of the most frequent local depositions of haemosiderin seen at autopsy is in the lungs, which is usually associated with high pulmonary venous pressure as in 'tight' mitral stenosis or left ventricular failure. Sometimes severe pulmonary haemosiderosis will be caused by immune injury of the Gell and Coombes type 2 variety. This is accompanied by acute immune-mediated injury to the glomerular basement membranes and is known as Goodpasture's syndrome.

Generalized haemosiderosis

If the body is overloaded with iron, haemosiderin is formed in excessive amounts and deposited in a wide range of tissues. The total quantity of iron normally present in the body is 4 to 5 g and this level appears to be controlled by powerful homeostatic mechanisms.

Normal Western-style diets contain 10 to 15 mg of iron per day and only about 10% of this is absorbed. There is a normal loss of about 1 mg per day through shedding of cells from the gastrointestinal tract, skin, etc. Females lose about 200 to 300 mg per year as a result of menstruation.

There are two basic morphological patterns for the deposition of the excess haemosiderin: firstly, parenchymatous deposition and, secondly, deposition in the cells of the reticuloendothelial system. This latter pattern is seen following parenteral iron administration or repeated blood transfusion.

The possible mechanisms which might account for the accumulation of excess iron in the body are:

1. Increased absorption of iron
2. Decreased excretion (although there is no evidence for this as yet)
3. Impaired utilization
4. Excess breakdown of haemoglobin with release of iron

Haemochromatosis

The disorder known as **haemochromatosis** can be characterized as a syndrome in which the following occur:

1. Cirrhosis of the liver, which is associated with heavy deposits of iron. Over 50 g of iron have been extracted from the livers of patients who have come to autopsy
2. Pancreatic fibrosis and siderosis which are usually accompanied by diabetes mellitus
3. Siderosis of other organs
4. Skin pigmentation, which is due to excess melanin

In its classic form the combination of skin changes and diabetes has led to the use of the term '**bronze diabetes**'. The pathogenesis of this condition remains one of the most controversial areas in medicine.

Many workers consider that it represents an inborn error of metabolism which is inherited as an autosomal dominant. It has been postulated that the basic defect is some abnormality in the mechanisms regulating the absorption of iron from the gastrointestinal tract which leads to excess absorption (2–3 mg daily) and that over the years the body accumulates large stores of haemosiderin. Many of the relatives of patients with this disorder do show increased iron absorption.

Haemochromatosis most commonly affects men. Presumably this is due to the protection afforded by menstruation against accumulation of very large amounts of iron.

Morphologically, the most striking feature of the disease complex is hepatic cirrhosis accompanied by heavy siderosis. The liver is usually markedly enlarged, nodular and a dark chocolate brown in colour. On histological examination it is apparent that the haemosiderin is deposited within the parenchymal cells as well as in the Kupffer cells.

Apart from the intrinsic dangers of liver failure and portal hypertension which this pathological picture in the liver represents, there is a not inconsiderable risk in these patients of primary carcinoma of the liver. The plasma iron levels are high and transferrin saturation is almost complete.

Pigments associated with fats

This group of endogenous pigments are termed the **lipofuscins** (Latin *'fuscus'* = dark or sombre). These are often also spoken of as 'wear-and-tear' pigments since they appear to accumulate as a manifestation of ageing.

Lipofuscins are yellowish-brown granular pigments which appear within atrophic parenchymal cells, particularly in the liver and heart of old people. When present in large amounts they impart a brown colour to the affected organ or tissue. Such organs are spoken of as showing **brown atrophy.** These pigments are deemed to represent the breakdown products of membranes of 'worn out' organelles. With ageing of cells, autophagic vacuoles are formed in increasing number as active metabolic organelles become 'redundant'. Within these autophagic vacuoles the lipid portions of the membranes tend to resist lysosomal digestion. These lipid remnants undergo auto-oxidation to form a variety of lipoperoxides and aldehydes which have a yellow colour. The pigment remains within lysosomes and appears to produce no ill-effects on the tissues.

Exogenous pigmentation

Exogenous pigmentation can occur, but tends to be of social rather than pathological significance. The commonest example is to be found in tattoo marks of the 'Alf loves Flo' type. Occasionally the long continued use of external medications containing metals, e.g. silver-containing ear drops, produces pigmentation.

Heterotopic Calcification

Heterotopic calcification is the deposition of calcium salts in tissues other than osteoid and enamel. There are two main varieties: **dystrophic calcification** and **metastatic calcification.**

Dystrophic calcification

In dystrophic calcification, serum calcium levels are normal and the calcium salts are deposited in dead or degenerate tissues. This occurs in the following sets of circumstances:

1. Caseous necrosis (calcification is the hallmark of old caseation)

2. Fat necrosis
3. Thrombosis
4. Haematomas, e.g. subdural haematoma or myositis ossificans
5. Atherosclerotic plaques
6. Chronic inflammatory granulation tissue, e.g. constrictive pericarditis
7. Mönckeberg's sclerosis of the medial coat of muscular arteries
8. Degenerate colloid goitres
9. Cysts of various kinds
10. Degenerate tumours, e.g. uterine leiomyomas

Metastatic calcification

Here the fundamental defect is an elevated blood calcium level. This may result from the removal of calcium from the bones as, for example, in hyperparathyroidism or from excess calcium derived from the gut. Occasionally, as in renal osteodystrophy, the precipitating factor appears to be a high blood phosphate.

This type of calcium deposition occurs in a variety of sites:

1. The **kidney**. Deposition occurs round the tubules and damages them. Ultimately this may lead to renal failure. These patients often show an inability to acidify their urine. Stone formation in the renal pelvis and ureter is very often associated with nephrocalcinosis.
2. The **lung**. Calcium is deposited in the alveolar walls.
3. The **stomach**. The calcium is deposited around the fundal glands. It has been suggested that since these glands secrete hydrochloric acid, the tissues are left relatively alkaline and this is said to favour calcium deposition.
4. **Blood vessels**. The coronary arteries are most affected.
5. The **cornea**

Causes of metastatic calcification

There are five common causes of metastatic calcification:

1. Hyperparathyroidism, either as a result of primary or secondary hyperplasia, or as a result of neoplasia (parathyroid adenoma), the commonest type of parathyroid hyperactivity
2. Excessive absorption of calcium from the bowel, which may be due to hypervitaminosis D or vitamin D sensitive states such as idiopathic hypercalcaemia of infancy or even through excessive milk drinking

3. Hypophosphatasia
4. Destructive bone lesions
5. Renal tubular acidosis

The last three causes are much less common.

Identification of heterotopic calcification

On histological examination calcium salts appear as granules which stain a deep blue colour with haematoxylin. They typically form encrustations on such structures as elastic fibres in the lung or in arteries.

Calcium salts can be stained with alizarin red which stains them a magenta colour. More commonly the von Kossa method is used, in which silver impregnation forms the basis of the stain. What it shows is, in fact, phosphate and carbonate, but since these are almost always associated with calcium when in its particulate and insoluble form, it constitutes quite an effective method for the demonstration of calcium.

Chapter 24

Neoplasia: Disorders of Cell Proliferation and Differentiation

In communities where undernutrition, malnutrition and infectious diseases are no longer a major problem, neoplastic disease comes second only to cardiovascular disease as a cause of death. In the UK it will kill over 100 000 people in the next 12 months.

Definitions

The term **neoplasia** is derived from two Greek words: '**neos**' meaning 'new' and '**plassein**' meaning 'to mould'. This is usually translated as **new growth**, though this phrase begs certain important questions as to the essential nature of neoplasia. Neoplasia is, in fact, not easy to define; many pathologists regard the best available definition as that suggested by Willis:

'A neoplasm is an abnormal mass of tissue, the growth of which exceeds and is uncoordinated with that of the normal tissues, and which persists in the same excessive manner after cessation of the stimulus which has evoked the change.'

If we attempt to analyse this definition in operational terms it becomes clear that there are at least three types of disturbance of cell behaviour inherent within it, each of which deserves separate consideration. This approach enables us to regard neoplasia in terms of a set of disorders showing:

1. A disturbance in cell proliferation
2. A disturbance in cell differentiation
3. A disturbance in the relationship between cells and their surrounding stroma

A disturbance in cell proliferation

There is a disturbance in those mechanisms which normally maintain a given cell population within relatively narrow limits. This escape from normal control gives rise to a population of dividing cells which, in a sense, is **immortal** in that cell division continues for a far greater number of times than in a normal cell line. The end result is a focus made up, in most instances, of one type of cell in numbers which are totally inappropriate for the anatomical location. This will lead to the formation of a mass or tumour.

A disturbance in cell differentiation

Differentiation is the sum of the processes by which the cells in a developing multicellular organism achieve their **specific set of functional and morphological characteristics.** The cells which share a set of such characteristics become organized into tissues, and these in turn may be arranged as organs. A fertilized ovum contains *all* the genetic information required for that organism and is, thus, totipotent in terms of future structure and function. A differentiated cell such as a muscle cell or a liver cell obviously expresses only a small part of the genetic information; thus differentiation must involve a progressive **restriction** of genomic expression. Impairment of differentiation of the cell line involved is extremely common in the formation of a neoplasm. At a practical level, the degree of differentiation in a neoplasm may, in many but not all instances, give useful information as to the likely natural history of the disease. In general terms, the poorer the degree of differentiation, the worse the behaviour of the neoplasm is likely to be. Loss of the ability to differentiate fully may lead to the acquisition of functional characteristics quite foreign to the mature differentiated cell. This may be expressed in the form of secretion by the neoplastic cells of fetal proteins or of hormones inappropriate for that particular cell type (**ectopic hormone production**) (see p. 419).

A disturbance in the relationship between cells and their surrounding stroma

There is a disturbance in the relationship between the cells which make up the neoplasm and the normal tissue which surrounds them. In many instances the cells of a neoplasm grow as a compact mass in an expansile fashion (**benign neoplasms**); in others the constituent cells **invade** the surrounding tissues and may spread to distant sites (**malignant neoplasms**).

The Classification of Neoplasms

In theory, neoplasms might be classified in a number of different ways. Some of the criteria which have been tried in the past include:

    aetiology
    embryogenesis

organ of origin
histogenesis or cytogenesis (tissue or cell of origin)
biological behaviour

On a practical day-to-day level, the most useful of these are the cell type from which the neoplasm has originated and the biological behaviour. The latter is obviously of particular importance in determining the outcome of the disease in an individual. The pathologist who examines tissue removed in the course of either biopsy or excision of a neoplasm will try to predict the biological behaviour on the basis of the morphological appearances.

Histogenesis and cytogenesis

As already stated, the cell and tissue types from which neoplasms arise constitute the basis of the most commonly used classifications (Table 24.1). At the simplest level these tissues of origin can be divided into two: epithelia and connective tissues. However, a much greater degree of subdivision is both possible and desirable. It is worth bearing in mind that, even at the basic level of grouping neoplasms as being either of epithelial or connective tissue origin, certain difficulties may arise in correct attribution of a given neoplasm to one or other of these categories. For instance, neoplasms arising from mesothelial cells which line serosal cavities may show morphological characteristics suggestive of both epithelium and connective tissue. A more frequent problem in practice is that the cell population of a neoplasm may be so poorly differentiated as to make it very difficult or even impossible for the pathologist to identify the original cell type. In this situation, the use of immunological methods applied at the slide level to identify either specific antigens or specific cell products may be helpful (Fig. 24.1).

Biological behaviour

From the point of view of the patient, the most important characteristic of a neoplasm is its behaviour pattern. Essentially, all neoplasms, with only a few exceptions, are divided on this basis into two main groups: **benign** and **malignant**. Malignant neoplasms which arise from **epithelia** are called **carcinomas** and those which have their origin from **connective tissue elements** are called **sarcomas**. While this division into benign and malignant relates to the behaviour of a given neoplasm in operational terms, the behavioural characteristics, as stated above, are reflected to a considerable extent in the morphological appearances of the lesion.

Table 24.1 A classification of tumours.

	Behaviour		
Tissue of origin	*Benign*	*Intermediate*	*Malignant*
Epithelium			
Covering and protective epithelium	Squamous, transitional and columnar cell papilloma		Squamous and transitional cell carcinoma; adenocarcinoma
Compact secreting epithelium	Adenoma: if cystic—cystadenoma; if papillary and cystic—papillary cystadenoma		Adenocarcinoma: if cystic—cystadenocarcinoma
Other epithelial neoplasms		Basal cell carcinomas; salivary and mucous gland neoplasms; carcinoid tumours (argentaffinoma)	
Connective tissue			
Fibrous	Fibroma		Fibrosarcoma
Nerve sheath	Neurilemmoma Neurofibroma		Neurofibrosarcoma
Adipose	Lipoma		Liposarcoma
Smooth muscle	Leiomyoma		Leiomyosarcoma
Striated muscle	Rhabdomyoma		Rhabdomyosarcoma
Synovium	Synovioma		Synoviosarcoma
Cartilage	Chondroma		Chondrosarcoma
Bone			
Osteoblast	Osteoma		Osteosarcoma
Unknown		←—— Giant cell tumour ——→	
Mesothelium	Benign mesothelioma		Malignant mesothelioma
Blood vessels and lymphatics			Angiosarcoma
Meninges	Meningioma		Malignant meningioma

Tissue	Benign	Malignant
Specialized connective tissue		
Neuroglia and ependyma		◄─── Astrocytoma, oligodendroglioma ───►
		Ependymoma
		Malignant variants
Chromaffin tissue	Carotid body tumour; phaeochromocytoma	
Lymphoid and haemopoietic tissue	Myeloproliferative disorders	Malignant lymphoma of varying degrees of differentiation; Hodgkin's disease; plasmacytoma; multiple myeloma syndrome; Waldenstrom's macroglobulinaemia; leukaemias
Melanocytes		Malignant melanoma
Fetal trophoblast	Hydatidiform mole	Choriocarcinoma
Embryonic tissue		
Totipotential or pluripotential cell:	Benign teratoma	Malignant teratoma
Kidney		Nephroblastoma
Liver		Hepatoblastoma
Unipotential cell:		
Retina		Retinoblastoma
Hind brain		Medulloblastoma
Sympathetic ganglia and adrenal medulla	Ganglioneuroma	Neuroblastoma
Unipotential embryonic cells in pelvic organs		Juvenile rhabdomyosarcoma (sarcoma botryoides)
Embryonic vestiges		
Notochord		Chordoma
Enamel organ	Ameloblastoma	
Parapituitary residues	Craniopharyngioma	

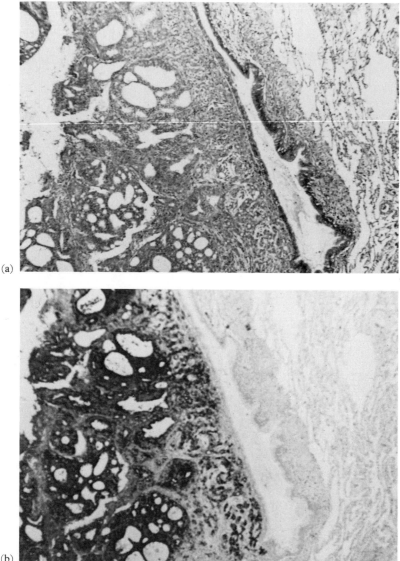

(a)

(b)

Fig. 24.1   (a) A section of a metastatic deposit in the lung of a prostatic adenocarcinoma stained with haematoxylin and eosin. (b) An adjacent section of the same lesion which has been treated with antibody against prostatic specific antigen. The characteristic dark staining of many of the tumour cells by the immunoperoxidase method indicates that the primary site is likely to be the prostate.

Benign Neoplasms

The use of the word 'benign' does not imply that such neoplasms are clinically unimportant or that they may not constitute a serious hazard. In the context of neoplastic disease, the word **benign** means that the cells which make up the neoplasm **show no tendency to invade the surrounding tissue** and, by the same token, *never* **spread to distant sites** (**metastasis**).

The growth pattern of a benign neoplasm is an expansile one, often associated with the formation of a capsule derived from the surrounding connective tissue and with some pressure atrophy of surrounding parenchymal elements. The growth rate is often low and few, if any, cells undergoing **mitosis** are seen.

The cells of the neoplasm and the way in which they are arranged often bear a close resemblance to what obtains in the parent tissue; such neoplasms are spoken of as being **well differentiated.**

Malignant Neoplasms

The absolute criterion of malignancy is **invasiveness.** Instead of the expansile growth pattern characteristic of benign neoplasms, malignant

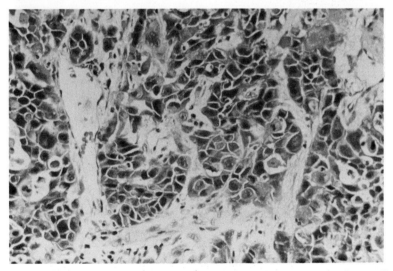

Fig. 24.2 Invasive squamous carcinoma of the bronchus. While the tumour cells can still be recognized as being of squamous origin because of their shape and the type of relationship to one another, they show features of malignancy both cytologically and in the form of breaching of the basement membrane and invasion of the subepithelial tissue.

cells separate from one another and grow out in an irregular pattern into the surrounding tissue (Fig. 24.2). In many instances the malignant cells gain access to vascular channels — either lymphatics, blood vessels, or both. Once such vascular invasion has occurred, groups of malignant cells can be carried in the blood or lymph until they impact at some distance from the primary growth. From the site of impaction the malignant cells emigrate into the extravascular compartment and may form new deposits of neoplastic tissue (**secondary deposits** or **metastases**). The mechanisms which are involved in tumour spread are discussed in Chapter 27.

From the morphological point of view, malignant cells and the structures which they form tend to show evidence of increased cell turnover and incomplete differentiation.

The first of these is expressed in the form of an increased number of **mitoses**. Not infrequently these mitoses are abnormal in appearance, with tripolar, quadripolar or annular spindles (Fig. 24.3). Poor differentiation shows itself both at the level of the individual cells and in the relationship of the cells to each other. Malignant cells tend to be larger than their normal counterparts and tend to show a much greater degree of **variation in size and shape** than normal cells of the same origin. Nuclei are especially prominent both as regards their size and

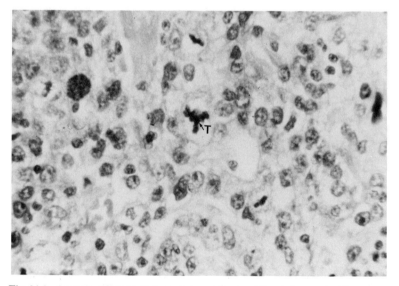

Fig. 24.3 A poorly differentiated squamous carcinoma of the uterine cervix. The tumour cells are barely recognizable as being of squamous origin (compare with Fig. 24.2). Atypical mitoses are present, including a tripolar one (T) in the centre of the field.

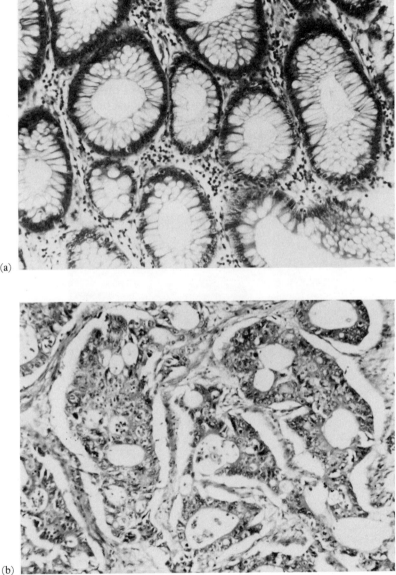

Fig. 24.4 (a) Normal fully differentiated rectal glands seen in an operation specimen. (b) Carcinoma of the rectum. This tumour was close to the normal rectal mucosa shown in (a) and is shown to emphasize the contrast between the fully differentiated glands in normal mucosa and the poor differentiation seen in the tumour.

their staining reaction with nuclear stains such as haematoxylin. The nuclei occupy a much greater proportion of the total cell volume than is normal; this is termed an increase in the nuclear/cytoplasmic ratio. The DNA content of the nuclei of malignant cells may be much greater than normal, and chromosomal analysis not infrequently shows loss of normal ploidy.

As stated above, loss of differentiation involves the patterns of cell arrangement as well as the morphology of individual cells. The normal orderly relationships between cells tend to disappear and the structures, such as ductules or glands, which the malignant cells may form differ considerably from their normal non-neoplastic counterparts (Fig. 24.4). In other instances the neoplasm may be so poorly differentiated that no recognizable structures are formed and the malignant cells grow in disorganized sheets or islands.

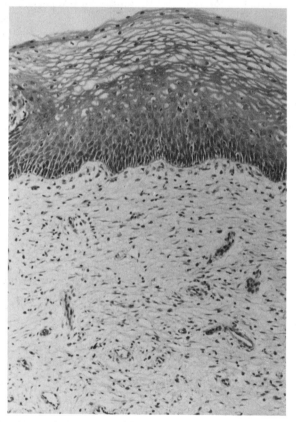

Fig. 24.5a

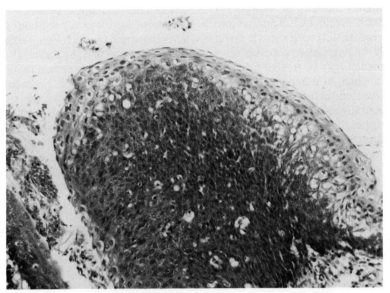

(b)

Fig. 24.5   (a) Section of uterine cervix showing normal maturation of squamous cells from base to surface. (b) Section of uterine cervix from same patient as in (a) showing intra-epithelial neoplasia. There is marked dysplasia in the squamous covering of the cervical tissue, with much variation in nuclear size and staining and some loss of the normal relationship of the squamous cells one to another.

Dysplasia

The morphological features described above in relation to malignancy may be found, especially in epithelia, at a stage when no invasion of the surrounding tissue is evident. This is termed **dysplasia** (from the Greek **dys** = 'bad'). The finding of dysplastic epithelia suggests that some irreversible and heritable change has taken place in the genome of the affected cells, but that full phenotypic expression of malignancy, in the shape of the ability to invade surrounding tissues, has not yet occurred. The finding of dysplastic changes sounds a warning note to the clinician that full-blown malignancy may, in the future, develop at the site of the dysplasia and that careful observation of the patient is required. Dysplasia is particularly common in squamous and transitional epithelia, such as those of the uterine cervix, the skin and the urinary bladder.

Dysplasia of the uterine cervix can usually be diagnosed by microscopic studies on cells which are exfoliated from the epithelial surface and can be collected on a spatula ('cervical smear cytology'). Such cytological diagnoses can be confirmed histologically by taking very small biopsies under direct vision (colposcopic biopsy) (Fig. 24.5). If the dysplastic process is severe and widespread within the cervix, the patient may be treated by a wide cone-shaped excision of cervical tissue in which, it is hoped, all the dysplastic epithelium is removed. Freedom from epithelial dysplasia in the lines of excision is checked for by histological examination. In some cases of epithelial dysplasia, the whole thickness of the epithelial covering shows dysplastic change; for these situations, the term **carcinoma in situ** is often used. Dysplasia represents a continuum of change which, as already stated, may end in frank malignancy. For this reason many pathologists prefer to label all cervical dysplasias as examples of **cervical intra-epithelial neoplasia** (**CIN**) of different grades of severity. It is difficult to predict the outcome for the individual patient with cervical intra-epithelial neoplasia, since some will remain more or less static and others progress at different speeds, but it is safe to assume that a considerable proportion of the cases with severe degrees of change will evolve into invasive carcinoma. Those patients in whom a diagnosis of dysplasia has been made, whatever the site, should be followed-up carefully.

Some Lesions Which May Be Confused With True Neoplasms

Hamartoma

The term **hamartoma** is derived from the Greek '*hamartanein*' which means 'to make an error'. Hamartomas are tumour-like masses which may grow to a considerable size but which lack the autonomy and the persistence of the excessive growth which is characteristic of the true neoplasm. In a hamartoma the elements which make up the lesion are fully differentiated and are normally found in the organ or tissue in which the hamartoma occurs. However, the way in which these elements are put together differs considerably from what is found in normal tissues. These lesions may be found in a wide range of anatomical situations and may consist of a wide variety of differentiated tissue elements. The lung is a not uncommon site for the development of a hamartoma; in this situation, well-demarcated masses of cartilage measuring up to 2–3 cm in diameter may be found. On histological examination, such lesions show the presence of small slits within the cartilage which are lined by bronchial type epithelium. Thus the lesion consists of some of the elements of the normal bronchial wall. In such easily inspectable tissues such as the skin, where hamartomatous lesions are common, it is clear that a hamartoma may be present at birth, but its growth phase may not occur until much later. The commonest hamartoma is vascular in type. There is a wide range of these from the flat 'portwine stain' to large, raised, complex masses of abnormal vascular spaces. Hamartomas may form part of some inherited syndromes. An interesting example is the Peutz–Jeghers syndrome in which multiple hamartomas involving the glands and muscle of the intestinal wall may be present. Because of the peristaltic contractions, these masses tend to be pushed out into the gut lumen in a polypoid fashion and may lead to intestinal obstruction due to intussusception. Associated with the tendency to form masses of abnormally arranged intestinal glands and muscle is a curious dark pigmentation of the lips, often most marked at the junction between the skin and the vermilion. The presence of this circumoral pigmentation may be a useful diagnostic pointer to the true nature of the problem in cases of acute intestinal obstruction.

Heteroplasia

Heteroplasia is the differentiation of part of an organ or tissue in a way which is quite foreign to the part. It can be distinguished from metaplasia since there is no change from one fully differentiated form to another. Instead the anomalous differentiation takes place from the stem cell stage. For instance, one might find gastric mucosa within the wall of a Meckel's diverticulum in the distal part of the ileum or in the gallbladder wall. Similarly, anomalous masses of pancreatic tissue sometimes occur in the wall of the small intestine; it is of interest that these consist of ductal and acinar tissue only, islets of Langerhans not being seen.

Occasionally heteroplasia may be expressed in the form of quite large and complicated masses in which several differentiated tissues may be seen. For example, a large mass on a patient's face has been described which contained ectopic liver, pancreatic tissue, and gut epithelium. Such heterotopic masses have been termed **choristomas.**

Some Structural Features of Common Neoplasms

Benign epithelial neoplasms

Epithelial neoplasms show two basic growth patterns which are largely, though not entirely, dictated by their own anatomical relationships. The first of these is where the neoplastic epithelial cells tend to grow in sheets covering a surface. Very often this mass of cells has a wavy

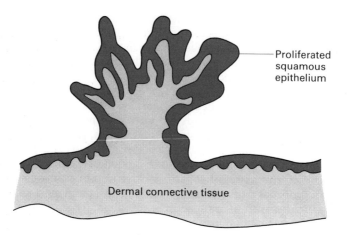

Proliferated
squamous
epithelium

Dermal connective tissue

Fig. 24.6 A papilloma of the skin.

irregular outline and is called a **papilloma** (Fig. 24.6). The second basic
pattern is where the cells grow as solid islands or masses, these being
separated from each other by stromal connective tissue. This growth
pattern is often seen in those neoplasms derived from ductal or
glandular epithelium and is known as an **adenoma.**

The genesis of a papilloma

The description of the development of a papilloma in *Muir's Textbook of
Pathology* is so masterly that it is quoted here in extenso:

'Inherent in the production of any neoplasm is a marked increase in the
cell population at that site. If one tries to visualize a covering epithelium
as a sheet of cloth which is pinned down at the edges and then increased
in area, it is obvious that it will be thrown into folds. If the increase is in
one dimension only, the folds will be regular pleats, but, since in a
benign epithelial neoplasm it occurs in two dimensions, simple folding
cannot occur and the result is an irregular mass of peaks and hollows.
Where the epithelium is raised into peaks, a core of connective tissue
and blood vessels is drawn into it, so that adequate nutrition to the
epithelium is maintained. The resulting mass of folds and projections is
the papilloma.'

Three main types of papilloma are described, these being consonant
with the three main varieties of covering epithelia: **squamous,
transitional** and **columnar.**

The genesis of an adenoma

Benign neoplasms arising from duct or gland epithelium are termed adenomas. The basic structure of adenomas is based on the tendency of the proliferating cells to form small groups which usually surround a lumen. In many instances this lumen is reduced to an inconspicuous slit and it may be impossible to see any lumen at all on light microscopy. This latter appearance is particularly common in adenomas arising within endocrine glands. The neoplastic acini have no draining duct systems. This absence of drainage, if combined with active secretion by the cells of the tumour, may lead to accumulation of the secretions, with distension of the lumina and eventual **cyst** formation. Such a neoplastic cyst derived from acinar or ductal epithelium is called a **cystadenoma**. If the formation of the cyst is accompanied by continued proliferation of the lining cells, the increase in the area of the lining will result in the appearance of papillary infoldings which project into the lumen — a so-called **papillary cystadenoma**. Such neoplasms are frequently encountered in the ovary but may occur at many other sites.

The macroscopic appearances of a typical adenoma are those of a clearly demarcated and usually rounded mass, often with a thin fibrous tissue capsule and with some compressed normal tissue around it. If the acinar or ductal lumina are small it appears solid when cut into, and it is usually paler and more homogeneous in texture than the surrounding tissue. If the gland or duct lumina are large and secretion has been a marked feature, this is usually easy to see when the lesion has been sectioned; either a single large cyst or many small ones may be present.

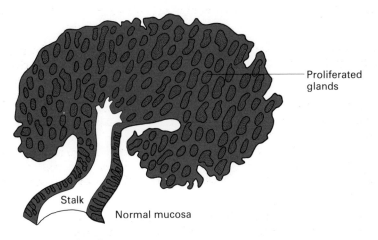

Fig. 24.7 A colonic polyp.

One of the commonest sites for adenoma formation is the large intestine. Because of peristaltic contraction, the localized islands of proliferated colonic glands tend to be pushed out into the lumen. In the early stages of this process, the small mass of glands will appear as a small lump standing a little proud of the surrounding mucosal surface. As the process continues, the mass of glands may be pushed out into the lumen, dragging with it a pedicle containing blood vessels and connective tissue. Such a lesion is termed a **polyp** (Fig. 24.7).

Chapter 25

Non-neoplastic Disturbances in Cell Growth and Proliferation

Not all quantitative changes in a given cell population are neoplastic. Indeed many such changes, involving both increases and decreases in the cell population, occur under both physiological and pathological circumstances. What distinguishes these from the changes in cell growth and proliferation occurring in neoplasia is that in the latter, **normal mechanisms of control do not operate.**

The cell cycle

Cells proliferate essentially by **mitosis.** However, the process of mitotic division occupies only a small part of the cell cycle (Fig. 25.1). The length of the cell cycle will determine, to an extent, the characteristics of a tissue in terms of its cell kinetics. After mitosis (M phase), which usually takes about one to two hours, the daughter cells enter a gap phase which is known as G_1. The length of this phase differs from cell type to cell type and varies greatly. The cell then enters a phase in which DNA is synthesized (the S phase); during this, the content of

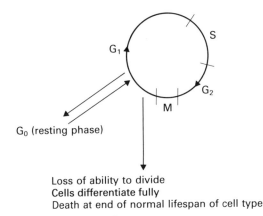

Fig. 25.1 The normal cell cycle. S = period of DNA synthesis; G_2 = pre-mitotic interval; M = mitosis; G_1 = period between mitosis and the start of DNA synthesis.

377

DNA is doubled. This S phase lasts from seven to twelve hours. After synthesis of DNA is complete, there is a second gap phase, known as G_2, which lasts, as a rule, from one to six hours. In human tissues, the M, G_2 and S phases are relatively constant in length, and the differences in cell cycle time which characterize different tissues are a function of variations in the length of G_1, which may last for days or even years. In cell culture models, arrest of the cell cycle occurs only in the G_1 phase. This finding implies that once a cell has passed out of the G_1 phase the cell cycle proceeds to completion. In fact, the **point of no return** occurs late in the G_1 phase and is known as the **restriction point**. This point in the cycle probably corresponds with the genetically programmed switching on of DNA polymerase synthesis.

In any given tissue, not all the cells are actually within the cell cycle; most fully differentiated cells **opt out**. When a cell leaves the cell cycle, the commonest event is an advance down the pathway of differentiation which must end, in most cases, in obsolescence and cell death. For instance, a daughter cell arising in the course of mitotic division in the basal layer of the epidermis migrates upwards into the malpighian layer where it begins to synthesize keratin. Eventually it moves to the horny layer of the epidermis and dies, being shed from the skin surface as a flake of keratin. There is, however, an alternative. Cells can leave the cycle **temporarily** and, under certain circumstances, re-enter it much later. Such 'resting' cells are said to be in G_0, though clearly it is not easy to distinguish between such cells and those in which there is a very long G_1 phase. That part of the cell population which remains within the cell cycle is known as the **growth fraction**. The proliferative activity in any tissue is a function both of the length of the cycle time and the size of the growth fraction.

Hypertrophy and Hyperplasia

Excess growth with **no** escape from normal control mechanisms may be expressed in two ways (Fig. 25.2):

1. In **hypertrophy** the increase in the bulk of tissue or organ results from an increase in the **size** of the individual cells of which the tissue is composed. In pure hypertrophy there is **no increase** in the **number** of cells.
2. In **hyperplasia** there is an increase in the **number** of cells making up a given tissue. An increase in cell size is not infrequently seen as an associated feature.

Hypertrophy and hyperplasia can, in most instances, be recognized as being caused by some specific stimulus. Once the stimulus is removed,

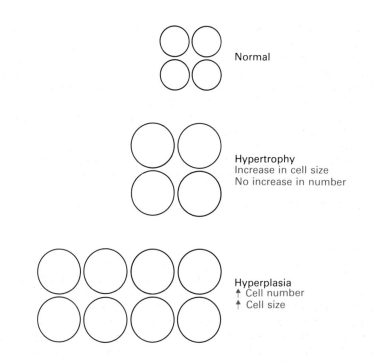

Fig. 25.2 Hypertrophy and hyperplasia.

there is a reversion to normal. This stimulus is often a physiological one, such as an increased demand for function which will lead either to an increase in cell number, cell size or both. Both can be regarded as **adaptation phenomena.**

Hyperplasia

In many instances, hyperplasia constitutes a **demand-led** physiological event, the increase in cells being the response to an increased functional need. This is seen, for example, in such tissues as the breast and thyroid at the time of puberty or pregnancy. The negative feedback mechanisms which appear to control these phenomena will act in a wide range of circumstances, even when the circumstances themselves are pathological.

Operation of this negative feedback is seen quite commonly in the field of **endocrine hyperplasia.** Some examples are given below.

Congenital adrenal hyperplasia (Fig. 25.3)

The clinical pictures associated with congenital adrenal hyperplasia make themselves apparent in infancy and early childhood. They are characterized by masculinization in the female and precocious puberty in the male; a salt-losing state may also be part of the syndrome. The basic defect is a deficiency in the cells of the adrenal cortex responsible for the synthesis of cortisol and aldosterone. These cells lack either a

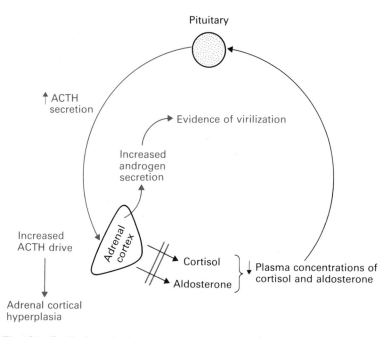

Fig. 25.3   Feedback mechanisms in congenital adrenal hyperplasia. ACTH = adrenocorticotrophic hormone.

C21 or a C11 hydroxylase and as a result there is a block in the pathways which normally lead to the synthesis of cortisol and aldosterone from cholesterol. The abnormally low concentrations of these hormones in the plasma lead to increased secretion of adrenocorticotrophic hormone (ACTH) by the pituitary and the adrenal cortex responds by increasing the number of functional cells. However, the block in hormone synthesis persists, the dammed back precursors are diverted to another metabolic pathway in the cortex, and large amounts of androgenic steroids (which are responsible for the virilization) are formed.

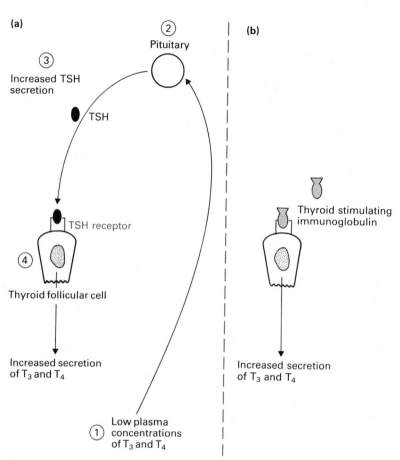

Fig. 25.4   Thyroid hyperplasia (a) due to increased drive controlled by negative feedback, and (b) due to abnormal drive (in the form of thyroid stimulating immunoglobulin). TSH = thyroid stimulating hormone; T_3 = triiodothyronine; T_4 = thyroxine.

Thyroid hyperplasia (Fig. 25.4)

This may occur either as a result of the operation of normal negative feedback mechanisms which control the levels of **thyroid stimulating hormone (TSH)** or as the result of the existence of abnormal stimuli. Many cases of hypothyroidism are associated with the structural changes of hyperplasia irrespective of the mechanism behind the hypofunction. Abnormally low secretion of thyroid hormones may arise from:

1. A lack of secreting tissue (as in cretinism)

2. A lack of substrate

3. A lack of the enzymes required for the various steps in hormone synthesis (dyshormogenetic goitre)

In all of these, the low circulating levels of thyroxine will lead to an increased output of TSH from the pituitary and hence to hyperplasia of the thyroid tissue.

Similar morphological changes may occur in **hyperthyroid** patients being treated with thiouracil or carbimazole. These compounds block the synthesis of thyroxine and the pituitary responds by secreting more TSH. The patient becomes clinically and biochemically euthyroid on this treatment, but the gland itself may become more hyperplastic.

Endocrine hyperplasia can occur not as the result of an increased normal drive controlled by negative feedback, but through the operation of abnormal drives. An example of this is primary hyperthyroidism (Graves' disease) in which the abnormal drive is a thyroid stimulating immunoglobulin which binds to the TSH receptor on the surface of the thyroid acinar epithelium. Binding to the receptor is followed by activation of the adenylate cyclase system and a rise in the intracellular content of cAMP. This, in turn, probably activates a protein kinase, leading to the phosphorylation of certain proteins. A cascade of events is initiated that can give rise to the activation of key enzyme systems, increased RNA and protein synthesis and, in cells which have the potential to divide, to mitosis. There are conflicting data from cell culture systems as to the effect of cyclic nucleotides on cell growth. It seems likely that the discrepancies can be explained on the basis of whether the increases in the local concentrations of these nucleotides have been continuous (in which case cell growth appears to be damped down) or in the form of transient bursts in the G_1 phase of the cell cycle (which occurs in many cell types after a mitogenic stimulus). The thyroid becomes markedly hyperplastic with a significant increase in both number and size of the acinar cells. The increase may be so marked as to give rise to invaginations of the epithelium into the lumen of the acinus; this can give a false impression of papillary ingrowths and may raise unjustified suspicions of malignancy.

Pancreatic islet hyperplasia in infants whose mothers are diabetic

Maternal diabetes is a potent risk for perinatal mortality unless appropriate measures are taken. These infants tend to be fat, flabby and rather cushingoid in appearance. On histological examination of the pancreas, there is a striking degree of islet cell hyperplasia.

Initially this was viewed as the result of the operation of normal feedback mechanisms, the high maternal blood glucose concentrations being deemed to induce a greater than normal degree of insulin secretion by the fetal islets and, hence, hyperplasia. However, this is an oversimplification of a much more complex problem, since the islet cell hyperplasia seen in the infants of diabetic mothers is seen also in the stillborn infants of mothers who are destined to become diabetic, sometimes many years later, a state known as prediabetes.

Hyperplasia in the target organs of hormones

Breast. An increase in the size of the breasts in the female is a normal, indeed welcome, feature of puberty, and also occurs during pregnancy and lactation. These changes are hormone-induced and consist of an increase in both the epithelial elements and the rather specialized connective tissue elements which surround the breast ducts and demarcate the breast lobules from the interlobular connective tissue. One of the most important factors in this change is oestrogen.

In clinical practice, breast hyperplasia of a rather different sort is common. This may manifest as a localized lump within the breast or as a generalized lumpiness in a fairly large area of the breast. It is not infrequently spoken of as **chronic mastitis**, a very poor term since the process is not inflammatory in nature. It is, instead, a mixture of hyperplastic and involutionary changes which are probably due to hormonal imbalance. The structural changes are basically an increase in fibrous tissue, both within and between the lobules, an increase in the number of ducts within individual lobules (this is called **adenosis**), and an increase in the number of cells lining individual ducts with a consequent 'heaping up' of the epithelial cells (so-called '**epitheliosis**'). In any single case the histological appearances will depend on the relative proportions of these three changes and the secondary effects (such as cystic change) which result from them.

Prostate. Enlargement of the prostate is an extremely common event in males over the age of 60. Both the fibromuscular and ductal elements are involved. The enlargement is confined to the middle and lateral lobes and gives the gland a nodular appearance. Not infrequently, nodules project into the urethra and can cause a ball-valve type of obstruction. Such evidence as is available suggests a strong hormonal influence on this process. In the male dog, which is the only other species which appears to develop prostatic hyperplasia, the process only occurs in animals with intact testes. The nodules of hyperplastic tissue contain larger than usual amounts of dihydrotestosterone, though the plasma concentrations of testosterone are no higher in dogs or men with prostatic hyperplasia than in controls. These data suggest that there may be an increased rate of receptor-mediated binding in those prostates in which hyperplasia is encountered.

Non-specific reactive epithelial hyperplasia

The lining epithelia of the skin, mouth, alimentary and respiratory tracts frequently become hyperplastic when any persistent irritant is applied to them. The irritant can be simple trauma, for example when a corn develops in response to the rubbing of ill-fitting shoes. Similarly, an incorrectly fitted denture can produce marked thickening of the squamous epithelium of the alveolar margin. Chronic inflammatory disease of the skin is often associated with thickening of the epidermis, and epidermal hyperplasia of a very marked degree can develop in response to the presence of certain intra-dermal lesions such as insect bites. At times this reactive epidermal hyperplasia may be so extreme as to raise suspicions that the process is neoplastic rather than reactive. It is humiliating to have to confess that the nature of the mitogenic stimulus in these quite common situations is not understood.

Hypertrophy

Isolated hypertrophy occurs only in muscle. Clearly the stimulus which elicits this response is an increased work load. This is seen in relation to **smooth muscle** in a number of pathological circumstances, particularly where there is partial obstruction to the normal progress of the contents of any hollow muscular organ. Some examples are given below.

The urinary bladder

Any obstruction of the outflow of urine as, for example, in post-inflammatory urethral strictures or with enlargement of the prostate will lead to an increase in size of the muscle fibres and a considerable degree of thickening of the bladder wall. Because of the orientation of the muscle in the bladder, this leads to a woven or trabeculated pattern being seen when the mucosal lining of the bladder is inspected at cystoscopy.

The gastrointestinal tract

The gut, an archetype of a muscular tube, shows muscle hypertrophy proximal to chronic obstructions arising from any cause. In the **oesophagus** this is seen in association with:

post-inflammatory scarring
carcinoma
obstruction due to disorders of innervation (cardiac achalasia)

In the **stomach**, muscle hypertrophy may not only result from some obstructive lesion but may also cause obstruction. This is seen in **congenital hypertrophic pyloric stenosis**. In this condition, affected infants, the vast majority of whom are male, present soon after birth with projectile vomiting shortly after feeding. On deep palpation of the abdomen, a small lump may be detected. At operation this is seen to be a thick ring of muscle round the pyloric opening. It is treated by dividing the muscle from the serosal aspect without damaging the mucosal lining. In this way the hypertrophied muscle ring is opened up and the obstruction is relieved.

The heart

Cardiac hypertrophy is commonly encountered in clinical practice. It is due to an increased work load. It may be of two types each of which is mirrored in the appearance of the heart (Fig. 25.5). In **high pressure overload**, such as is seen in aortic valve stenosis, systemic hypertension or, much more rarely, in coarctation of the aorta, there is a marked

High pressure overload
Aortic valve stenosis
Systemic hypertension
Aortic coarctation

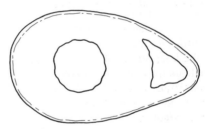

Normal or small LV cavity

High volume overload
Aortic valve incompetence
Mitral valve incompetence

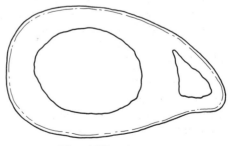

Dilated LV cavity

Fig. 25.5 The two types of increased work load that lead to left ventricular hypertrophy. LV = left ventricle.

degree of left ventricular hypertrophy which is associated with a left ventricular cavity which is either normal in size or smaller than normal. In the case of **high volume overload**, the increased work load stems from an increase in end-diastolic volume (such as occurs in aortic or mitral incompetence); this is inevitably associated with a large capacity left ventricular cavity.

Atrophy

Just as there may be an increase in the bulk of a tissue or organ as a result of hyperplasia or hypertrophy, there may also be a decrease. If the diminution in bulk is acquired, it is spoken of as **atrophy** and this, as with hyperplasia and hypertrophy, may occur as a more or less physiological phenomenon or in abnormal or pathological circumstances.

Physiological atrophy

This can occur at any time of life including the gestation period, but is particularly associated with early life. In the fetus, many structures are formed during embryonic development which undergo regression during the later stages of gestation. These include the notochord, the branchial clefts and the thyroglossal duct. Persistence of these structures to a greater or lesser degree may occur, and patients may present (in the case of the last two) with masses in the neck, the true nature of which is revealed on histological examination after surgical removal.

In the neonatal period, the ductus arteriosus and the umbilical vessels either disappear completely or remain merely as cords of fibrous tissue. Similarly, the fetal adrenal cortex undergoes a considerable degree of atrophy soon after birth.

Atrophy of the thymus occurs normally as adult life is entered, and in late middle and old age there is a significant decline in the amount of lymphoid tissue.

In the same way that increased functional demand can lead to hypertrophy and/or hyperplasia, a decrease in demand will lead to a degree of atrophy. This can be seen to a very marked extent in voluntary muscle if a limb is immobilized, as, for example, after a fracture. Muscle bulk decreases very rapidly indeed, and when the period of immobilization is over a considerable degree of exercise may be required to restore it to normal. Similarly, starvation is associated with some degree of atrophy of the gut, with particular emphasis on the enterocyte lining.

Osteoporosis

A common and important example of generalized atrophy is osteoporosis. This has been defined as a condition in which the mass of bone tissue per unit volume of 'anatomical' bone is reduced, with a decrease in the number and size of the trabeculae in cancellous bone. There is no defect in the mineralization of such osteoid matrix as is present, in contradistinction to **osteomalacia**, where the bone tissue mass is normal but the degree of mineralization is subnormal. Osteoporosis is usually generalized but is most severe in the spinal column and pelvis. The commonest association is with increasing age, in particular with the menopause. Other causal associations are:

1. Cortisol excess either as a result of hyperactivity of the adrenal cortex or because of prolonged administration of large doses of corticosteroids
2. Severe thyrotoxicosis
3. Acromegaly
4. Prolonged recumbency

Clinical effects of osteoporosis

As the most severely affected areas are the spine and pelvis, the symptoms are usually related to these parts of the skeleton. The patients complain of chronic backache, and the collapse of individual vertebrae may occur and produce acute exacerbations in the pain. A reduction in the patient's height secondary to the vertebral collapse is a common feature. Fractures may complicate the general picture, the commonest of these involve the lower part of the forearm and the proximal part of the femur.

Localized atrophy

Localized atrophy may occur in the following circumstances:

ischaemia
pressure
denervation

Chapter 26

Cell Proliferation in Relation to Neoplasia

In the examples of non-neoplastic expansion of cell populations thus far considered, all share one common feature: the cessation of increased cell proliferation following the removal of the stimulus which has evoked it. In contrast, the proliferation of cells seen in neoplasia appears to be autonomous; it is in no way demand-led and a continuous application of an exogenous drive towards cell division is not present.

The characteristics of transformed cells in culture

Much of the data on the growth characteristics of neoplastic cells are derived from cell culture systems. While these are useful, one must be careful not to extrapolate too uncritically from these to the in vivo situation.

Transformed cells show loss of contact inhibition

When normal cells are grown in a monolayer, their proliferation ceases once the culture has reached confluence. In other words, once each cell is in contact with a neighbour, cell division ceases. This is known as **contact inhibition.** In contrast, monolayer cultures of neoplastic cells of the same type (e.g. fibroblasts) do not show this characteristic. Instead of cell division coming to an end once the cells have reached confluence, it continues and the cells heap up in a multilayered fashion.

How does contact between normal cells cause them to stop proliferating? It has been suggested that cells of a certain line **recognize** each other, that they exchange information which regulates cell division, and that they adhere to one another. Recognition of cells by their homologues certainly does occur: if two types of embryonic cells are mixed in culture, each type will segregate itself from the other. However, there are no hard data to indicate that failure of recognition is an important factor in the loss of contact inhibition which occurs with neoplastic cells.

Transformed cells differ from their normal homologues in respect of their surface membranes

Neoplastic transformation appears to be associated in most instances with changes in the surface membrane glycoproteins. One variety of these changes can be detected by the use of a family of proteins known as **lectins**. These proteins, which are derived from a very wide range of sources, are able to bind to different sugars on cell surfaces with exquisite specificity. One of these, **wheat germ lectin**, has the ability to agglutinate neoplastic cells in suspension but cannot do this to their normal homologues. This change in lectin agglutinability is associated with binding to the sugar N-acetyl-glucosamine on cell surface membranes. Since transformed cells do not appear to synthesize more N-acetyl-glucosamine than their normal counterparts, it seems reasonable to suggest that something has been lost from the surface of the transformed cells with resulting exposure of the lectin-binding sugars. This view finds support from two studies. In the first, normal cells were treated with trypsin to remove some of the surface protein. They then became agglutinable by wheat germ lectin. In the second, transformed cells in culture were treated with a monovalent wheat germ lectin which bound to the N-acetyl-glucosamine residues, thus, in a sense, masking them. When cells treated in this way were cultured in a monolayer, contact inhibition was shown to be restored.

Possible Mechanisms for Autonomous Growth

The loss of contact inhibition shown by transformed cells in culture may be an expression of disordered regulation of growth, but it still does not tell us how the cells have escaped from the normal mechanisms of growth control.

As in the case of regeneration, two basic possibilities exist: first, there may be a **failure in some inhibiting mechanism which normally restrains excessive cell proliferation**, or, second, the abnormal growth may represent **a response to growth factors**.

The former situation could arise from a decrease in the production of the putative inhibitory chemical messenger or some change in the cells capable of division which renders them unresponsive to the inhibiting signal given by this molecule or **chalone**. The possible role of chalones has been discussed earlier (see p. 89). There is little doubt that in some normal epithelial populations, such as the squamous epithelium of the epidermis, some sort of negative feedback control is implicated in preserving a steady state in so far as the epidermal cell population size is concerned. Extracts from epidermis have shown effects both on the G_1

and G_2 phases of cell cycles. However, the assay methods which have been employed do not command universal approval and there has been controversy as to the purity of the preparations used. The chalone hypothesis is an attractive one in biological terms, but convincing evidence for a determining role for chalones in neoplastic cell proliferation is still lacking.

'Autocrine' growth factors and autonomous neoplastic cell proliferation

In addition to their escape from the mechanisms normally controlling cell proliferation, which is fundamental in neoplasia, transformed cells also require fewer exogenous growth factors for optimal growth and multiplication than do their normal counterparts. This has been explained by the suggestion that autonomous growth (and indeed some other phenotypic characteristics of malignant transformation) are due to the production of polypeptide growth factors which act on the same cells that produce them by binding to appropriate receptors on the surface membrane. This process, in which the secretory cells are activated by their own secretion products, has been called **'autocrine secretion'** (Fig. 26.1) and may well become a central concept in malignant transformation.

Many types of tumour, when cultured, have been shown to release polypeptide growth factors (one of which inhibits cell proliferation) into

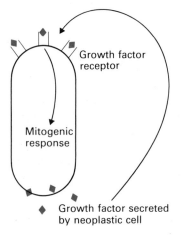

Growth factor
receptor

Mitogenic
response

◆ Growth factor secreted
by neoplastic cell

Fig. 26.1 'Autocrine' control of neoplastic cell proliferation. Transformed cells secrete growth factors which bind to receptors on the surface membrane of the same cell. Binding to these specific receptors generates a mitogenic signal.

their culture media, and these same cells often possess specific receptors for the released peptide. The peptides so far identified as functioning in this 'autocrine' fashion, include:

1. Type alpha transforming growth factor (which is structurally related to, but separate from, **epidermal growth factor**)
2. Peptides related to **platelet-derived growth factor** (PDGF)
3. Bombesin

Each of these acts on a specific membrane receptor, which in turn, probably through protein phosphorylation, transduces the signal generated by binding between the peptide and its receptor into a mitogenic response.

Theoretically, this signalling system might be modulated in three ways:

1. By the level of expression of the growth factor
2. By the level of expression of the membrane receptor
3. By the level of expression of the post-receptor signalling pathway

The autocrine action of a growth factor in malignant cells was first described in rodent cells transformed by either the Kirsten or the Molony mouse sarcoma viruses. The peptides identified are structurally related to epidermal growth factor (see p. 90) but are distinct from it. They have been named **alpha transforming growth factors** (**TGF alpha**) and have been shown to be released by a number of human neoplasms.

There is a very close relationship between the release of these TGF alpha peptides and the transformed state. This can be demonstrated using a temperature-sensitive mutant of the mouse sarcoma virus as the transforming agent. If the target cells are not cultured at a temperature suitable for the mutant virus, transformation does not take place and there is **no** release of the TGF into the culture medium.

Molecules showing a considerable degree of homology with **platelet-derived growth factor** (**PDGF**) are released by a number of neoplasms. In humans these include malignant connective tissue neoplasms of bone (**osteosarcoma**), malignant neoplasms of glial cells in the brain, and a cell line derived from human bladder cancer. In animal cell lines these molecules are released after transformation by a variety of RNA viruses. Many of these cell lines also possess receptors for PDGF. Antibodies against PDGF block tritiated thymidine incorporation into cells transformed by the simian sarcoma virus, and transformed cells which secrete small amounts of PDGF form only small tumours when inoculated into nude (athymic) mice. In contrast, those which secrete large amounts of the growth factor into culture media produce large masses in the nude mouse model.

Similar data come from studies of another growth factor known as **bombesin**. This is a tetradecapeptide which is produced and released by most human small-cell carcinomas of the lung ('**oat cell carcinoma**'). Monoclonal antibodies which are specific for the C-terminal end of the bombesin molecule prevent bombesin from binding to its receptor and inhibit the growth of small-cell lung cancer, both in culture and in xenografts in nude mice.

An increase in the output of the effector peptide may not be necessary for increased autocrine activity. An increase in the number or the binding affinity of the **receptors** will increase the autocrine effect of the peptide in the absence of any increase in its synthesis or secretion. Thus, human squamous carcinomas derived from the head and neck have been shown to have very large numbers of receptors for the epidermal growth factor (EGF) on their surface membranes and, in some tumour cell lines, the affinity of these receptors is very high. In at least one instance, where transformation occurs through the activation of a cellular gene known as **erb B** (see p. 474), the gene codes for a truncated version of the EGF receptor. This abnormal receptor cannot bind its ligand at the cell membrane, but appears to be able to generate a mitogenic signal independent of ligand binding. Other growth factor receptors also appear to be able to act as tyrosine kinases (and thus as initiators of mitosis) in the absence of their appropriate ligands.

Autocrine peptides can inhibit growth

At least one peptide has so far been identified which has a negative effect on cell growth. This is **beta transforming growth factor**, which is released from normal monkey kidney cells in culture and which appears to regulate their growth by binding to a receptor on the same cells. Whether this takes place in transformed cells is not yet known, but it is possible that such negative autocrine factors play a physiological role in regulating cell population size, and that transformation might lead to a situation where the inhibitory effects of such peptides are blocked with a **loss of negative growth control.**

Neoplasia and Disordered Cell Differentiation

Cancer is a set of diseases which arise in the first instance from normal cells in the body which, by one means or another are **transformed**. But from which normal cells? Since one of the cardinal features of neoplasia is the ability of a given cell population to go on proliferating in a relatively autonomous manner, the cells from which the neoplasm arises must have the ability to respond to mitogenic signals (normal or abnormal) and divide. In most normal cell populations, cells which have this characteristic are found in the **stem cell compartment** and hence, by implication, are undifferentiated cells. When a stem cell divides, one of its daughter cells may well retain the ability to divide while the other, by mechanisms which are not understood, becomes committed to differentiation and, ultimately, to death. By definition, the process of differentiation requires that for each type of differentiated cell, a **heritable** pattern of **read-out** of the genome must exist. Since all the cells in the body possess the same genetic information, differentiation similarly implies that in each type of cell, genes are expressed which are not expressed in other cell types.

Differentiation is also affected by the microenvironment of the cell

While genetic factors in the form of heritable patterns of gene transcription and translation undoubtedly play a major role in differentiation, the process may be affected in other ways as well. For instance, interaction between mesenchymal and epithelial elements is important in the development of many organ systems, including the pancreas, lung, kidney, salivary glands, breast, pituitary and liver. Pancreatic epithelium cultured from the developing rat pancreas will not differentiate. If the same cells are seeded onto a filter on the other side of which are mesenchymal cells in culture, then differentiation occurs. This suggests that a chemical differentiating signal is released from the mesenchymal cells. The effect of mesenchymal cell extracts is destroyed by trypsin and periodate oxidation, but not by ribonuclease or deoxyribonuclease. The factor is therefore presumably a glycoprotein. In cell culture systems, alteration of the medium may be sufficient to bring about profound changes in differentiation. Such a medium change may cause, for example, cartilage cells which synthesize type II collagen to revert to fibroblasts which secrete type I collagen. The mechanism responsible for this switch is not known.

Cell–cell interactions also appear to play a role in differentiation. If mixed embryonic cells are cultured, cells of each type will segregate. It may well be that some growth factors play a part in differentiation as well as in regulating the cell population size. For example, **epidermal growth factor** causes granulosa cells from the ovary to differentiate into luteal cells.

Changes in differentiation patterns do not necessarily imply neoplastic transformation

A complete change in differentiation from one fully differentiated form to another fully differentiated form occurs not infrequently in cells (mainly epithelial cells) subjected to chronic irritation or to changes in the hormonal milieu. This is known as **metaplasia**. One of the commonest forms is a change from cuboidal or columnar epithelium into squamous epithelium. Such metaplastic change may occur under the following circumstances:

1. The pseudo-stratified ciliated columnar epithelium of the bronchi may change into squamous epithelium. This occurs in cigarette smokers, patients with chronic bronchitis, and in chronic abscess cavities in the lung which can become lined by epithelium.
2. Squamous metaplasia is common in chronic cervicitis. The metaplastic epithelium may spread down into the cervical glands and fill the lumina. This process is called 'epidermidalization' by some, and may be mistaken for invasion by squamous carcinoma by the inexperienced.
3. The transitional epithelium of the renal pelvis and urinary bladder may undergo squamous metaplasia in the presence of chronic infection. This is seen very often in Egypt where schistosomal cystitis is very common. The presence of stones seems to increase the likelihood of metaplasia.
4. The columnar cell lining of the gallbladder sometimes undergoes squamous metaplasia in the presence of gallstones and chronic inflammation.
5. Prostatic ducts, which are normally lined by columnar epithelium, undergo squamous metaplasia in patients treated with oestrogens for prostatic carcinoma.
6. A deficiency of vitamin A may be associated with squamous metaplasia of the nose, bronchi and urinary tract. In addition, keratin formation is accelerated and increased in amount in the skin and conjunctiva.

Is there any identifiable mechanism that causes metaplasia?

Recent experiments on cultured cell lines suggest that metaplasia can be caused by agents which interfere with DNA methylation, and this supports the idea that such methylation plays a part in keeping the state of expression of genes stable. If cells are grown for a few cycles in the synthetic nucleotide analogue 5-aza-cytosine, the analogue becomes incorporated into the DNA in place of some of the cytosine residues. The 5-aza-cytosine is incapable of being methylated and also inhibits the action of the methylating enzyme. This breaks the chain of events in which the pattern of DNA methylation of a gene is passed from one cell generation to the next. When cultured cells resembling fibroblasts are treated in this way, they differentiate into a variety of cell types including skeletal muscle cells, to which they would never give rise under normal circumstances.

Cellular differentiation in malignant neoplasms

Cancer cells are cells that are **not fully differentiated.** Since fully differentiated cells are unlikely to be able to 'go backwards' so far as differentiation is concerned, it seems likely that the cancer cells are blocked at some stage in the maturation process. Unlike most normal cells that have progressed down the pathway toward full differentiation, these partly differentiated cells **still retain the capacity to divide.** The

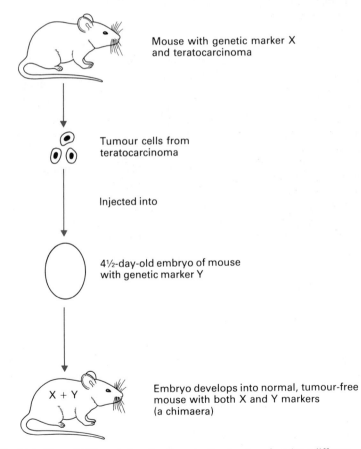

Mouse with genetic marker X and teratocarcinoma

Tumour cells from teratocarcinoma

Injected into

4½-day-old embryo of mouse with genetic marker Y

X + Y

Embryo develops into normal, tumour-free mouse with both X and Y markers (a chimaera)

Fig. 26.2   Normal differentiation of malignant cells when transferred to a different microenvironment.

degree of differentiation in neoplasms may be related to the precise point at which transformation occurs in the time-dependent sequence of events in which different genes are switched to the 'on' and 'off' positions after the stem cell has divided. This is particularly applicable to the liver, where there is a marked heterogeneity in respect of differentiation in neoplasms induced by chemical carcinogens. Such neoplasms vary from very well differentiated lesions in which the constituent cells can be distinguished only with difficulty from those of normal liver, to highly malignant, very poorly differentiated neoplasms in which the hepatic origin is difficult to determine.

The microenvironment in which malignant cells grow is involved in the maintenance of the malignant state

Malignant teratomas are neoplasms arising from multipotent cells and can express a variety of differentiation patterns. The commonest site of origin is in the gonads. Strains of mice exist in which malignant teratoma occurs in about 1% of the males. If cells from such a neoplasm are injected into the peritoneal cavity of unaffected mice of the parent strain, large cystic bodies develop. These are called embryoid bodies and contain both cancer cells and differentiated cells, suggesting that both the differentiated and cancer cells arise from a single precursor.

If teratoma cells from mice with certain genetic markers are injected into four-and-a-half day old embryos of mice with a different set of genetic markers, the embryos develop into **completely normal mice** which express the genetic markers both of the embryo and of the teratoma cells (a **chimaera**) (Fig. 26.2). None of these chimaeras develops teratocarcinoma. This shows that the microenvironment of the embryo is able to convert the **neoplastic** teratoma cells into fully differentiated normal cells. If, on the other hand, single teratocarcinoma cells are injected subcutaneously into adult mice, large neoplasms regularly develop at the injection site. Thus the differentiation signals provided by the embryo are lacking in the adult subcutaneous tissue.

Chapter 27

The Relationship of Neoplastic Cells with their Environment: Tumour Spread

The ability of malignant tumours to invade and destroy surrounding tissues has been recognized since the time of Hippocrates. Indeed, the term 'cancer' was derived from the crab-like, macroscopic appearance of certain malignant neoplasms in which processes of tumour tissue can be seen to penetrate the surrounding stroma. While a number of morphological and behavioural characteristics are used to differentiate between **benign** and **malignant** neoplasms, the only *absolute* criterion is the ability of a malignant neoplasm to invade surrounding tissue and to colonize distant sites (metastasis).

Malignant neoplasms can spread:

1. **Directly** through the tissues adjacent to the primary growth
2. Via the **lymphatics**
3. Via the **bloodstream**
4. Through body cavities (**transcoelomic**)

Direct Spread

Direct spread involves the invasion of the tissues adjacent to the original lesion; such spread occurs more or less in continuity with that lesion (Fig. 27.1). The infiltrating malignant cells are shed from the original mass. This implies that cell-to-cell adhesiveness in malignant neoplasms is reduced to comparison with normal cells of the same type. Normal epithelial cells, for example, develop well established points for anchorage with each other (desmosomes), but these appear to be either totally lacking or partially deficient in malignant cells. Another mechanism which has been suggested as playing a part in the reduced adhesiveness of malignant cells is an increase in the nett negative surface charge of the tumour cells. This could result from synthesis of abnormal amounts of a negatively charged sialomucopeptide or of normal amounts of a strongly negatively charged molecule of the same type.

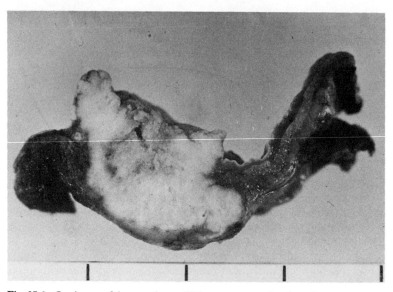

Fig. 27.1 Carcinoma of the oesophagus. This transverse section through the oesophagus shows an ulcerated tumour mass with everted edges protruding from the epithelial surface. The invasive nature of the neoplasm is shown by the deep extension of white tumour tissue through the submucosa and the muscle layer of the oesophageal wall.

In order for direct spread to take place, the tumour cells must cross certain connective tissue barriers which normally separate the tissue compartments from each other. Several suggestions have been made to account for their ability to do this. The invading cells tend to follow paths where the resistance is least and spread along natural clefts or within tissue planes. This can be seen in cancer of the alimentary tract where, once the invading cells have reached the main muscle layers, the infiltrating columns of cells tend to avoid the muscle itself and pass instead through the connective tissue septa which separate the muscle fibres. On naked eye examination, this gives the muscle a curiously segmented appearance, as if the muscle fibres were bricks and the intervening tumour-infiltrated septa, the mortar. On the basis of these patterns of spread, it has been suggested that invasiveness can largely be accounted for by mechanical factors. If quick-setting dental plastic is injected into tissue samples, the plastic spreads along the zones of least resistance in a manner similar to that seen in some tumours. Such simple mechanical models do not, however, appear to explain the very rapid invasive behaviour of some malignant neoplasms. In addition, in cell culture systems, invasiveness can be shown to occur even though there is no mechanical pressure.

The extracellular matrix which must be crossed by tumour cells in the course of invasion consists of two types: basement membranes and interstitial stroma. If distant spread is to occur, the invading cells may have to cross several such barriers in the course of their journey from the primary focus to and then through the lymphatic or vascular systems to the point where they leave these preformed systems and establish colonies in some other organ.

Neoplastic changes in the extracellular matrix

Malignant cells can alter the extracellular matrix in three ways:

1. Destruction of the matrix by tumour cells
2. Increased production of matrix by the host ('desmoplasia')
3. Synthesis of matrix by tumour cells

The first of these appears to bear most directly on tumour spread.

Matrix destruction

The malignant cells may degrade the matrix in order to penetrate it. Such degradation is probably localized to those areas where active invasion is taking place. It is of particular importance in relation to the penetration of basement membranes, loss or disorganization of basement membranes being a general finding in malignant neoplasms. It marks the transition from purely intra-epithelial malignant change (**carcinoma in situ**) to invasive carcinoma and is thus an important feature in the histological diagnosis of cancer.

Basement membrane loss may, in theory, be due to reduced synthesis, increased turnover, or destruction by enzymes. Many types of malignant cells can degrade basement membrane in vitro, and human breast cancer cells have been shown, by immunohistochemical methods, to contain collagenase capable of degrading type IV collagen (the type found in basement membranes).

A first step in penetrating the connective tissue matrix may be some form of attachment of the tumour cell to one of the constituents of the matrix. Evidence is beginning to accumulate that the malignant cells may attach to **laminin**. This is a glycoprotein found only in basement membranes and is produced by the cells that normally rest on the basement membrane. Cells from malignant tumours with a marked tendency to produce metastases bind strongly to laminin and a saturable laminin receptor has now been identified in several malignant cell lines.

Collagenase activity. Following attachment, it is believed that the malignant cells degrade the matrix locally. Such a step seems an essential part of spread since the density characteristics of the matrix are such as to not otherwise allow the entry of invading cells (whether in inflammation or in neoplasia). Many tumour cell lines can be shown to contain collagenase activity in respect of both basement membrane and interstitial matrix collagens. Cartilage is a rich source of collagenase inhibitors and it is not without interest that cartilage is one of the most resistant of all tissues to invasion by malignant cells.

It is almost certainly too simple to equate invasiveness and metastatic potential with enzyme activity. The malignant cell probably needs many other qualities, such as motility and ability to resist the host's immunological defence mechanisms, in order to travel and to survive in a hostile environment. This having been said, the collagenase activity of malignant tissue is consistently higher than that of its benign counterpart. There is at least one study which equates the clinical aggressiveness of a series of squamous carcinomas of the mouth, pharynx and larynx with their collagenase activity, and for a number of tumour cell lines derived from a single parent cell, a quantitative relationship was demonstrated between the amount of type IV collagenase activity and the metastatic potential.

Other tumour-associated proteolytic enzymes. It has been known for 60 years that extracts from virally induced tumours in chickens lysed plasma clots. Human sarcomas have been shown to have similar fibrinolytic properties. This fibrinolytic activity is now known to be due to the production by the tumour cells of **plasminogen activator**, a phenomenon which occurs in many cell lines following malignant transformation. There is some evidence to suggest that the acquisition of the ability to produce plasminogen activator is associated with the ability to invade extracellular matrix. In this connection it must be remembered that some normal cells also produce plasminogen activator. Some of these cells (such as macrophages, polymorphs, and trophoblastic cells) travel through the connective tissue matrix, while others (such as breast epithelium, Sertoli cells in the testis, thyroid and parathyroid epithelium, and beta cells in the islets of Langerhans) are fixed.

Desmoplastic response

The amount of stroma associated with malignant neoplasms determines, to a very considerable extent, their consistency. The extreme hardness and 'gritty' feel of some tumours is due to the high proportion of fibrous tissue within them. The ancient Greek physicians recognized this phenomenon and coined the term 'scirrhous' (rock-like) for such lesions. The biological purpose of desmoplasia is not clear. Its presence is certainly not necessary for invasion to occur; some invasive tumours have very little stromal response, while others, notably breast, stomach and bile duct tumours, show a marked desmoplastic reaction.

Synthesis of matrix

Some controversy also exists as to the origin of the fibrous tissue related to malignant tumours. Some workers, studying the stromal response to breast cancer cells, maintain that the new collagen is synthesized and secreted by the invading tumour cells. The results of other studies support a role for the host cells. Recently, myofibroblasts, which are not normally present in breast stroma, have been identified in the stroma of some breast cancers, and it has been suggested that malignant cells may, in some unknown way, either recruit or stimulate the formation of myofibroblasts, which then produce the excess connective tissue matrix found in tumours with a marked desmoplastic response.

Other phenotypic characteristics of malignant cells which may contribute to invasiveness

Loss of anchorage dependence

With the exception of lymphocytes and haemopoietic cells, normal cells, when cultured, will grow only on a firm surface such as glass, plastic or solid agar. This type of growth is spoken of as **anchorage dependent**. Many cell lines derived from malignant neoplasms or from cells which have undergone malignant transformation in culture can grow in suspension or in semi-solid soft agar. This growth feature in cell culture systems, more than any other, correlates with the ability of the cultured cells to produce malignant tumours when injected into animals of the appropriate species ('tumourigenicity').

Loss of fibronectin from the cell surface

Fibronectin is a glycoprotein which has been identified as a component of the extracellular matrix of many cells in culture. It is also found in basement membranes and interstitial stroma in many animal and human tissues and circulates in the blood (where it was originally called cold-insoluble globulin). Fibronectin can be found on the external surface of many cells, where it forms a fibrillary meshwork around and between them. It acts as an adhesive protein in cell-to-cell binding and in the binding of cells to their substratum. Malignant transformation is accompanied by a loss or marked reduction of cell surface fibronectin. The loss of this surface protein (and presumably the decreased adhesiveness which follows) may be an expression either of an increase in degradative enzymes on the surface of the malignant cell (see p. 400) or of a disturbance in the cytoskeleton, more particularly the microfilaments beneath the cell surface.

Lymphatic Spread

The invasion of lymphatic channels at an early stage of the infiltrative process is a characteristic property of carcinoma (malignant epithelial neoplasm). Malignant tumours derived from connective tissue cells (sarcomas) show a much greater tendency to invade the small blood vessels.

Invasion of the lymphatics may be made easier by the fact that the basement membranes do not contain any type IV collagen or laminin. Because of this difference, it is possible, using appropriate antibodies, to determine whether the small vascular channels in tissue sections showing invasion by tumour are lymphatics or venules.

Little is known as to the actual mechanics of invasion. In certain experimental models, tumour cells have been seen to line up alongside the lymphatic channels and to enter the lymphatic by first pushing cytoplasmic processes between the endothelial cells and then travelling through the inter-endothelial gap in a reverse direction to that seen when leucocyte emigration occurs in inflammation.

Once the malignant cells have gained access to the lymphatic vessel, they can grow along the lumen as a continuous cord which permeates the lymphatic drainage in that area and may extend quite widely. The presence of such intra-lymphatic tumour in a tissue section is, of course, an indicator of possible spread to regional lymph nodes. However, in some cases the presence of intra-lymphatic tumour in the absence of lymph node deposits may have an even more ominous prognostic significance, since it has been reported that patients with breast cancer in whom there is evidence of lymphatic permeation by tumour but no regional node deposits have an **increased risk** of developing distant metastases.

Lymphatic permeation is a particularly prominent feature of **carcinoma of the breast**. Lymphatic blockage occurs quite frequently in this situation. This results in diversion of lymph flow and may be accompanied by a similar diversion of groups of tumour cells which may impact within the lymphatic drainage of the breast, causing satellite tumour nodules. Lymphatic blockage also causes lymph-oedema of the tissues caudal to the block. In patients with carcinoma of the breast this produces an appearance of the skin which has been aptly termed **peau d'orange**. In the lung, extensive lymphatic permeation by tumour, often from a breast or gastric primary, produces the condition known as **lymphangitis carcinomatosa**. On chest x-ray the lung shows a curious reticulated appearance. This is mirrored by the outlining of the subpleural lymphatic channels seen when the lung is removed at post-mortem examination.

Malignant melanoma is another of the neoplasms which tends to permeate local lymphatic drainage. If the tumour cells are producing melanin, the cord of cells permeating the lymphatics may be seen as a black streak in the subcutaneous tissue.

Tumour cells enter the regional nodes and gain access to the subcapsular peripheral sinus in the first instance. From here, the cells extend to involve the sinuses in the centre of the node. Within the node, tumour cells may be destroyed, may remain dormant for long periods, or may establish a growing focus with partial or total replacement of the node. For the last of these, acquisition of an adequate blood supply is important. Normal nodes have a dual blood supply, partly from hilar vessels and partly from transcapsular anastomoses. If the tumour nodules invade intra-nodal vessels, haemorrhage and necrosis may occur within the secondary deposit.

Tumour cells within lymph nodes may gain access to the bloodstream in a number of different ways. These include invasion of small intra-nodal blood vessels, invasion of extra-nodal blood vessels by nodal deposits which have breached the lymph node capsule, opening up of small lymphatico-venous communications and, finally, via the thoracic duct. These connections between the lymphatic channels and the bloodstream work in both directions. If radioactively labelled tumour cells are injected into a peripheral vein of a rat, tumour cells can be recovered from lymphatics within an hour. Thus malignant cells within the bloodstream are not always trapped in the first capillary bed they encounter, but can escape into the lymphatic system.

Blood Spread

Apart from the connections between the lymphatic system and the blood vessels mentioned above, malignant cells may enter the bloodstream either by invading small new vessels within the substance of the tumour itself or by invading the host blood vessels near the growing edge of the tumour. The vessels within the tumour are derived from the host vessels in the surrounding stroma, the ingrowth of new vascular channels being elicited by angiogenic factors secreted both by the tumour cells and, possibly, by macrophages within the tumour.

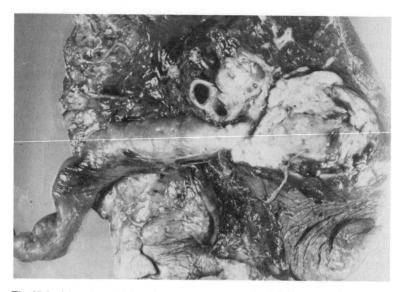

Fig. 27.2 A large bronchial carcinoma which has invaded the main pulmonary vein. The vessel is virtually occluded by a mixture of tumour and thrombus which, at operation, was found to extend into the right atrium.

These newly-formed vessels often have defective basement membranes and may lack normal perivascular connective tissue. Sarcomas often contain large, irregular blood-filled channels, the linings of which consist partly or entirely of malignant tumour cells; these lining cells can, of course, be shed directly into the bloodstream. This may, in part, account for the predilection for blood spread which is shown by the sarcomas.

Permeation in continuity along invaded venous channels may be seen in certain malignant tumours. These include carcinomas arising from renal tubular epithelium (so-called **hypernephroma**) and carcinoma of the bronchus (Fig. 27.2). In the case of renal adenocarcinoma, venous invasion may occur quite early and the tumour cells extend as a solid mass along the course of the renal vein. In rare instances, the inferior cava may be involved and cases have been recorded where the tumour has grown up into the right atrium. When the left renal vein is involved in this way, the first clinical evidence of this occurrence may be the appearance of a left-sided scrotal mass consisting of dilated spermatic veins (**varicocele**). This is said to be due to the fact that the spermatic veins on the left side drain directly into the left renal vein. If the latter becomes blocked by tumour, the hydrostatic pressure rises in the spermatic veins and they become distended.

Metastasis

A growing colony of malignant cells which becomes established at a point distant from the original or primary lesion and with no continuity between the primary lesion and new deposit is termed a **metastasis**. The majority of metastases arise as a result of invasion of lymphatics or blood vessels, but in some instances they owe their existence to 'seeding out' of malignant cells across serosa-lined spaces such as the pleural and peritoneal cavities.

Metastasis is, fundamentally, an **embolic** process. It may be viewed as a series of events which occur sequentially. Some of these have already been discussed. These events are:

1. The **liberation** of cells from the primary tumour mass
2. The **invasion** of blood vessels or lymphatics
3. Their **transfer** as tumour emboli to distant sites
4. **Migration** from the vessels in which the emboli have impacted
5. **Survival** at the new site
6. **Multiplication** and **growth** to form secondary tumours

As already stated, metastatic spread occurs as a result of invasion of lymphatic channels, the bloodstream and serosal cavities.

In carcinomas, deposits of tumour in the regional nodes is a common occurrence. If the efferent channel is invaded by the tumour cells, the stage is set for further extension to the next set of nodes, which may also become wholly or partly replaced by tumour. The extent of such nodal invasion is important in assessing the prognosis of patients with cancer and, despite the introduction of a number of new criteria in recent years, the presence or absence of lymph node metastases remains one of the more reliable indicators of the natural history of an individual patient with cancer. For instance, in one of the commonest malignant neoplasms encountered in clinical practice — carcinoma of the breast — absence of lymph node metastases after a careful search of the axillary contents is associated with a five-year survival rate of 75–80%. The presence of lymph node deposits reduces this figure very considerably, perhaps to approximately 50%.

A combination of assessment of direct spread and lymph node metastases gives valuable prognostic information in carcinomas of the colon and rectum, and forms the basis of the Dukes' staging scheme for these tumours. If a colonic or rectal carcinoma penetrates the bowel wall no further than the main muscle coat (Dukes' stage A), the five-year survival rate should be 80–90%. Penetration of the bowel wall by tumour through the muscle to reach the subserosa (Dukes' stage B) reduces the five-year survival rate to approximately 50%. If the tumour is associated with lymph node deposits (Dukes' stage C) the five-year survival rate is reduced to about 30%.

The occurrence of blood-borne metastases is the feature of malignant disease which is responsible for death in most fatal cases. It is obvious when considering an accessible tumour such as carcinoma of the breast, which can apparently be completely excised with relative ease, that it is the presence of **occult** metastases at the time of primary excision which will determine the outcome for that patient.

Much of our knowledge of this process comes from experimental systems such as transplantable breast cancers or malignant melanomas in mice. Once a transplantable tumour has grown to a few grams in weight, it starts to release several million malignant cells into the blood every day. Fortunately the presence of malignant cells in the blood (or lymph) does not mean that metastases will inevitably develop. An overwhelming majority of the tumour cells released into the blood die very quickly. In studies carried out using radioactively labelled malignant melanoma cells, it was found that only 1% of the injected cells survived for 24 hours. After two weeks only 0.1% had survived. However, at this stage deposits of secondary tumour could be seen in the lungs. While in the bloodstream the malignant cells may adhere to other tumour cells to form clumps, they may adhere to platelets or lymphocytes, and when they enter the capillary bed in which they may impact, they can adhere to the capillary endothelium. The greater the degree of clumping of tumour cells, the more likely is impaction and the greater the chances of a secondary deposit forming. After impaction in a small vessel, some tumour cells stimulate the production of fibrin; it has been suggested that this fibrin tends to protect the clump of malignant cells and enables them to proliferate. In animal models of the metastatic process, administration both of plasmin and of anticoagulants were shown almost 20 years ago to reduce the number of metastases consequent on intravenous injection of malignant cells.

After impaction in small vessels, the malignant cells must emigrate from the vascular compartment into the perivascular tissues. It has been shown in experimental tumours that endothelial cells retract, leaving cell-free spaces through which the tumour cells can escape. Within the extravascular tissues, a new and suitable microenvironment must be established if the colony of tumour cells is to grow and flourish. If the colony is to grow to a significant size, a new blood supply must become available both for the nutrition of the tumour cells and for carrying away cellular waste products. The new blood vessels, as mentioned earlier, are derived from the host's vasculature. Ingrowth of these vessels is stimulated by the secretion of a large molecule which has been termed **tumour angiogenesis factor**. If tumours are implanted into the cornea of animals, initially tumour growth is slow. After about a week small capillaries begin to grow out from the iris into the cornea and when these vessels reach the tumour, a marked spurt of tumour growth occurs. Implantation of normal tissues does not have this effect. Extracts from tumours applied to the chorio-allantoic membrane of a fertilized chicken egg also show a considerable angiogenic effect. However, this tumour angiogenesis factor has not yet been purified, and it is known that certain other, non-neoplastic cells, as well as other growth factors such as epidermal growth factor, can also stimulate the ingrowth of blood vessels.

Are malignant cells homogeneous in respect of their tendency to metastasize?

Only a small fraction of the malignant cells released into the circulation from a primary tumour survive to establish secondary deposits. Does this mean that the cells which are successful have some special properties not shared by the other cells of the tumour?

This hypothesis has been tested in the mouse melanoma model. Malignant melanoma in humans frequently develops lymphatic and blood-borne metastases; non-human melanomas behave in much the same way. Murine B16 melanoma, which arises spontaneously in a certain strain of black mice, can be transplanted from one animal of the strain to another and the cells can be grown in culture with relative ease. When B16 cells are implanted into the subcutaneous tissue of mice, the melanoma metastasizes at a low or moderate rate. In order to quantify the phenomenon of metastasis it is customary to inject a known number of tumour cells into the mouse tail vein and then count the number of lung metastases. If the metastatic deposits are harvested and cultured and these cultured cells then injected into mouse tail veins, the yield of metastases is greater. After, say, 10 cycles a cell line will have been established which has a very much greater metastatic potential than the cells from the original tumour line. These data suggest that the original tumour cell population was not homogeneous in respect of the qualities needed to establish metastases.

This model may also throw some light on the common clinical observation that particular primary tumours metastasize preferentially to certain sites. For example, breast cancers commonly spread to lung, liver, bone and brain; lung tumours often spread to the brain and adrenals, and prostatic cancers frequently spread to bone. About 80 years ago, Ewing and Paget suggested that different patterns of metastasis were due to the fact that different tumour cells would thrive in certain '**biological soils**' but not in others. More recently the use of experimental models has suggested that properties of the malignant cells themselves also influence the pattern of their metastasis.

For instance, is the pattern of metastasis solely due to anatomical factors such as the vascular bed first encountered by tumour emboli? If radioactively labelled B16 melanoma cells are injected into the tail veins of a batch of mice and also into the left ventricles of other mice, the initial distribution of the radioactivity suggests that the cells have indeed impacted in different sites. Within 24 hours, however, the distribution and number of surviving cells is the same, irrespective of the site of injection, and after two weeks the numbers of metastases in the lungs are the same in both cases. These results suggest that tumour cells destined to form secondary deposits in a particular organ can detach themselves from their initial impaction site and 'home' onto the favoured tissue. By cell selection procedures similar to those described previously, it has been possible to isolate a subpopulation of B16 cells which metastasizes *only* to one area of the brain, and another which preferentially colonizes the ovaries. While the nature of this 'homing' mechanism is unknown, it appears to be related to the nature of the surface membrane of the malignant cell. A lung-metastasizing line of B16 cells was found to shed small membrane-bound vesicles into the culture fluid. These vesicles can be fused with a line which metastasizes poorly to the lung using polyethylene glycol. The cells enriched with vesicles now produce very large numbers of pulmonary metastases. Each of the melanoma cell lines which produce preferential metastases has been shown to have a specific pattern of cell surface proteins. How far these observations relate to the behaviour of malignant tumours in humans is unknown, though there is increasing evidence that human tumours are heterogeneous with respect to features such as karyotype and DNA content, the presence of hormone receptors, antigenic determinants and cell surface constituents, pigment synthesis (in the case of malignant melanoma), drug sensitivity, and growth in nude (immunosuppressed) mice.

Some common patterns of metastasis in human tumours

The liver

The liver is the site in which blood-borne metastases occur most frequently. Gastrointestinal and pancreatic tumours regularly metastasize there, which is not surprising in view of their venous drainage via the portal system. Other primary tumours which commonly metastasize to the liver are carcinomas of the lung, breast and the genito-urinary system, malignant melanoma (Fig. 27.3), and various sarcomas. Rare examples of transplacental metastases have been recorded in the liver.

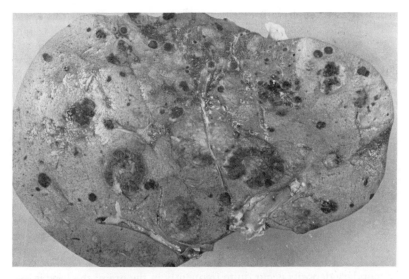

Fig. 27.3 Liver showing numerous, discrete darkly pigmented tumour masses. These are metastatic deposits from a malignant melanoma arising in the skin.

The lung

Tumours commonly producing metastatic deposits in the lung are carcinoma of the breast, carcinoma of the stomach, and sarcomas. Blood-borne metastases in this tissue may be single or multiple and tend to occur as well-demarcated rounded masses. Sometimes it may be difficult to distinguish between a single secondary deposit and a peripherally situated primary carcinoma of the lung. In a city dweller, whose lung tissue is usually laden with carbon pigment, the absence of pigment from the centre of the tumour, which is characteristic of secondary deposits, may be helpful.

The skeleton

After the liver and the lungs, the skeleton is the most frequent site for metastatic deposits to occur. The site of origin of the primary is commonly lung, breast, prostate, kidney or thyroid. Bony metastases may either elicit the production of new bone (**osteoblastic**) or destroy bone (**osteolytic**). In the former, the secondary deposits are very hard as a result of the abundant new bone formation and on x-ray appear as radio-opaque shadows. Plasma alkaline phosphatase levels are high, reflecting active osteogenesis. Serum calcium and phosphate concentrations are usually normal. Such osteosclerotic secondaries are commonly seen in association with carcinoma of the prostate. When this is the case, plasma concentrations of acid phosphatase (of tumour cell origin) are also much elevated. Osteolysis shows itself on x-ray examination by the presence of zones of radiolucency. Clinically, it draws attention to itself by pain or because of pathological fractures (fractures occurring after only slight trauma). If bone destruction has been extensive, hypercalcaemia may be present.

The mechanisms of tumour-mediated bone destruction are not well understood. Many tumours contain collagenase capable of degrading type I collagen. In organ culture systems where portions of breast cancer are incubated together with small pieces of mouse skull, osteolysis can be detected. This osteolysis can be inhibited by adding cyclo-oxygenase inhibitors such as aspirin to the culture medium. This suggests that the release of prostaglandins may play some part in mediating bone destruction.

The brain

Secondary deposits occur quite frequently in the brain; the lung is one of the commonest primary sites. Often neurological and/or psychiatric disturbances produced by the metastasis are the first indication of the presence of cancer in these patients.

The adrenal

Of all endocrine organs, the adrenal is the most frequently involved by metastatic tumour. The medulla is the most favoured site for metastases but nodules of secondary tumour may also be seen in the cortex. Common primary sites for adrenal secondaries include the lung and the breast.

Transcoelomic Spread

The term **transcoelomic spread** is applied to the sequence of events which follows the invasion of the serosal lining of an organ by malignant cells. A local inflammatory response usually develops in relation to the infiltrating tumour cells and the malignant cells may become incorporated into the inflammatory exudate on the serosal surface.

These small groups of cells become detached from the main colony of tumour cells and can be swept away by the fluid portion of the exudate and float out into the serosal cavity. They settle on the walls of such a cavity, where some of them proliferate and set up small secondary deposits. These may elicit the formation of more exudation and the serosal cavity may, in time, come to contain a large volume of fluid.

This type of spread is most commonly seen in the peritoneal cavity in cases of gastric, colonic and ovarian carcinoma. The greater omentum may be so massively infiltrated that it becomes converted to a thick, firm, often rather gelatinous mass, which some, rather infelicitously, refer to as 'omental cake'. Deposits arising from gravitational seeding are especially common in the pouch of Douglas.

From time to time, gastric or colonic carcinoma may be associated with a highly individual pattern of transcoelomic spread in which the ovaries become preferentially involved. The ovaries become grossly enlarged and have smooth capsular surfaces and slightly mucoid cut surfaces. Much of the enlargement can be seen, on microscopic examination, to be due to a desmoplastic response in the ovarian stroma to the presence of the relatively scanty cancer cells. The classical jargon term for these ovarian deposits is 'Krukenberg' tumours.

Chapter 28

Both benign and malignant neoplasms can produce a wide variety of effects on the host. While the term 'malignant' rightly has ominous prognostic overtones, 'benign' lesions, while not invasive and having no metastatic potential, may have serious or even lethal consequences.

Local effects due to mechanical pressure or obstruction

In many cases the effects of neoplasms on their host will depend on the interaction between the **site** of the tumour and its **size**. A large number of such instances exist and only a few examples will be given in the following section; no pretence of completeness is made.

In the gastrointestinal tract, the clinical presentation of a neoplasm is frequently related to the fact that the lesion may cause obstruction, which is usually, though not invariably, **chronic.** For example, in the case of a colonic or rectal tumour, the patient may complain of an alteration in the bowel habit. The obstruction may be due to the actual bulk of the neoplasm itself, but more often it is caused by the fibrous tissue response elicited by the presence of the cancer cells (desmoplasia). In a few instances, a polypoid tumour mass may lead to intussusception (see p. 337).

Obviously the anatomical site of a neoplasm will play a major role in determining whether or not obstruction will occur. A small neoplasm in an unfavourable anatomical location can produce very serious obstruction. For instance, carcinomas in the common bile duct or in the head of the pancreas will produce a severe degree of cholestatic jaundice, this being associated with marked dilatation of the biliary passages above the obstruction and, not infrequently, with dilatation of the gallbladder as well.

From the point of view of mechanical disturbances, one of the most serious locations for neoplasms to occur, apart from any question of their inherent malignancy, is within the cranium. One of the commonest intracranial tumours arises from the meninges (**meningioma**). The overwhelming majority of these are benign, but they can cause serious or fatal consequences as a result of the rise in intracranial pressure which they produce and the distortion of normal anatomical relationships that follows.

In some cases the types of obstructive phenomena are determined by the **pattern of spread** of the neoplasm. This is seen very strikingly in carcinoma of the uterine cervix. Here the direct spread of the tumour within the pelvis often involves the lower portions of the ureters, these being encased in a rigid sleeve of tumour and associated fibrous tissue. The obvious sequel is ureteric obstruction and in due time, if the obstruction cannot be relieved, chronic renal failure.

Another example of the role of anatomical location in determining the clinical picture may be seen, from time to time, in carcinomas of the lung occurring at the apices of the upper lobes. If such a neoplasm extends directly beyond the anatomical confines of the lung, it may involve either the brachial plexus or the sympathetic chain. In either instance there may be striking local neurological consequences with a unilateral Horner's syndrome being produced in the case of sympathetic involvement.

Local effects related to the destruction of tissue

Destruction of tissue may occur either as a result of pressure or as a result of the aggressive invasive properties of the tumour. Examples of the former may be seen in the erosive effects of a benign adenoma of the pituitary, which may be associated with destruction of part of the pituitary fossa, or in the mucosal ulceration which can occur over benign connective tissue tumours of the bowel wall such as smooth muscle tumours (leiomyomas) or tumours of nerve sheath (neurilemmomas).

Destruction of bone due to the presence of deposits of tumour is not infrequent and leads to a great deal of distress for the patient. In addition to the pain which may be produced by bony secondaries, the actual loss of tissue may lead to so-called **pathological fractures.** These are manifested in the vertebral column as collapse of infiltrated vertebrae. The presence of multiple bony deposits may be associated with extensive osteolysis leading to hypercalcaemia. Skeletal metastases are responsible for many cases of hypercalcaemia, but hypercalcaemia can also occur in the presence of certain neoplasms **without secondary tumour being present within the skeleton.**

Non-metastatic hypercalcaemia

If plasma calcium levels are elevated it seems reasonable to assume that the excess calcium has been released from bone, and, in the absence of primary or secondary tumour actually within the bone, some other calcium-releasing mechanism must be invoked.

Studies exist in which some tumours (not of the parathyroid) have been found to secrete parathyroid hormone (PTH). This particular example of **ectopic hormone production**, which is considered in more detail later in this chapter, has been especially noted in tumours of the lung and kidney. However, tumour-related hypercalcaemia can occur both in the absence of bony metastases and in the absence of raised PTH concentrations. Extracts of the tumours from these patients have an osteolytic effect in vitro. At least part of this effect is now thought to be due to prostaglandin (PG) production, either by the tumour cells or by cells associated with them. In a number of animal tumours, secretion of PGE_2 was noted and the hypercalcaemia could be prevented by the administration of a cyclo-oxygenase inhibitor such as indomethacin. PGE_2 can be shown to have a marked capacity for causing bone resorption in studies carried out in vitro. Several studies in humans also indicate that increased secretion of PGE_2 is causally associated with hypercalcaemia.

Substances other than prostaglandins capable of inducing resorption of bone have also been found in association with certain tumours. Cultured cell lines of plasma cell tumours and from Burkitt's lymphoma (a B lymphocyte-derived tumour believed to be associated with infection by the Epstein–Barr virus) produce a non-prostaglandin, non-PTH, soluble factor which can stimulate osteoclasts to resorb bone in vitro. In addition, some breast cancer cell lines have been shown to contain an osteolytic substance which does not appear to act by stimulating osteoclasts and which is not blocked by indomethacin.

Haemorrhage

Most neoplasms involving surfaces lined by epithelium or lying subjacent to such surfaces will undergo a certain degree of ulceration, with resulting haemorrhage. In most instances the bleeding is slow and unspectacular, though none the less dangerous. The chronic blood loss may well produce a severe microcytic anaemia of the type associated with iron deficiency. Occult bleeding of this type and degree is not infrequently seen in cancers of the right side of the colon or of the caecum. Indeed, the symptoms of vague ill-health associated with anaemia of this type may be the first and, for a long time, the only indication of the presence of the neoplasm. Occasionally, ulceration of a tumour may result in torrential haemorrhage. One of the situations in which this occurs is in smooth muscle tumours of the stomach or intestine, from which bleeding may be so severe as to necessitate replacement of the total blood volume several times over.

Infection

Infection in relation to malignancy is common and may be the determining factor in the timing of a patient's death. Local infection tends to occur in any situation where the presence of a neoplasm causes obstruction to a drainage system with retention of secretions behind the obstruction. An example of this may occur in bronchial carcinoma, where narrowing or total blocking of the bronchus may cause damming back of the secretions derived from more distal parts of the bronchial tree. The retained secretions constitute an advantageous medium for the growth of organisms and this, coupled with the collapse of lung parenchyma distal to the obstruction, tends to lead to episodes of bronchopneumonia which may be severe.

The role of malignant disease in promoting susceptibility to infections through immunosuppression has already been alluded to (see p. 146) and will be considered further later in this chapter.

Fever

Episodes of fever are extremely common in patients with malignant disease, even in the absence of recognizable evidence of infection. Fever is particularly common in malignant diseases involving the lymphoid system such as malignant lymphomas, the leukaemias and Hodgkin's disease, though it also occurs in cases of disseminated, solid, epithelial tumours. Some cultured cell lines derived from lymphoid tumours have been found to contain factors capable of inducing fever (**pyrogens**), but the majority of cases of fever unrelated to infection are difficult to account for. Occasionally fever may be the presenting feature of a neoplasm. This is seen most notably in renal adenocarcinoma (hypernephroma), a tumour which seems particularly prone to produce non-metastatic systemic disturbances.

Cachexia

Marked weight loss and wasting of tissues, especially muscle, is a well-recognized feature of the later stages of the natural history of many malignant neoplasms. This state is known as cachexia and understanding of its pathogenesis is still far from complete. Processes which have been canvassed as playing a role in the production of cachexia include:

1. **Anorexia.** Loss of appetite is a conspicuous feature in certain malignant disorders and appears not to be related to tumour bulk or location. Many reasons have been advanced to account for this, but none can be shown to operate in all instances of tumour-related anorexia.

2. **Malabsorption.** This may occur in association with neoplasms, such as medullary carcinoma of the thyroid, which secrete products which increase gastrointestinal motility. In most cases where malabsorption is present, the mechanism producing it is not known.

3. **The metabolic processes of the neoplasm.** In some experimental tumour models, the tumour gives the impression of 'growing at the expense of its host'; force-feeding of these animals results in tumour growth being stimulated in the absence of any weight gain in the host. However, when the dietary **constituents** are manipulated, a situation can be brought about in which tumour growth is minimal and the host animal's weight is maintained. This is alleged to be because the metabolism of many tumour cells appears to be dominated by anaerobic glycolysis, for which appropriate substrates are required. If such substrates are deficient in the diet, the rate of tumour progression slows down. There is little to suggest that these data, none of which are very recent, can be readily applied to the human situation.

4. **Is some toxic product liberated from the neoplasm?** From time to time the suggestion has been made that some toxic product liberated from the neoplasm could be responsible for the nutritional changes seen. Decreased hepatic catalase activity can be shown to occur both in certain patients with malignant disease and in animals with ex-perimentally-induced tumours; this decline in catalase activity can be reproduced in animals injected with a polypeptide extractable from human gastric or rectal carcinoma. This extracted material also produces changes in plasma iron concentrations, increases the levels of protoporphyrin in the liver, and may cause thymic involution. In a rat hepatoma, substances have been identified which uncouple oxidative phosphorylation in normal liver mitochondria and this could, in theory, be responsible for considerable weight loss. These data are interesting, but there is still no good evidence that mechanisms of this type are responsible for weight loss in the human situation.

The effect of neoplasms on the immune system of the host

Patients with malignant disease, especially if this is related to the lymphoid system, appear to have their immune defences compromised and, as a result, are more prone to infection than expected. Depression of the defensive abilities of phagocytes is often present and patients, especially those in whom there is bone marrow involvement, quite commonly show a decline in the number of granulocytes. Both humoral and cellular immune mechanisms may be depressed, a decline in the latter being associated with an increased liability to tuberculous, fungal and viral infections. It should not be forgotten that, in addition to the disease itself, treatment may cause a decline in the efficiency of the host's defences against infection, since both chemotherapy and irradiation have an immunosuppressive effect.

In addition to the immunosuppression associated with some cases of malignant disease, an association with autoimmunity has also been recognized. Many patients can be shown to develop non-organ-specific autoantibodies directed against such 'self' components as smooth muscle, nuclei and nuclear fractions. Immune complex formation may also occur and some patients with malignant neoplasms present with an immune complex mediated nephrotic syndrome (massive proteinuria, hypoalbuminaemia and oedema).

Haematological effects of neoplasms

Anaemia

Many patients with cancer show a diminished red cell mass at some stage in their illness. Clearly a number of possible mechanisms may be invoked to explain the presence of anaemia in any individual patient.

Iron-deficiency anaemia may result from occult blood loss associated with ulceration of a neoplasm involving an epithelial surface. A poor nutritional state may be associated with a decreased folate intake, and if malabsorption is present, such folate as is present may not be absorbed adequately, and a **macrocytic anaemia** may result. Excess red blood cell destruction may occur as a result of an **autoimmune haemolytic anaemia**, with autoantibodies directed against components of the patient's own red cells. This tends to occur in association with neoplasms of the lymphoreticular system such as Hodgkin's disease and non-Hodgkin malignant lymphomas. Why such an autoimmune reaction should occur is not understood. Lastly, anaemia may occur in association with malignant disease as a result of a relatively decreased level of erythropoietin secretion. Marrow cells from such patients appear to respond quite normally to erythropoietin in culture and the defect does not, therefore, appear to be a failure of response on the part of red cell precursors.

Increased red cell production

An increase in red cell mass is encountered not infrequently in certain neoplastic states. This has been reported as occurring most notably in **renal adenocarcinoma, cerebellar haemangioblastoma, uterine fibroleiomyoma,** and **liver cell carcinoma,** and less frequently in ovarian carcinoma, adrenal tumours and carcinoma of the lung. The abnormal drive for red cell production seems to be due to the ectopic secretion of erythropoietic substances by the tumours.

Effects on platelets and clotting

In some patients with malignant disease there is a significant decrease in the number of circulating platelets and thrombocytopenic purpura may be seen. In some of these instances there is an immune-mediated destruction of the platelets, but this is by no means always the case.

In contrast, an increase in clotting is quite often seen. This, of course, may itself contribute to the decrease in the platelet count. Evidence of continued intravascular coagulation may be found in some patients by determining the level of fibrinopeptide A (FPA) in the plasma. In one recent study, 60% of a group of patients with advanced cancer showed such evidence of intravascular coagulation. In these patients, serial determinations of FPA revealed an upward trend which appeared to be related to the progression of the neoplastic disorder. This intravascular clotting could be inhibited by giving oral anticoagulants such as warfarin. It was stated earlier that, in experimental tumour models, agents which promote clotting tend to promote tumour growth, while those which inhibit one or more aspect of the clotting process are associated with tumour regression. A clinical trial of anticoagulants in patients with small-cell carcinoma of the lung reported prolonged survival of these patients. This is an area which may well reward further study.

Some malignant tumours are associated with a curious syndrome in which **recurrent migratory thrombophlebitis** occurs. Episodes of venous thrombosis involving both superficial and deep veins occur and are recurrent in nature. Carcinomas of the bronchus, pancreas, stomach and female genital tract are most frequently implicated and the thrombophlebitis may, in some instances, be the first indicator of occult malignancy.

Endocrine effects of neoplasms

Hormonal effects associated with neoplasms fall into two main groups. In the first the neoplasms, whether benign or malignant, occur in endocrine glands and the hormones produced are appropriate in relation to the location of the tumour. For example, the fact that an adenoma of the beta cells of the islets of Langerhans produces large amounts of insulin surprises no-one. Such tumours retain the normal biosynthetic pathways for the production of the hormones and differ from normal cells only in their escape from normal 'feedback' controls. Examples of this type of situation are given below:

1. **Acidophil adenoma of the pituitary** produces growth hormone. This results in gigantism if the tumour has been present before the time of epiphyseal fusion and acromegaly in adults.

2. **Basophil adenoma of the pituitary** produces adrenocorticotrophic hormone (ACTH) with resulting adrenal cortical hyperplasia and excess output of cortisol. This results in Cushing's syndrome.

3. **Chromophobe adenoma of the pituitary** produces excess amounts of prolactin; this may cause amenorrhoea, galactorrhoea or impotence.

4. **Adrenal cortical adenomas**, depending on their cell type, may produce either excess amounts of cortisol or excess amounts of aldosterone. In the first case, the patients present with Cushing's syndrome; in the second, with Conn's syndrome (hypertension, muscle weakness and hypokalaemia).

5. **Parathyroid adenoma** produces excess amounts of parathyroid hormone, with resulting hypercalcaemia.

6. **Islet cell tumours of the pancreas** (which may be benign or malignant) may secrete a wide variety of hormones. The commonest are **insulin** and **gastrin**. In the former case the patients may present with a history of episodes of highly uncharacteristic and aggressive behaviour, fits and loss of consciousness, all as a result of hypoglycaemia. Excess secretion of gastrin leads to intractable peptic ulceration, the so-called Zollinger–Ellison syndrome.

Ectopic hormone production by neoplasms

The second way in which hormonal effects may be experienced by patients with various forms of neoplasm is when hormones are secreted by the cells of tumours arising in **tissues not normally associated with hormone production**. This is termed **ectopic hormone production** and was first described in 1928 in a patient with a small-cell bronchial carcinoma who developed diabetes, hirsutism, high blood pressure and bilateral adrenal cortical hyperplasia (i.e. Cushing's syndrome). However, it was not until more than 30 years later that it was proved that the reason for the appearance of such syndromes in patients with tumours arising outside the endocrine system was secretion of ACTH by the tumours. Though only a small percentage of patients with bronchial carcinoma of the small-cell variety show the clinical features associated with excess ACTH secretion, radioimmunoassay of extracts of such tumours show ACTH to be present in the majority. The disparity between the number of tumours which contain immunologically identifiable ACTH and those secreting 'active' ACTH is due to the fact that, in most cases, the hormone exists in the form of an inactive precursor or 'big' ACTH, which has less than 5% of the biological activity of ACTH secreted by the pituitary.

A wide variety of such **'paraendocrine'** syndromes have now been described. Some examples are given in Table 28.1.

Table 28.1 Ectopic hormone production by tumours.

Hormone	Principal tumours	Chief effects
Adrenocorticotrophic hormone	Bronchus Pancreas Thymoma Thyroid Ovary	Hypokalaemic alkalosis, weakness, thirst, polyuria
Antidiuretic hormone	Bronchus Duodenum Lymphoma Prostate Thymoma Ewing's tumour	Dilutional hyponatraemia
Thyroid-stimulating hormone	Lung Breast Choriocarcinoma	Hyperthyroidism
Melanocyte-stimulating hormone	Bronchus	Abnormal pigmentation
Parathyroid hormone	Bronchus (squamous) Kidney Liver Adrenal	Hypercalcaemia, vomiting, constipation, psychotic behaviour
Human chorionic gonadotrophin	Breast Bronchus Testis Stomach Pancreas Liver Ovary	Gynaecomastia; precocious puberty
Luteinizing hormone	Trophoblastic Malignant teratoma Bronchus	Gynaecomastia
Growth hormone	Lung Stomach Ovary Breast	Acromegaly; hypertrophic pulmonary osteoarthropathy
Glucagon	Kidney	Hyperglycaemia, etc.
Prolactin	Bronchus Breast	Galactorrhoea

Why are ectopic hormones produced by 'non-endocrine' tumours? One hypothesis suggests that the tumour cells involved in ectopic hormone secretion are derived from cells with potential endocrine functions that are normally present in many tissues and that would normally secrete amines such as serotonin and catecholamines.

Two groups of cells might fill this role. The first is made up of the neuroendocrine cells which are widely distributed in many tissues. The argentaffin cells in the gut, which can secrete serotonin and from which **carcinoid** tumours can arise, might be taken as an example. The second is a group of cells characterized by Everson Pearse as the **APUD** series. The acronym APUD stands for **A**mine **P**recursor **U**ptake and **D**ecarboxylation, this name describing some of the outstanding characteristics of these cells. Associated with these is the ability to produce biologically active amines and peptide hormones. Such cells are present in small numbers in any individual location and could produce the 'ectopic' substance continuously. Clonal expansion of such a cell population, as would take place in tumour formation, would obviously be associated with an increase in the total amount of hormone produced, this being sufficient in some instances to produce a recognizable biological effect. It has been suggested that APUD cells are derived originally from the neural crest and migrate from there, principally to organs formed in the course of the development of the foregut. Support for this comes from the fact that a number of the active substances secreted by so-called APUDomas are also secreted within the brain and that many APUD cells and the tumours which arise from them express markers such as **neurone-specific enolase,** which would support a neural origin. This is no longer believed to apply to all cells and tumours in this group, some of which are thought more likely to have an endodermal origin. An example of an APUD cell is the parafollicular or C cell of the thyroid. This cell secretes the calcium-mobilizing hormone, **calcitonin.** The tumour arising from these C cells is known as a **medullary carcinoma.** It may occur as one of the genetically determined syndromes which can affect more than one endocrine organ simultaneously (see p. 438) or as an isolated phenomenon. Most medullary carcinomas have amyloid in the stroma and the amyloid protein contains amino acids 9 to 19 of calcitonin (see p. 239).

The **'oat cell carcinoma'** is an archetype of APUD tumours. It is one of the small-cell tumours which occur in the bronchi; the cells are arranged in a ribbon-like pattern in close relation to sinusoidal blood vessels. Electron microscopy shows the presence of dense-cored neurosecretory granules. These tumours are not only associated with a number of paraendocrine syndromes (see Table 28.1), but with some other systemic manifestations as well. The APUD concept has made a very considerable contribution to our understanding of this area of pathology, but clearly cannot account for all cases of ectopic hormone secretion by neoplasms, such as the secretion of PTH by squamous carcinoma of the bronchus or renal adenocarcinoma.

A complementary suggestion that has been made is that some instances of ectopic hormone production are due to the presence of large amounts of mRNA coding for the ectopic product in the tumour cells. In some cells which are not known to make significant amounts of a polypeptide hormone, very small amounts of the inappropriate product may be found, suggesting that some transcription of the responsible gene may be occurring. Some workers have referred to this phenomenon as 'leakiness' of the gene. The difference between this situation and one in which large amounts of an inappropriate product are secreted by a neoplasm may be merely quantitative. Indeed, there is a considerable degree of homology between the mRNAs of normal cells and their neoplastic counterparts. The secretion of significant amounts of an 'ectopic' hormone may therefore simply represent an increase in gene expression via increased transcription.

Non-metastatic osseous and soft tissue changes

Clubbing

Clubbing of the fingers was first described more than 2000 years ago by Hippocrates. The angle between the nail and the cuticle becomes filled in and the nail appears to 'float' on the nail bed. The curvature of the nail itself is altered, the nail being curved from front to back and having a rather 'beaked' appearance. In more severe instances, the periosteum over the terminal phalanges, wrists and ankles becomes thickened and new bone is formed from stem cells within the periosteum. In its most severe form, the complex of soft tissue and bony changes is termed **hypertrophic pulmonary osteoarthropathy (HPO)**. Clubbing and HPO occur in association with a number of disease states. These include the cyanotic forms of congenital heart disease, chronic pulmonary sepsis, infective endocarditis, mesothelioma of the pleura, and carcinoma of the bronchus.

The pathogenesis of this curious change is still far from clear. Some studies suggest that in affected patients the blood flow to the limbs is increased. Dividing the vagus nerve above the hilus of the affected lung relieves the condition in some instances, and this is certainly associated with a reduction in blood flow to the affected part. Other studies suggest that there may be ectopic secretion of growth hormone in some cases of tumour-related hypertrophic pulmonary osteoarthropathy.

Interestingly enough, in view of the many systemic manifestations of small-cell carcinoma of the bronchus, HPO shows a strong *negative* correlation with this tumour. The commonest thoracic neoplasm to be associated with this syndrome is mesothelioma of the pleura. However, squamous carcinoma and adenocarcinoma of the bronchus have both been recorded as being the cause of HPO.

Non-metastatic changes in nerve and muscle

Neuromyopathic changes associated with neoplastic disorders have been separated into three groups:

1. **Encephalomyeloneuropathy**, where degeneration of ganglion cells in the central nervous system is the dominant pathological feature
2. **Myopathies** with or without features of myasthenia
3. **Demyelinating** disorders

In the first two there is no constant relation between the progress of the neoplasm and that of the neurological condition. Indeed, neurological abnormalities may precede the diagnosis of tumour by up to three years or, at the other end of the spectrum, may appear after the tumour has been removed. The primary tumours most frequently implicated are carcinomas of the bronchus, breast, ovary, uterine cervix and colon.

The cause of these neurological complications is unknown. They are not uncommon, an overall prevalence of neurological change of this type being recorded in 14% of patients with carcinoma of the bronchus (chiefly of the small-cell variety).

Some cutaneous manifestations of malignancy

Polymyositis and dermatomyositis

This rather uncommon condition, encountered chiefly in the fifth and sixth decades of life, is associated with malignancy in 25–30% of cases. The muscular symptoms include pain and weakness, especially of proximal muscles such as those of the shoulder and hip girdles. Joint pain and stiffness are quite common. If the disorder is confined to muscle it is termed **polymyositis**, but the full clinical picture may include a striking rash as well. This ranges from a barely perceptible flush to a red or violaceous eruption, usually over the malar areas and the flush areas of the chest, back of neck and extensor surfaces of the arms and legs. Fine telangiectases (dilated small blood vessels) are almost always present on the cuticles. If the disease appears when the patient is more than 40 years old, there is a one-in-two chance that it is associated with malignancy. The neoplasms associated with dermatomyositis are often those of the gastrointestinal tract, but carcinomas of the bladder, the bronchus and other endodermally-derived tumours are not rare in this context. In cases associated with tumour, complete eradication of the tumour, where this is possible, cures the dermatomyositis.

Acanthosis nigricans

In this condition, there is increased pigmentation of the skin, especially of the axilla, the back of the neck, and the peri-areolear region of the breast. In the early stages, despite the name **acanthosis**, there is little or no thickening of the skin, though itching is often present. Later, the skin becomes thick, velvety and pigmented; the process may extend to involve quite large areas of skin. Acanthosis nigricans associated with malignancy appears most often in middle age when the age-related incidence of tumours is rising. About two-thirds of the tumours associated with this skin lesion are carcinomas of the stomach.

Erythema gyratum repens

This is a rare but highly characteristic dermal accompaniment of malignancy. It appears as wavy, irregular bands of red macropapules which coalesce to form a 'snake-skin' or 'wood-grain' pattern across the affected area of skin. This condition has been reported in patients with adenocarcinoma of the bronchus, small-cell carcinoma of the bronchus, carcinomas of the breast, uterine cervix, tongue and gastrointestinal tract. In the case of some of these tumours, such as 'oat cell' carcinoma of the bronchus, the eruption usually occurs after obvious metastases have been diagnosed.

Some biological markers of malignancy

The alterations in gene expression, whether qualitative, quantitative or both, that are part of the spectrum of malignant transformation may be associated either with the secretion of inappropriate substances or the expression of new antigens. Such biological markers can be helpful in diagnosis or in monitoring the progress of certain neoplasms. They fall into three main groups:

hormones
isoenzymes
tumour-associated antigens.

The first of these categories has already been described earlier (see p. 419).

Isoenzymes

Acid phosphatase. An association between raised acid phosphatase concentrations in the plasma and carcinoma of the **prostate** has been known for many years. High plasma levels are particularly likely to be found in patients whose carcinomas have already metastasized, especially where secondary deposits are present in the skeleton.

Carcinoplacental alkaline phosphatase. This enzyme was discovered in the blood of a patient named Regan who had a carcinoma of the bronchus and it is termed by some workers the **Regan isoenzyme.** It is similar to the alkaline phosphatase found in the human placenta.

The Regan isoenzyme may appear in the blood of 3 to 15% of patients with malignant neoplasms. Primary tumours include carcinomas of the bronchus, colon, pancreas and liver. Germ cell tumours may also express this enzyme.

The use of the Regan isoenzyme as a diagnostic test for the presence of malignant disease has proved disappointing. Its elevation tends to occur late in the natural history of malignancy. False positives have also been recorded in patients suffering from certain chronic inflammatory bowel diseases such as ulcerative colitis and also in patients with cirrhosis of the liver. Low levels of the enzyme can be found in the plasma of some normal subjects.

Tumour-associated antigens

Alterations in the antigenic state of transformed cells will be discussed further in Chapter 29. In some instances transformation and tumour growth may be associated with the appearance of antigens on tumour cells which are characteristic of the stage of *fetal* development and which are not present in fully differentiated adult cells. Such antigens are spoken of as **oncofetal antigens.**

Alpha-fetoprotein. Alpha-fetoprotein (AFP) is an alpha-1-globulin which is secreted in embryonic life, first by the yolk sac and later by the fetal liver. Secretion in the liver is established by the sixth week of embryonic life and reaches a peak of 3–4 mg/ml in the plasma by the thirteenth week of intrauterine life. From this time on, the levels of AFP fall rapidly and in normal adults, the amounts which can be detected in the plasma by immunoassay are only about one-millionth of the amount present in fetal plasma. In 1963 it was discovered that adult mice with transplantable liver cell tumours had high concentrations of AFP in their plasma. This observation was extended to humans with liver cell cancer two years later and the presence of elevated plasma concentrations of AFP has proven to be a fairly useful marker for this tumour. Subsequent studies have shown that AFP may appear in the plasma in up to 50% of patients with **malignant teratomas,** there being a strong correlation between the presence of elevated concentrations of AFP in the plasma and teratomas which contain elements histologically recognizable as showing **yolk sac** differentiation.

Carcinoembryonic antigen (CEA) This substance was discovered in 1965 to be present in fairly large amounts in malignant tumours of the large bowel. It is normally found in the gastrointestinal tract, liver and pancreas during the first six months of embryonic life. CEA is a water-soluble glycoprotein with a molecular weight of about 200 000. It is intimately associated with the glycocalyx on the cell surface membranes and can be localized to the luminal surface of the neoplastic cells which express it. Early studies suggested that the presence of elevated plasma concentrations of CEA was specific for neoplasms derived from the endoderm. However, it has now become obvious that this is not correct. Increased levels of CEA can be found in association with neoplasms of different histogeneses and may also occur in association with some non-neoplastic conditions. This last factor clearly limits the usefulness of CEA as a **diagnostic** marker. A further disadvantage is that CEA levels tend to be correlated with the extent of spread of certain neoplasms; before such spread has occurred, CEA concentrations may not be raised significantly. For example, in carcinoma of the colon or rectum, localized (Dukes' stage A) tumours are associated with increased CEA levels in only 40% of cases. In those cases of colorectal carcinoma where metastasis has occurred, 80–95% of the patients have elevated CEA levels.

The main application for the determination of CEA levels in the plasma is in the follow-up of cancer patients after surgery and in monitoring the effects of therapy. After successful removal of a tumour which is associated with elevated CEA concentrations in the plasma, the CEA concentration tends to fall to normal over a period of two to four weeks. If there is no recurrence of tumour, these normal levels persist. A subsequent rise in the plasma concentration of CEA probably indicates either the presence of metastases or a local recurrence of tumour. Such a rise in plasma CEA may precede, by several months, clinical evidence of metastatic or recurrent disease.

The Ca 1 antigen. In 1982 some studies reported the discriminatory ability (between malignant and non-malignant cells) of a monoclonal antibody prepared against an extract of a human laryngeal carcinoma cell line. This antibody was found to distinguish between malignant and non-malignant hybrid cells and was called **Ca 1.**

Ca 1 is an IgM antibody which reacts with two components from cell extracts which together have been termed the **Ca 1 antigen.** These components are glycoproteins and their antigenicity is destroyed by neuraminidase (which removes sialic acid) and by proteolysis. The Ca 1 antibody reacts with a wide range of human tumours, even though the tissue samples have been embedded in paraffin wax which involves treatment with organic solvents and heating. The original reports suggested that the Ca 1 antibody was a reagent which could distinguish with complete reliability between malignancy and non-malignancy in a given tissue (such as the breast). However, the Ca 1 antibody has now been found to react with a number of normal tissues including:

transitional epithelium of the bladder
collecting tubules of the kidney
luminal epithelium of the fallopian tube
epithelium of apocrine glands
trophoblast of the developing fetus
type 2 pneumocytes in the alveoli of the lung

The absence of Ca 1 antigen from some malignant tumours, its focal distribution in others, and its presence in a number of normal tissues as well as in benign tumours such as fibroadenomas of the breast suggest that the antibody is unlikely to play a major role in distinguishing malignant from non-malignant epithelia (something that is by no means always as easy as one might think).

The antigen itself seems to be the same as a certain mucin which can be extracted from human urine and which binds peanut lectin. In cultured tumour cell lines the production of Ca 1 can be induced by exposing the cells to lactate. In view of the protective action of mucins in relation to epithelial surfaces it may well be that Ca 1 antigen serves a similar function in respect of those tumour cells which produce it, perhaps in response to the local increases in lactate associated with anaerobic glycolysis.

Chapter 29

The Effect of the Host on Neoplasms

Essentially, the effect of the host on the neoplasm must be deemed to reside in the interaction between the host's immune system and the tumour, since it is difficult to think of any other mechanism through which resistance to the progression of malignant disease might be mediated. There are a number of ways in which this question might be examined:

1. Is there direct evidence that immune mechanisms modulate the behaviour of human neoplasms?
2. Is there histological evidence that human neoplasms excite an immune response?
3. Is there any increase in the frequency of neoplastic disease in patients with immune deficiency states?

The first of these is extremely difficult to prove. It is true that in some instances malignant neoplasms regress, this having been noted most frequently in neuroblastoma and malignant melanoma. However, there is no direct evidence that such tumour regression is brought about by immune mechanisms, though in some cases of malignant melanoma which remain localized for a long time there may be antibodies in the plasma which are cytopathic for that patient's tumour cells in culture.

Other clinicopathological oddities such as the prolonged survival of some patients with malignant disease, the frequency of clinically occult tumours found at necropsy, and the occasional regression of metastases after removal of the primary tumour have all been cited as possible expressions of an immune response. However, proof of the validity of this view is lacking.

Histological features suggesting an immune response to the presence of tumour

On histological examination, some tumours are seen to be infiltrated by lymphocytes, macrophages and plasma cells, this being especially common in carcinomas of the breast. In addition, a marked degree of hyperplasia of the macrophages lining the sinuses of lymph nodes draining a tumour may be seen, as well as epithelioid cell granulomas.

There is some evidence from prospective studies that the presence of these histological features may correlate positively with an improved prognosis, this evidence being strongest in the case of breast cancer.

Immune deficiency states and malignancy in humans

If it were true that immune reactions mounted by the host play a significant part in inhibiting the development and growth of malignant neoplasms, then one would expect an increased frequency of malignant disease in patients with immune deficiency. Up to a point, this is true: patients with inborn deficiency syndromes such as **ataxia telangiectasia**, the **Wiskott–Aldrich syndrome** and the **Chédiak–Higashi syndrome** all show an increased frequency of malignant disease as compared with their peers. However, most of these neoplasms primarily involve the lymphoid system.

In cases of iatrogenic immunosuppression, such as in patients who have received renal allografts, there is also an increase in the frequency of malignant disease; again, the vast majority of these are of the lymphoid system. There have been occasional reports, however, where recipients have received kidneys from patients dying with malignant disease. Although the donor kidneys were macroscopically free from tumour, tumours with the histological characteristics of the donor's primary are said to have grown in some of these kidneys. In two cases the withdrawal of the immunosuppressive drugs on which the patient had been maintained was reported to have led to regression of the tumour. These observations, scanty as they are, suggest that immunosuppression creates a favourable milieu for tumour progression.

An interesting epidemiological experiment of nature which tends to support this view is to be found in relation to Burkitt's lymphoma, a B lymphocyte derived neoplasm believed to be caused by a herpesvirus, the Epstein–Barr virus (see p. 460). This virus is ubiquitous but appears to be associated with malignant lymphoma chiefly in certain parts of Africa where malaria is holoendemic. The possession of the sickle cell trait by some inhabitants of these areas, which confers protection against malaria, also appears to confer protection against developing this lymphoma. It has been suggested that chronic malarial infestation has an immunosuppressive effect, chiefly on the T cell arm of the immune system.

Tumours can be rejected by animal hosts

The possible role of cell-mediated immunity in controlling tumour growth can be studied most easily in relation to animal tumours induced by certain viruses. The most fully studied example is **polyoma virus**, which is a small DNA virus that infects many laboratory and wild mouse colonies. When large doses of the virus are injected into adult mice, no tumours result. Inoculation of the virus into **newborn** mice of the same susceptible strain produces large numbers of tumours. If, however, newborn mice are thymectomized and, when they have grown to adulthood, are inoculated with the polyoma virus, tumours occur in fairly large numbers. This type of experiment therefore provides good evidence that adult mice are protected against the oncogenic effect of the polyoma virus because they can mount an effective cell-mediated response. The same sort of events are seen when mice of the C57BL strain, which are resistant to the oncogenic effect of the polyoma virus, are studied. Neonatal thymectomy or the use of repeated injections of antilymphocyte serum can make young mice of this strain develop polyoma-induced tumours.

While there is some evidence that cell-mediated rejection of some virally induced tumours can occur, the picture is by no means a simple one. If T cell mediated immunity plays a major role in **immune surveillance** against tumour development, one would expect a high frequency of spontaneous tumour development in the '**nude mouse**' which is athymic. This is not so, though this mouse has been used with some success in studying transplantable tumours.

Tumour-associated transplantation antigens

A number of experiments in inbred strains of mouse indicate that tumour rejection can occur as a result of the expression of certain antigenic determinants on the surface of the tumour cells which have nothing to do with the histocompatibility antigens coded for by the major histocompatibility complex.

In general, tumours which have been induced by irradiation or chemicals have unique antigenic determinants on the cell surface which function as **transplantation antigens** (**TATA — tumour-associated transplantation antigens**) and can thus elicit rejection. Even two tumours produced by the same carcinogen in a single animal will have distinct transplantation antigens. Tumours caused by viruses, however, show new antigens on the cell surface which cross-react with those on other tumours induced by the same virus. These virally induced TATA appear not to be typical viral structural proteins.

Unfortunately, spontaneous tumours arising both in animals and humans show much less tendency to develop transplantation antigens on their cell surfaces, though some neoplasms appear to elicit a cell-mediated immune response which cannot be ascribed to allogeneic rejection mediated through the major histocompatibility complex.

Tumours of this class include malignant melanoma, renal carcinoma, and astrocytomas in the brain. In melanoma, which has been studied in most detail, three classes of cell surface antigen have been identified. The first of these is distinct for the particular patient's tumour. The second is specific for malignant melanoma cells, but may be shared with cells of other malignant melanomas. The third is found on both tumour cells and some normal cells.

Mechanisms by which the immune system can combat tumour growth

A number of possible effector arms of the immune system may play a role in destroying tumour cells. These include:

the macrophage system
effector T cells
antibodies which can promote antibody-dependent cell-mediated cytotoxicity
natural killer cells

Macrophages

In culture systems, macrophages can be shown to destroy tumour cells. The precise mechanism is not clear, but does appear to involve cell-to-cell contact. The macrophages can be activated in two ways: firstly, by contact with tumour antigen and secondly as a result of the release of the lymphokine **macrophage-activating factor** (MAF) from T cells which have been stimulated by contact with tumour antigens. Activation by MAF is associated with an increase in the number of Fc receptors on the surface of the macrophage and it is possible that coating of tumour cells by antibodies may help, through the binding of Fc to Fc receptors, to bring the macrophage into close contact with the tumour cell.

Effector T cells

Cell killing by the T cell arm is presumably carried out by cytotoxic T cells in a manner analogous for that described in relation to the macrophage. The helper T cell may also play a part through its stimulatory effect on the cytotoxic subgroup. The relative proportions of T helper and T suppressor cells may have some influence on the immune status of the host in respect of tumour cells. In certain transplantable tumours in animals, tumour growth is increased if there is a large population of T suppressor cells. It has been suggested that this comes about through an autoimmune reaction against the specific clone of cytotoxic T cells which bind to the tumour cells. This reaction is mediated by T suppressor cells, which recognize surface markers of a certain idiotype on the cytotoxic T cells and are themselves specifically cytotoxic for cells bearing that idiotype. In this way, the cytotoxic T cells are prevented from destroying the cells of the tumour.

Antibodies

Theoretically, as outlined earlier, humoral immune mechanisms could act in two possible ways in the destruction of tumour cells. Firstly, they could bind to tumour cells and initiate complement-mediated cell lysis. Such evidence as we possess suggests that this is not a significant mechanism in tumour control. Secondly, they may adhere to the surface of tumour cells and thus attract potentially cytotoxic cells which have Fc receptors on their surface. These include macrophages, T lymphocytes and so-called **natural killer cells.**

Natural killer (NK) cells

The natural killer cell constitutes a subset of the lymphocyte population which is believed by some workers to be derived from clones of immature pre-T lymphocytes. They are non-adherent, non-phagocytic and have Fc receptors on their surfaces. Their ability to kill tumour cells does not depend on the host being immunized against determinants on the tumour cells. It has been suggested that the natural killer cell can itself recognize several different types of determinant on cells which may exhibit cross-reactivity and that this may explain its broad range of cytotoxic activity. The activity of natural killer cells is stimulated by interferon, which is released, in this context, by T effector cells and by NK cells themselves, the latter constituting a positive amplification loop.

Does immune surveillance exist?

The original concept of immune surveillance was that malignant transformation of cells occurs frequently and that these cells are eliminated by immune mechanisms before clonal expansion can take place. In respect of 'spontaneously arising' neoplasms, this mechanism must clearly be deemed to fail in every case where a clinically or pathologically apparent neoplasm arises. However, in chemically or virally induced tumours in experimental animals, immune protection can be shown to be reasonably effective and it is possible that, in humans, immune mechanisms may be responsible for the fact that most people infected with the Epstein–Barr virus develop a self-limiting illness (infectious mononucleosis) and not a malignant lymphoma.

If immune protection is not effective in spontaneously arising neoplasms, how do the malignant cells which survive and form tumour masses evade the potential cytotoxicity inherent in immune effector mechanisms? It may be that many malignant cells are poor immunogens and natural selection processes would favour the survival of such cells in an antigenically heterogeneous tumour cell population. It is known, however, that it is possible for the host to develop an immune response to malignant cells but be unable to kill them. This 'blocking effect' appears to be associated with the presence in the host plasma of tumour-specific antibodies. It has been suggested that in such instances the tumour cells constantly shed surface antigens which bind to the appropriate antibodies to form immune complexes. The circulating complexes can bind to any killer cells which have Fc receptors for the tumour antibody and thus prevent them from having a cytotoxic effect on the tumour cells.

Another factor which determines the effectiveness or otherwise of an antitumour immune response appears to be the actual physical bulk of the tumour. Small tumours are much more likely to yield to efforts to improve a host's immune response, and removing much of a host's tumour load, either by surgery or by other means, appears to be associated with an improvement in the effectiveness of the antitumour response.

Chapter 30

Oncogenesis

The many epidemiological data relating the risk of developing one or another malignant neoplasm to a variety of environmental factors indicate that there is no such thing as a single cause of malignancy, though the number of final mechanisms involved in malignant transformation, at the molecular level, may be rather small.

Genetic Factors

The occasional clustering of certain types of malignancy in families and the presence of malignant neoplasms as part of some well-recognized inherited syndromes suggest that the genotype of an individual may play a part in determining susceptibility to malignant disease. An increase in the liability of any individual to develop a malignant neoplasm may be inherited as part of a clinical syndrome which may have diagnostic features of its own apart from the increased risk of malignancy. This may make it possible to recognize the individuals who are at risk and to take appropriate measures to reduce the chances of malignancy. However, an increased likelihood of tumours developing may, though rarely, be the only manifestation of a single gene abnormality.

The inherited syndromes associated with an increased risk of malignancy may be divided, essentially, into two groups:

1. Chromosomally determined syndromes
2. Syndromes apparently determined by a single gene abnormality. These may be associated with an immunological defect, as in **ataxia telangiectasia** (see p. 142), or there may not be any identifiable defect in immunity.

Chromosomally determined syndromes

Three such syndromes associated with malignancy have been described:

1. Down's syndrome (mongolism)
2. Klinefelter's syndrome (a type of male hypogonadism associated with the presence of an extra X chromosome)

3. Gonadal dysgenesis in patients with a female phenotype and a male genotype

Patients with Klinefelter's syndrome show an increased tendency to develop tumours of the male breast and those with gonadal dysgenesis are more likely to develop tumours of the gonads. However, this increased risk may be the secondary result of the interaction between an abnormal hormonal milieu and an unresponsive target organ rather than a primarily genetically determined type of carcinogenesis.

In the case of Down's syndrome, the increased risk of developing acute leukaemia (myeloblastic: lymphoblastic = 1:2) appears to be an integral part of the syndrome.

Single gene abnormalities

Since the syndromes associated with immune deficiencies of one sort or another have been considered already (see p. 142), only some outstanding examples of those with no evidence of an immunological defect will be mentioned here.

Xeroderma pigmentosum

This rare condition, inherited in an autosomal recessive fashion, was first described by the famous dermatologist Kaposi in 1874. It is characterized by hypersensitivity to ultraviolet light and by a marked tendency to develop malignant skin tumours during childhood and adolescence. The skin of affected children appears normal at birth, but repeated exposure to sunlight results in a dry scaly skin with many areas of hyperpigmentation. These skin changes are followed within a few years by the appearance of a variety of skin tumours, some of which are malignant, such as squamous carcinoma. It is important for our understanding of this condition to note that **unexposed** skin remains normal. Precise prevalence data are not available, but estimates of the frequency of xeroderma pigmentosum vary from 1 in 65 000 to 1 in 250 000 live births. The condition is most commonly encountered in North Africans. Protection from sunlight either by suitable clothing or by barrier creams against ultraviolet light can reduce the risk of tumours developing; these are important measures to institute once the condition has been diagnosed.

Lack of the enzymes responsible for excision and repair. Xeroderma pigmentosum is, happily, rare, but the nature of the intrinsic defect in affected individuals is of great interest. The main target for ultraviolet light within the cells of the epidermis is DNA. Absorption of photons by DNA results in the formation of a variety of new products, of which the most important are dimers formed by adjacent pyrimidine bases (usually thymine). Under laboratory conditions this phenomenon can be shown to occur in the DNA of cultured fibroblasts and of bacteria. Normally the abnormal portion of the DNA which contains the thymine dimers is excised by an **endonuclease** and replaced by a new length of DNA some 100 nucleotides in length. In xeroderma pigmentosum, the endonuclease responsible for initiating this process of 'excision and repair' is lacking and the change in DNA induced by the ultraviolet light is permanent. Other syndromes in which DNA repair appears to be defective, and in which there is an increased risk of malignancy, are **ataxia telangiectasia** and **Fanconi's anaemia**, in which there is an increased risk of leukaemia, and **Bloom's syndrome**, which is also characterized by hypersensitivity to sunlight. In this condition, unlike xeroderma pigmentosum, the increased risk of malignancy is not confined to the skin. The defect in repair, at the molecular level, has not been characterized in these three conditions. The implication which can be obtained from these four rare syndromes is that **non-reparable alterations to the DNA of a target cell, however they may be caused, constitute one of the initiating mechanisms for carcinogenesis.**

Familial adenomatous polyposis coli and related disorders

This syndrome, which is due to the inheritance of an autosomal dominant gene, is rare and accounts for only a small proportion of the deaths due to colorectal cancer. Theoretically if one parent were to be affected, half the children could be expected to develop the disease. In practice, the penetrance rate is only about 80%, so that 40% of the children would show the features of this disease. The polyps are not present at birth and, as a rule, only begin to make their appearance between the ages of 10 and 20 years. The rather small polyps are frequently present in their thousands but, in some patients, there may be as 'few' as 200. The lesions are distributed fairly evenly through the large bowel, but the greatest concentration is to be found in the rectum, which is always involved. In their pre-malignant phase, the lesions show the features of adenomas on microscopic examination, each lesion being in no way different, at this stage, from the common solitary adenomatous polyp.

Of the patients with polyposis who present with symptoms attributable to their polyps, about 65% already have cancer of the large bowel. The average age at which cancer is diagnosed in these patients is 40 (which is about 20 years younger than in the non-polyposis population). Death as a result of colorectal cancer also occurs at a much younger age in these patients than in the general population. The precise frequency with which patients suffering from polyposis coli develop colorectal cancer is not easy to assess, but some writers maintain that by the age of 60 years, 100% of the victims of polyposis will have developed cancer of the large bowel. This gloomy prospect places a heavy burden of decision on the medical attendant of such a patient, since the only means of avoiding malignant transformation of one or more of the polyps is to undertake a prophylactic resection of the whole of the large bowel, including the rectum.

Other inherited, multiple colonic polyp syndromes are **Gardner's syndrome** and **Turcot's syndrome.**

In Gardner's syndrome, also inherited in an autosomal dominant manner, there are multiple colonic polyps associated with tumours in skin, subcutaneous tissue and bone. The likelihood of a sufferer developing colorectal cancer is about 100%.

Turcot's syndrome consists of a combination of colonic polyps together with brain tumours. It is inherited in an autosomal recessive manner. There appears to be an increased risk of colorectal cancer, but the magnitude of this risk has not been established.

Increased risk of neoplasia may be inherited alone

An increased risk of certain neoplasms developing may be inherited in the absence of any recognizable 'pre-malignant' or 'pre-neoplastic' syndrome such as polyposis or xeroderma pigmentosum. It is only rarely that these neoplasms occur in a pattern suggesting a major role for inheritance. They include retinoblastoma and phaeochromocytoma.

Retinoblastoma. This malignant neoplasm affects the retina in young children and spreads to involve the optic nerve. It may be inherited as an autosomal dominant, some 40% of retinoblastomas falling into this group. In children born with this genetic abnormality, the likelihood of their developing a retinoblastoma is about 95% and in these circumstances the neoplasm not infrequently affects both eyes. The increase in risk for such a person is of the order of 100 000 times. Patients with this inherited form of retinoblastoma may show deletion of chromosome 13q.

Phaeochromocytoma. This neoplasm arises wherever chromaffin cells are present, being most common in the adrenal medulla. The tumour cells secrete noradrenaline and adrenaline and the patients may present with systemic hypertension. About 5 to 10% of these tumours are malignant. Most phaeochromocytomas occur sporadically, but it is thought that 10 to 20% are familial; these occur in association with one of a number of syndromes.

1. An **autosomally dominant tendency for phaeochromocytomas to occur.** These often occur in childhood and more than 50% are bilateral.
2. **Multiple endocrine neoplasia syndrome type IIa** (Sipple's syndrome), which consists of a combination of phaeochromocytoma, medullary carcinoma of the thyroid and parathyroid adenoma or hyperplasia. This syndrome is thought to be inherited as an autosomal dominant with a high degree of penetrance. The phaeochromocytomas occur between the ages of 30 and 40 years and there is an increased tendency for them to be malignant.
3. **Multiple endocrine neoplasia syndrome type IIb.** In this variant there is phaeochromocytoma, medullary carcinoma of the thyroid and neuromas affecting mucosal surfaces. It is also transmitted as an autosomal dominant.
4. An **association between phaeochromocytoma and neurofibromatosis**

These are uncommon situations. One common and major neoplasm in which heredity plays a role is **carcinoma of the female breast.** A women whose mother has had such a carcinoma is three to four times more likely to suffer from the same disease as one whose mother did not have breast cancer.

Chemical Carcinogenesis

Epidemiological studies dating back more than 200 years have established that many types of malignant neoplasm occurring in man are causally related to environmental factors. Any such factor which can increase an individual's risk of developing a malignant neoplasm is spoken of as a **carcinogen**, though it might be more precise to refer to it as an **oncogen**. Such factors may be chemical, physical or viral. This section is concerned with the first of these.

The history of this field of oncological research starts with the observation, made in 1775 by Percivall Pott, a noted London surgeon, that there was a high prevalence of cancer of the scrotal skin in chimney sweeps' boys. Anyone who has read *The Water Babies* by Charles Kingsley, a work of more than usually revolting sentimentality, will recall that these hapless children were sent up into the chimneys to clean them and were consequently covered with soot. Pott's writings were said to have inspired a ruling made by the Danish Chimney Sweepers' Guild in 1778 that its members should bathe daily. That this simple measure was effective is suggested by a study carried out by Butlin a century later, in which he showed that scrotal cancer in chimney sweeps was comparatively rare outside England and attributed this to the habit of wearing protective clothing and bathing daily.

During the earlier phases of the industrial revolution, a similarly high prevalence of skin cancers was found in association with a number of occupations. Mule spinners in the Lancashire cotton mills, the front of whose garments were often soaked with lubricating oils, frequently developed cancer of the skin of the abdomen and of the scrotum; workers engaged in the extraction of oil from shale appeared to be similarly at risk. All these observations, relatively crude as they were, suggested that coal tar or one of its constituents might be responsible for the induction of such skin cancers and this led, ultimately, to the recognition of **polycyclic hydrocarbons** as a group of compounds with considerable carcinogenic potential.

Remote, proximate and ultimate carcinogens: carcinogenicity and mutagenicity

Many of the substances which we call carcinogens on the basis of their ability to produce tumours in certain animal species are not themselves carcinogenic, but become so only after metabolic conversion in the body of the host to forms which are more active biologically. In current terminology the parent substance is called a **remote carcinogen** or pre-carcinogen. Its metabolites with greater carcinogenic potential are called **proximate carcinogens**, and the final molecular species which interacts with the host DNA is termed the **ultimate carcinogen** (Fig. 30.1). This is of obvious importance when one tries to identify the carcinogenic potential of new compounds before they are marketed.

Normal cells transformed by carcinogens show permanent alteration of their phenotypes. This alteration is inherited from generation to generation of the cell line and we can infer from this that a permanent alteration to the genome of the transformed cell has occurred. Such an alteration falls within the definition of a mutation. It is now known that most of the carcinogenic chemicals so far identified are also mutagens, though not all mutagens are carcinogenic. Nevertheless, the demonstration that a given compound is mutagenic sounds a warning that it may also be carcinogenic. In testing for mutagenicity, the possibility that the test compound may be only a remote carcinogen must, therefore, be taken into consideration.

Most tests for mutagenicity employ submammalian species. These include bacteria, bacterial viruses (bacteriophages), fungi and insects. All of these are useful because they have relatively small genomes and reproduce themselves quickly. A commonly used test is the Ames test in which the effects of the test compound on the histidine-requiring mutant of **salmonella typhimurium** is assessed (Fig. 30.2). Reversion

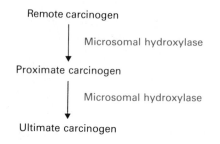

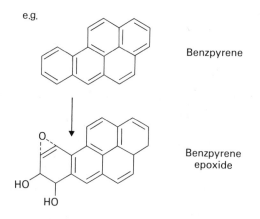

Fig. 30.1 Activation of potentially carcinogenic compounds.

of this strain, produced by a single base-pair substitution or insertion of a single base-pair, can be detected quickly and easily. The possibility that metabolic conversion is needed before mutagenicity is expressed can be taken care of by pre-incubation of the test compound with liver microsomes.

The polycyclic hydrocarbons

Despite the recognized association between exposure to coal tar derivatives and skin cancer, it was not until 1915 that the experimental induction of coal tar related neoplasms in animals was first carried out. By repeated applications of coal tar to the inside of rabbit ears,

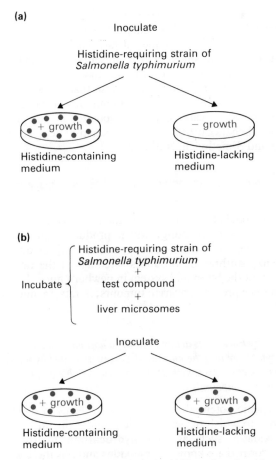

Fig. 30.2 Testing for mutagenicity using bacteria. (a) Normal results with a histidine-requiring strain of *Salmonella typhimurium*. (b) The presence of colonies in medium lacking histidine indicates mutation of some bacteria to a state of histidine independence.

Yamagiwa and Ichikawa produced skin tumours in the areas of skin on which the tar had been painted. The next step was to be the isolation of the substances in the tar which were responsible for the tumours. It was found that the compounds responsible were present in the higher boiling fractions obtained during the fractional distillation of coal tar. The fluorescence spectra of these fractions resembled that of the polycyclic hydrocarbon 1.2-benzanthracene.

This compound is only weakly carcinogenic in the skin-painting model but, using its characteristic fluorescence spectrum as a guide, Sir

Ernest Kennaway and his colleagues were able in 1930 to isolate 50 mg of the powerful carcinogen 3.4-benzpyrene as the end product of the fractional distillation of two tonnes of tar. This compound is a major constituent of cigarette smoke and is present in the exhaust fumes of petrol engines. Many other hydrocarbons have been tested since then. Not all are carcinogenic, and among those that are there are distinct differences in their ability to induce tumours in experimental animals. Moderate or powerful carcinogenic compounds in this group include 7,12-dimethylbenz(a)anthracene, 3,4-benzpyrene, 1,2,5,6-dibenzanthracene and 3-methylcholanthrene.

The site of application of oncogenic hydrocarbons and the species used affect the type of neoplasm produced

The classical model of experimental induction of tumours by polycyclic hydrocarbons is skin painting, which produces squamous tumours locally. However, the subcutaneous injection of 7,12-dimethylbenz(a)anthracene produces sarcomas in the rat, and malignant tumours of the lymphoid system in newborn mice. Intraperitoneal injection in mice produces ovarian tumours; in rats, mammary tumours result.

Carcinogenic hydrocarbons act by binding to host macromolecules both within the cytoplasm and the nucleus. They are activated by mixed function oxidases to form epoxides which are more water soluble and more reactive than the parent compounds

The carcinogenic potential of hydrocarbons seems to reside in certain double bonds to which oxygen is added (under the influence of mixed function oxidases such as **aryl hydrocarbon hydroxylase**). The compounds formed are known as **epoxides** and it is these which appear to have the ability to bind to DNA as well as to macromolecules in the cytoplasm of the target cells. This binding tendency is related to the fact that the epoxides are **electrophilic** (i.e. they are positively charged molecules that form covalent bonds with the negatively charged nucleophilic atoms in DNA, RNA and proteins). The greater the degree of DNA binding, the greater the carcinogenic potential of the hydrocarbon.

Cigarette smoking and lung cancer

Almost certainly the most important of the polycyclic hydrocarbons in relation to neoplasms in humans is 3,4-benzpyrene, one of the more than 3000 components of cigarette smoke.

There is now a vast literature that supports the existence of a direct causal association between cigarette smoking and lung cancer (chiefly of the squamous variety). If one were to regard the risk of a non-smoker developing a carcinoma of the bronchus as an arbitrary level of 1, the relative risk to an individual who smokes 20 or more cigarettes per day may be as great as **32**. Giving up smoking reduces the chance of a carcinoma appearing in that individual and the longer the cigarette-free period, the greater is the reduction in risk. Clearly, not all smokers develop lung cancer (though about 10% do) and this raises the possibility that there may be some genetic contribution to the risk of an individual smoker developing cancer. This genetic component may be related to the inducibility of the enzyme **aryl hydrocarbon hydroxylase (AHH)** by the hydrocarbon substrate. It has been reported that differences exist in the inducibility of this enzyme, and those subjects in whom the enzyme is more readily induced may be at greater risk of developing a cigarette-related tumour. In another study, patients who had had bronchial and laryngeal tumours resected and who, at the time, were tumour-free were analysed in respect of their inducibility of AHH. The distribution of AHH inducibility was the same in the patients as in an equivalent group of controls. These conflicting reports may be due to the fact that AHH measures the sum total of oxidation due to a number of P450 cytochromes and that the conversion of benzpyrene to a carcinogenic metabolite may be a function of only some of these enzymes. High-pressure liquid chromatography shows that benzpyrene is converted to more than 40 metabolites. *One* of these, a diol epoxide, is highly mutagenic and carcinogenic and is found covalently bound to cell DNA.

The ways in which individuals metabolize drugs may also be useful in delineating groups who may be more or less at risk of developing cancer after exposure to carcinogens. In a recent study, a majority of the patients with lung cancer were shown to be rapid metabolizers of debrisoquine, the pattern of distribution suggesting that this trait was inherited as an autosomal dominant.

Lung cancer is not the only neoplasm which appears to be causally associated with smoking; carcinomas of the oesophagus, pancreas, kidney and urinary bladder are others which also seem to be more frequent in smokers.

Aromatic amines and azo dyes

2-Naphthylamine

As early as 1895, a high prevalence of carcinoma of the bladder was reported in men who had worked in an aniline dye factory in Germany. The causal nature of this association was soon confirmed and it is now known that several occupations carry an increased risk for the development of carcinoma of the bladder. These include aniline dye manufacture, the rubber and cable industry, the manufacture of certain paints and pigments, textile dyeing and printing, and certain categories of laboratory work.

The carcinogens identified in these situations are the **aromatic amines** 2-naphthylamine and benzidine. Only humans and dogs are said to be susceptible to the urothelial effects of the naphthylamine, though in at least one study bladder tumours have been produced in the rat bladder after naphthylamine feeding. In humans the bladder cancers occur on average about 15 years earlier than in the population not exposed to aromatic amines. The average latent period between exposure and the development of bladder tumours is about 16 years. The duration of exposure may be quite short.

The aromatic amines should be classified as **pre-carcinogens** since, while it is possible to produce bladder tumours in dogs by **feeding** 2-naphthylamine, the insertion of pellets of this compound directly into the bladder has **no such carcinogenic effect.** To exert such an effect the amine must be converted into a biologically active form. This is achieved by hydroxylation in the liver, which yields the actively carcinogenic metabolite, 2-amino-1-naphthol. This is normally detoxified in the liver by conjugation with glucuronic acid and the resulting glucuronide is excreted by the kidney. This glucuronide is said to be non-carcinogenic. The susceptibility of human and dog urothelium is explained by the fact that the urothelial cells in these two species secrete the enzyme beta-glucuronidase, which splits the glucuronic acid from the 2-amino-1-naphthol, thus releasing the carcinogenic molecule.

2-Acetyl-aminofluorene

This amine has excited considerable interest as an experimental model of carcinogenesis. It was developed as an insecticide in the 1940s, but before marketing was found to be carcinogenic. Unlike 2-naphthylamine or benzidine, which appear to produce tumours only in the bladder, 2-acetyl-aminofluorene produces neoplasms in a wide range of tissues including the liver, breast, lung and intestine. As with naphthylamine, this compound is also a pre-carcinogen which undergoes hydroxylation in the liver to produce a proximate carcinogen of greater activity. The final step in the production of the ultimate carcinogen is probably esterification to form an N-sulphate ester, which is a highly reactive electrophilic compound.

Azo dyes

When Azo dyes such as butter-yellow and scarlet-red are fed to rats, liver cell tumours are produced with little evidence of liver cell necrosis.

These compounds are rather less effective in the mouse. In the rat, the carcinogenicity of azo dyes is enhanced by diets deficient in riboflavin. Azo dyes have been used commercially for colouring leathers and some foodstuffs, but there is, as yet, no evidence that neoplasms in humans have been caused by this group of compounds.

Nitrosamines and nitrosamides

The carcinogenic potential of this group of compounds has excited a great deal of interest since the discovery in 1956 that animals receiving dimethylnitrosamine in the diet at a dose level of 50 parts per million developed liver cell tumours after six to nine months' dosing.
   Nitrosamines have the general formula,

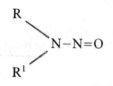

in which one of the R groups is an alkyl radical and the other either an aryl or alkyl radical. In the case of the **nitrosamides**, one R is an alkyl radical and the other an amide or an ester. The nitroso compounds, in animals at least, have proved themselves to be potent and versatile carcinogens producing tumours in a wide range of animal species and in many different tissues. An interesting feature of the individual compounds in this large group is their organotropy, many of them showing a marked degree of organ specificity.
   In the case of the nitrosamines, as with 2-naphthylamine, the parent compound is a remote carcinogen which requires metabolic activation. In the course of this activation, alkylating agents are formed and these bind to both the N7 and the O6 position on guanine, the latter probably being of more significance in so far as malignant transformation is concerned. Nitrosamines can be formed in the gastrointestinal tract by the interaction of nitrous acid, derived from nitrites, with secondary amines. It has been suggested that the frequency of certain tumours, notably gastric carcinoma, may be related to the dietary intake of nitrites, which are present in large amounts in pickled, salted and smoked foods.
   Nitrosamides do not require enzymatic activation in order to render them carcinogenic. Thus, instillation of methyl-nitroso-urea into the rat bladder at an appropriate dose level results in the production of urothelial tumours in the majority of instances. An interesting aspect of nitrosamide activity is displayed by the compound ethyl-nitroso-urea.

When this compound, which has a half-life of only a few minutes, is given to a pregnant rat after the eleventh day of gestation, the offspring develop malignant tumours of the brain at about the age of nine months. Samples of brain taken from the litter at different ages and grown in culture show a stepwise development of the phenotypic evidence of malignant transformation.

Direct-acting alkylating agents

Alkylating agents can bind to DNA without any need for prior activation. This group includes such compounds as mustard gas, beta-propiolactone and several agents used in the treatment of malignant disease, such as cyclophosphamide, melphalan and busulphan. While the interaction of these molecules with DNA makes them useful as antitumour agents, this property constitutes a double-edged sword since they also increase the risk of other neoplasms developing, most notably leukaemia and malignancies of the lymphoid series.

Some naturally occurring chemical carcinogens

The groups of chemical carcinogens considered thus far can hardly be looked on as natural environmental hazards, with the possible exception of nitrosamines derived in the gastrointestinal tract from dietary constituents. The marked influence which geographical factors appear to have on the prevalence of certain neoplasms such as carcinoma of the liver and carcinoma of the oesophagus suggests that these differences in tumour frequency may be affected by the existence of naturally occurring carcinogens in particular areas. In relation to carcinoma of the liver, which is comparatively rare in Europe and North America but common in Asia and in certain parts of Africa, an interesting potential candidate for the role of naturally occurring carcinogen is a group of toxins produced by fungi, most notably **Aspergillus flavus.** The toxins derived from this mould, which may contaminate cereal and ground nut crops, are known as **aflatoxins.** Aflatoxins were discovered in 1960 when a very large number of poultry, fed on ground nut meal imported from East Africa, died from extensive liver cell necrosis. When formal toxicological studies were carried out it was found that, at low dose levels, the toxin was capable of producing liver cell carcinomas. Like some other carcinogens, the aflatoxins bind covalently to guanine in cell DNA.

The frequency of liver cell carcinoma is high in those parts of the world where there is a poor, largely agrarian population heavily dependent on cereal crops for subsistence. Such crops may become contaminated by *Aspergillus flavus* and, indeed, there are epidemiological data which indicate a positive correlation between aflatoxin consumption and the incidence of liver cell carcinoma. For example, in Thailand, where the difference in aflatoxin intake between two areas of the country was of the order of nine times, there was a six-fold difference in the frequency of liver cell carcinoma.

While these data are very interesting, their impact is somewhat weakened by the fact that those populations most likely to be affected by aflatoxins are those in whom the infection rate by the **hepatitis B virus** is very high. Most patients with liver cell cancer are carriers of the hepatitis B virus and there are good reasons for supposing that this virus has a causal role in relation to liver cell tumours. It is possible that contamination of cereals by aflatoxins acts synergistically with the hepatitis B virus, but this cannot be proved at present.

Occupational carcinogens

The recognition that certain chemicals might be implicated in carcinogenesis stemmed directly from the observations of Pott and others (see earlier) that certain occupations carried a higher than normal risk for the development of certain neoplasms. A considerable number of occupational hazards of this kind is now known to exist (Table 30.1).

Table 30.1 Some occupational hazards in relation to neoplasia

Carcinogen	Site of tumour
2-naphthylamine	Bladder Renal pelvis Ureter
Arsenic	Lung Skin
Asbestos	Lung (squamous carcinoma) Mesothelium (mesothelioma)
Benzene	Bone marrow (leukaemia)
Ionizing radiations	Lung Bone Bone marrow
Bischlormethyl ether	Lung ('oat cell carcinoma')
Nickel (refining)	Lung Paranasal sinuses Larynx
Vinyl chloride monomer	Liver (angiosarcoma)
Hardwood dusts	Paranasal sinuses

While it is impossible to give a detailed account of the 'occupational' neoplasms which have been recognized, a few general points of principle are worth considering.

In general, a neoplasm related to an occupational hazard does not differ from its non-occupational counterpart, either in clinical or structural terms. In some instances there may be associated histological features which may provide a clue as to the occupational aetiology, such as the finding of asbestos bodies in the resected lung of a patient with squamous carcinoma of the bronchus.

Sometimes the clue may reside in the unusual nature of the tumour or in the fact that it is of a type which is unusual in that particular anatomical site. An example of the first is **mesothelioma**, a neoplasm, which, as its name implies, arises from the mesothelial cells of serosal linings. Mesotheliomas occur most commonly in the pleura, leading to a tremendous degree of thickening of the visceral pleura. They may show a biphasic pattern, the appearance in some areas resembling that of a spindle cell sarcoma, while in other areas the tumour cells resemble epithelium and are arranged in a ductal pattern. Asbestos bodies are found in the lung tissue of all patients with mesothelioma and similar neoplasms can be produced in experimental animals following intra-bronchial instillation of asbestos.

Asbestos is a series of fibrous silicates of which crocidolite is said to be the most oncogenic. Exposure occurs in the course of asbestos mining, pipe-lagging, ship building, etc., and the lag phase before the appearance of the mesothelial tumours may be very long (25–45 years). Asbestos exposure is also a major hazard in relation to squamous carcinoma of the bronchus, the latent period between exposure and the development of the neoplasm being much shorter than in the case of mesothelioma. Cigarette smoking acts as a very powerful synergistic factor in individuals who have been exposed to asbestos; the relative risk for the development of bronchial carcinoma in a non-smoker who has not been exposed to asbestos and a smoker who has been so exposed is 1:53.

An example of the second type of situation mentioned, where a tumour unusual in a particular anatomical site is encountered, is **adenocarcinoma of the paranasal sinuses** in hardwood workers. Such a tumour otherwise only occurs rarely in this site.

No general rule appears to operate in respect to the age at which occupationally related neoplasms occur. It appears to be a function of two variables: the age at which exposure begins, and the latent period characteristic of the particular carcinogen. In a study of occupationally related cancer of the urinary bladder, the mean age at exposure was found to be 29 years and the average latent period 16.6 years. Thus the tumours became obvious at a somewhat earlier age than is usual for bladder cancer.

Carcinogenesis as a multistep process: tumour initiation and promotion

In the late 1940s it was found that painting the skin with compounds such as croton oil, which are not themselves carcinogenic, greatly increased the yield of skin tumours in mice which had previously received a *sub-carcinogenic dose* of the carcinogenic polycyclic hydrocarbon benzo(a)pyrene (Fig. 30.3). Croton oil alone produced no tumours and if it was applied to the mouse skin **before** the hydrocarbon, **no** tumour enhancing effect was noted. The effect of the benzo(a)pyrene was described at that time as **the initiation of carcinogenesis** and the enhancing effect of the croton oil was termed

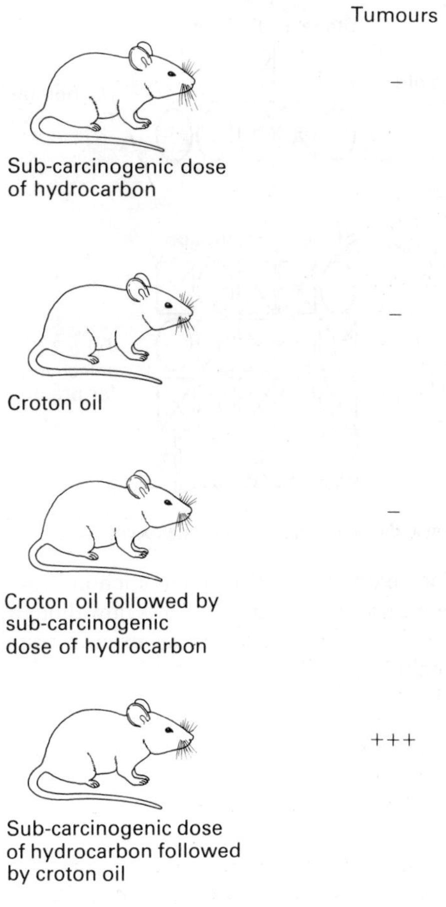

Tumours

Sub-carcinogenic dose
of hydrocarbon

−

Croton oil

−

Croton oil followed by
sub-carcinogenic
dose of hydrocarbon

−

Sub-carcinogenic dose
of hydrocarbon followed
by croton oil

+++

Fig. 30.3 Initiation and promotion of neoplasms in a mouse skin model.

Normal genotype
and phenotype

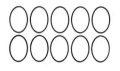

Initiation

Occasional cell with
altered genotype X

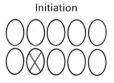

Stage 1. Promotion

Initiated cells acquire
new phenotype
(pre-neoplastic)

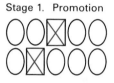

Membrane-bound promoter
reacts with protein kinase

Stage 2. Promotion

Expanded clone of
pre-neoplastic cells

Type 2 promoters
selectively mitogenic
for pre-neoplastic cells

Fig. 30.4 Initiation and promotion—a multistep process.

promotion. For many years this phenomenon was believed to be
confined to the mouse skin model, but it is now thought that two-stage
or multi-stage pathways in carcinogenesis exist in respect of a number
of neoplasms including:

liver
bladder
lung
breast
colon
oesophagus
pancreas

If the term **promotion** as originally defined in the mouse skin model is to have an application in the wider field of carcinogenesis, it is important that common features should be demonstrated in both **operational** and **biochemical** terms between the mouse model and other chemically induced neoplasms.

Chemical carcinogenesis can be regarded, in operational terms, as a series of processes in which a normal cell and its progeny are converted into malignant cells (Fig. 30.4).

Initiation

The **initiation** phase involves a change in the genome of the target cell, this change being inherited by the progeny of that cell. The change in the genetic material, as indicated previously, is usually associated with covalent binding of the active form of the carcinogen to DNA. While high doses of initiating compounds can cause tumours to develop without the assistance of any other factors, **a low dose of the initiator will not be expressed in the form of phenotypically altered cells and may induce damage in the genome of only a small number of target cells.**

Characteristically, initiation is a very rapid event, is produced in a dose-related fashion after a single exposure to an initiating carcinogen, and occurs in only a small proportion of the target cell population. The number of cells affected is increased if rapid proliferation of the target cells is taking place. Unless the damage is quickly repaired and provided that the target cell is a 'stem' cell and not a fully differentiated cell, the effect on the DNA is permanent and inheritable, even though there is no detectable change in the cell phenotype.

Promotion

The promotion phase in multistep carcinogenesis is brought about by agents which catalyse biochemical events in both normal and initiated cells, leading to an altered pattern of gene expression. In the case of the **initiated** cells, this results in the expression of cells with a new phenotype; these cells must be regarded as being **pre-neoplastic.** If exposure to the promoter is short-lived, the pre-neoplastic cells will not increase in number relative to their normal neighbours and the phenotypic changes which have occurred may not be identified easily since only a few cells are affected. If exposure to the promoting agent is continued or if the promoter is replaced by any other agent capable of causing an increase in cell turnover and hence hyperplasia, then there will be a concomitant increase in the number of the initiated and promoted (pre-neoplastic) cells and a histologically detectable tumour may develop. In the mouse skin model, such a tumour will be a benign papilloma.

It is believed that another event is necessary for the benign focus of pre-neoplastic cells to be transformed into an invasive neoplasm. This event will also produce an inheritable change in the genome of the affected cells and may either involve a further biochemical alteration of DNA, some transposition of genetic material, or activation of part of the genome to produce a portion of DNA capable of inducing malignant transformation (an oncogene) (see later in this chapter).

Promotion itself is not a single stage process. Promotion can be divided into two stages. There is an early phase (stage 1 promotion), which can be brought about by diterpene esters such as TPA (12-*o*-tetra-decanoylphorbol-13 acetate), and a later, less specific one (stage 2 promotion), in which other compounds such as turpentine are active. Specific inhibitors exist for each of these phases. In initiated skin, only a single exposure to promoters which have both stage 1 and stage 2 actions is required for tumours to develop. For the same result, multiple exposures to stage 2 promoters are necessary.

Promotion as a biochemical event. Different biochemical events underlie initiation, stage 1 promotion and stage 2 promotion (Fig. 30.5). Initiating carcinogens react with cell DNA, while the target for stage 1 promoters is the surface membrane of the cell. High-affinity receptors have been identified for TPA and other promoters on cell surface membranes in many tissues and in many species. The binding of a stage 1 promoter to such a receptor sets off alterations in membrane phospholipid metabolism and in the structure and function of the membrane. The binding site for TPA appears to be the specific calcium and lipid-binding protein kinase known as protein kinase C.

When TPA binds to this enzyme and activates it, phosphorylation of serine and threonine residues in specific cell proteins occurs. The state of phosphorylation of these proteins is the crucial factor mediating the activity of various hormone and growth factors. Thus TPA is acting on the cell surface membrane in much the same way as insulin, epidermal growth factor or platelet-derived growth factor, all of which bind to another protein kinase (tyrosine kinase). The effects of TPA on these processes take place very rapidly, but are not by themselves sufficient to bring about tumour development. For this, stage 2 events are also necessary.

Stage 2 promotion is dependent on prolonged exposure to the promoting compound and on sustained cell proliferation, which enables the growth potential of the latent tumour cells to be expressed. Stage 2 promoters **induce enzymes**, the products of which increase the speed of

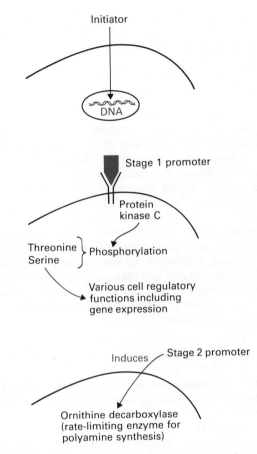

Fig. 30.5 Some of the biochemical events in initiation and promotion.

cell division. The enzyme that appears to be particularly concerned is **ornithine decarboxylase** (**ODC**), which is the rate-limiting enzyme for the synthesis of certain polyamines which have a role in the synthesis of DNA, RNA and protein. Further investigation has shown that most growth-promoting stimuli (e.g. growth promoting hormones, epidermal growth factor, partial hepatectomy) induce ODC and will also act as stage 2 promoters.

Not all enhancers of tumour development are promoters. Many factors other than stage 1 or stage 2 promoters can enhance the production of tumours. Some operate by increasing the efficiency with which the active metabolite of an initiating carcinogen is presented to the target cell, while others may modify the physiological response of the host to the presence of developing tumour cells. The latter include a wide range of factors, which may be nutritional or may affect immune surveillance mechanisms.

Initiation and promotion occur in tumour formation apart from the mouse skin model

In experimental bladder cancer, saccharin, cyclamates and some metabolites of tryptophan fulfil many of the criteria for labelling a compound as a promoter. Induction of ODC in cultured bladder urothelium has been shown after treatment of the cells with saccharin and these data suggest that mechanisms similar to those identified in the mouse skin model may act in this different situation.

The importance of retaining the concept of initiation and promotion in relation to human neoplasms rests chiefly on the realization that a long period of promotion may be part of the natural history of the development of many neoplasms. In some instances, the promotion process may be reversible and this may offer us the chance to deploy novel treatment strategies such as the use of retinoids (which inhibit stage 2 promotion) in order to modify the natural history of neoplasms such as carcinoma of the bladder.

Hormones and Neoplasia

Recognition of the possibility that the hormonal milieu might play some part in the natural history of cancer dates back to 1895, when Beatson in Glasgow removed the ovaries from a woman with recurrent breast cancer and found that the tumour regressed. This observation suggested that at least some breast cancers were oestrogen-dependent; this hypothesis has received considerable support from both human and animal studies.

A single dose of dimethyl-benz(a)anthracene given either intravenously or via a stomach tube produces carcinoma of the breast in rats. If the animal has been ovariectomized before the carcinogen is given, no tumour is produced. Ovariectomy has a similar inhibiting effect in relation to the tumours produced by the mouse mammary tumour virus. In addition, tumours occurring after administration of dimethyl-benz(a)anthracene regress following ovariectomy. In contrast, if prolactin levels in the rats are raised by giving them drugs of the phenothiazine group, there is an acceleration in the growth of the breast tumours. Data of this type suggest that this model of breast carcinoma is hormonally dependent, but do not rule out the possibility that the hormones mentioned may also act as promoters.

Human breast cancer

A link between ovarian function and human breast cancer is suggested by the increased risk encountered in those who had an early menarche, a delayed first pregnancy (or no pregnancies) and a prolonged period of menstrual activity.

While it is also true that ablation of ovarian function, whether by surgical, radiotherapeutic or pharmacological means, induces remission, at least temporarily, in a proportion of cases of breast cancer in humans, there is at best only conflicting evidence that patients (as compared with controls) have high circulating levels of either oestrogen or prolactin.

A relationship has been noted between urinary levels of aetiocholanolone (C19 steroids) and the natural history of patients with breast cancer. When the levels of these steroids excreted in the urine are low, the prognosis is, in general, poor; these patients also show a poor response to removal of the ovaries.

Of equal interest has been the recognition of oestrogen receptor sites on certain tumour cells. The oestrogen-binding protein is believed to form part of a two-step process in which oestradiol is bound in the cell and transported to the nucleus. Absence of these receptors from the majority of the cells in an individual breast cancer indicates that the response to endocrine therapy is likely to be poor.

Carcinoma of the endometrium

Many data suggest that the development of endometrial carcinoma is influenced by oestrogenic steroids:

1. Oestrogen-producing tumours of the ovary are frequently associated with endometrial hyperplasia and in some of these patients carcinoma of the endometrium supervenes.
2. Carcinoma of the endometrium and carcinoma of the breast occur in the same patient more frequently than would be expected if the association was a chance one.
3. There is an increased risk of endometrial carcinoma in obese females. It is said that 50% of patients with endometrial cancer weigh more than 82 kg (180 lb). This association is believed to be due to the fact that precursor steroids for oestrone, such as delta-4-androstenedione, are converted in adipose tissue. This conversion rate is twice as high in post-menopausal women as in those still in active reproductive life, and obesity has a marked incremental effect. Conversion of delta-4-androstenedione to oestrone is also increased in

diabetic females; here too the risk of endometrial cancer is greater than in non-diabetic, age and weight-matched peers.

It seems likely, therefore, that carcinoma of the endometrium can be regarded as one in which a certain degree of hormone dependency is present and in which oestrogenic steroids may also exert a promotional effect.

Other neoplasms in which hormones influence the natural history

Carcinoma of the prostate, like carcinomas of the breast and endometrium, is a neoplasm which has its peak incidence at a time when involution of the tissue could be expected. The prostate is clearly an endocrine-dependent organ. In primates, cells in the peripheral part of the prostate, where cancers develop, have been shown to have androgen receptors, and castration leads to atrophy of the normal prostate and to regression of prostatic carcinomas. The administration of oestrogens to patients with prostatic cancer also results in regression of the tumours.

Another interesting example of the influence of hormones on tumour genesis is the rather curious clear-celled adenocarcinoma of the vagina which occurred in the daughters of some women given diethylstilboestrol in the course of their pregnancies. The neoplasms only appeared in their daughters in late adolescent or early adult life. Some hundreds of cases of this sequence of events have been reported but, fortunately, only a small minority of the women treated with stilboestrol had daughters affected in this way.

Physical Agents in Oncogenesis

Ultraviolet irradiation

The association between skin cancers and exposure to sunlight was reported more than 100 years ago. Epidemiological observations suggesting a role for ultraviolet light as the responsible agent were supported by the induction of skin tumours in rats exposed to ultraviolet irradiation in 1928. Since ultraviolet light is a low energy form of emission and does not penetrate deeply, the skin absorbs most of the energy and hence is the primary target for this form of carcinogenesis.

Evidence of an aetiological role for sunlight in skin carcinoma is very strong. Most such neoplasms occur in exposed areas. They are relatively infrequent in dark-skinned races, in whom the ultraviolet radiation is filtered out by melanin, and are common in fair-skinned

people. The prevalence of malignant tumours of the skin in the
fair-skinned appears to be related to the intensity of solar radiation and
is increased in those regions close to the Equator. The mechanism
responsible for the induction of such neoplasms is likely to be
associated with the production of abnormal thymine dimers in the
DNA of the epidermal cells and perhaps the lack of efficient excision
and repair of the abnormal DNA, such as is seen in **xeroderma
pigmentosa** (see p. 435).

The most common sunshine-related neoplasms are **basal cell
carcinoma**, which may invade locally but almost never metastasizes,
squamous carcinoma, which may both invade the surrounding tissues
and metastasize, and **malignant melanoma**, which is often highly
malignant and is capable of spreading very widely.

Ionizing radiation

It has been recognized since the early part of the century that ionizing
radiation constitutes a risk factor for the subsequent development of
cancer. In man, this is seen under a number of different circumstances:

1. There was an increased prevalence of both leukaemias and skin
cancers in radiologists who, during the early days of diagnostic
radiology, were inadequately protected.
2. There is a greater than normal frequency of leukaemias and
carcinomas of the thyroid, breast and lung among the survivors of the
nuclear explosions over Hiroshima and Nagasaki.
3. There is an increased risk of carcinoma of the thyroid in people who
have had irradiation to the neck during childhood.
4. There is an increased risk of osteosarcoma following ingestion of
bone-seeking radioactive substances. This was first reported in the
1920s following the exposure to radium and mesothorium of 800 young
women employed in the painting of luminous watch dials in a factory in
Orange, New Jersey. In order to get a sufficiently fine tip on their
brushes, the workers wetted the brushes on their tongues, leaving
behind a deposit of the radioactive paint. Several years later a high
prevalence of osteosarcoma was reported in this group.
5. A thorium-containing contrast medium, **Thorotrast**, was used to
outline the margins of abscess cavities in the 1940s. The prevalence of
malignant tumours in patients investigated in this way was about twice
as high as would normally be expected, with a six-fold increase in
leukaemias and liver neoplasms.

The mechanisms by which ionizing radiation induces malignant
transformation are not clear. Irradiation causes free radical generation
(see p. 11) and these very active chemical species may well react with

elements in the target cell genome. Certainly irradiation can produce obvious changes in chromosome morphology and is mutagenic to cultured cells. In addition, in at least one model, a virus-induced leukaemia in the mouse, irradiation may activate viral oncogenes and bring about transformation in this way.

Malignancy induced by foreign materials

Certain foreign substances are capable of inducing the formation of connective tissue neoplasms when implanted, usually subcutaneously, into the tissues of a variety of animals. The precise physical form in which these foreign materials exist appears to be of fundamental importance in relation to tumour induction. For example, sheets of certain plastics evoke a brisk fibrous tissue response when inserted subcutaneously which eventually leads to the formation of low grade fibrosarcomas. If the same plastic sheeting is ground up and then inserted into the connective tissue of the same species, no tumours result. Similarly, if holes are made in the sheeting before insertion, the likelihood of tumour formation decreases, this diminution of risk appearing to be associated with the size of the holes. This has been studied using millipore filters as the tumour-provoking agent. If the filter has a pore size greater than 0.22 µm, no tumours appear. The mechanisms involved in this curious form of oncogenesis are not known and there is, as yet, no evidence that the prosthetic materials widely used in surgical practice confer any increase in the risk of neoplasia.

Viruses and Neoplasia

It has been known since 1908 that certain tumours in animals can be caused by viruses. It was recognized at that time that a variety of fowl leukaemia could be transmitted by cell-free extracts of tumour tissue. This discovery was followed by the pioneering studies of Peyton Rous, who found that cell-free extracts of chicken sarcomas produced identical tumours when injected subcutaneously into other chickens.

Those viruses which are capable of inducing neoplasms are known as **oncogenic** viruses. Oncogenic viruses are found among both the **DNA** and the **RNA** viruses.

DNA oncogenic viruses

The best authenticated DNA oncogenic viruses come from three groups:

the **papova** group
the **herpes** group
the **hepatitis** group

The papova group

The word **papova** is an acronym constructed in the following way:

pa from *pa*pilloma
po from *po*lyoma
va from simian *va*cuolating virus

Papilloma viruses. The first virally induced mammalian neoplasm to be recognized was the so-called Shope papilloma, a curious warty lesion on the tails of Kentucky cotton-tailed rabbits. This neoplasm can be passaged in the same way as the Rous sarcoma, but in the case of the Shope papilloma virus, the host response makes a considerable difference to the natural history of an infection. If wild cotton-tailed rabbits are infected with the virus, tumours grow slowly, are usually benign, and free virus can be harvested from the horny layer of infected skin. If, on the other hand, domestic strains of the rabbit are infected, the tumours are rapidly growing, some of them become frankly malignant, and free virus cannot be harvested from the cells. Thus cell-free extracts from tumours in the domestic strain cannot be passaged.

In man, the papilloma viruses are the only ones which have been **proved** without doubt to cause neoplasms. The lesions associated with wart virus infections are the common skin wart, and anal and genital warts (**condylomata acuminata**), and it is now believed that certain papilloma viruses are implicated in cervical cancer.

Polyoma viruses. Polyoma virus, a large DNA virus, causes a wide variety of neoplasms in a variety of small animals (mice, rabbits, rats, hamsters) when they are infected in the neonatal period. Adult members of susceptible species are immune unless they have been neonatally thymectomized, an observation which suggests an effective degree of T cell surveillance of cells transformed by the virus. A number of different tumours in various anatomical sites have been described as following infection with this virus, hence the name **poly**-oma. There is no evidence of any involvement of the polyoma viruses in the field of human neoplasia.

Simian vacuolating virus (SV40). This virus was discovered in 1960 in the kidney cell cultures used to produce the first polio vaccine. In the course of immunization against poliomyelitis, some thousands of people had also been inoculated with the SV40 virus. Later it was shown that the virus could induce tumours in newborn hamsters and that it could transform human cells in culture. However, no evidence has yet accrued that could lead to this virus being implicated in human neoplasia.

SV40 enters the affected cells through the action of its coat proteins; after uncoating, either the whole or part of the viral genome is inserted into the host DNA. Transcription of the viral DNA takes place in two waves, the earlier mRNA being derived from those codons responsible for transformation as well as for viral replication.

Herpesviruses in neoplasia

Viruses of the herpes group are certainly responsible for the production of at least one important malignant neoplasm in poultry and probably involved in two or more neoplastic diseases in humans.

In chickens, a herpesvirus causes a variety of malignant lymphoma known as **Marek's disease.** Infection with this virus can be economically disastrous unless the birds have been immunized with an attenuated form of the virus, since, unlike most oncogenic animal viruses, the virus of Marek's disease spreads horizontally and is very contagious. Though the cell which undergoes malignant transformation is almost certainly a T lymphocyte, the virus invades epithelial cells in the skin in association with the feather sockets and is shed from the skin.

Burkitt's lymphoma. This is a malignant lymphoma arising from B lymphocytes which was first recognized in Uganda by a British surgeon called Denis Burkitt. Burkitt's lymphoma occurs chiefly, though not exclusively, in children, the peak incidence being at about seven years of age. It is commonest in certain parts of tropical Africa, its geographical distribution being strikingly circumscribed to areas in which **malaria** is holoendemic and where climatic conditions favour the anopheline mosquito. In those areas in which malaria has been eradicated, there has been a significant decline in the prevalence of Burkitt's lymphoma.

In the course of culturing the lymphoblastic cells for a case of Burkitt's lymphoma, Epstein and Barr found herpesvirus-like particles within some of the cultured cells. They then went on to show that lymphoblastic cells in biopsies of the Burkitt tumour, while not containing viral particles (these only appear when tumour cells are cultured), do contain virus-associated antigens which react with antibodies in the serum of patients suffering from the disease. It was then discovered that the virus associated with the Burkitt lymphoma was identical with that which causes the widely prevalent disorder of B lymphocytes — **infectious mononucleosis** or glandular fever. Infectious mononucleosis occurs chiefly in adolescence and in early adult life. It is characterized by fever, malaise, sore throat, lymph node enlargement and the presence of large atypical T cells in the blood. In the vast majority of instances, infectious mononucleosis is a benign and self-limiting disease, though an X-linked syndrome does exist in which the T cell response which normally eliminates the infected B cells does not occur. In this case, B cell proliferation goes on unchecked and a leukaemia-like syndrome, which may be fatal, develops (Duncan's syndrome). Occasionally such a clinical picture develops sporadically.

If the Epstein–Barr virus (EBV) is as prevalent as epidemiological data would suggest, it seems remarkable that Burkitt's lymphoma should, on the whole, be so circumscribed. The data suggest that the difference is to be found in the host response to EBV infections and, in view of the fact that malaria is known to be immunosuppressive, it seems probable that Burkitt's lymphoma represents a malaria-related failure of immune surveillance. This view is strengthened by the observation that people who bear the **sickle cell trait**, and who are thus resistant to malaria, also have a reduced risk of developing Burkitt's lymphoma.

Nasopharyngeal carcinoma. An association has also been found between the EBV and a curious lymphoepithelial neoplasm found in the nasopharynx. Like Burkitt's lymphoma, this tumour shows a distinctive geographical distribution being prevalent in China (especially Southern China) and some other parts of south-east Asia. The clustering of cases of this tumour, not only within this area but within people originating from it, has been recognized for more than 300 years, and, indeed, has led to the disease being termed Kwantung tumour by some, since it is so prevalent in Kwantung province. On histological examination, the neoplasm is seen to consist of two cell lines, one of these being a poorly differentiated epithelial cell and the other a lymphoblastoid cell. The EBV can be found in cell lines cultured from both these components and the patients show high titres of EBV antibodies. Again the question arises as to why this widely prevalent virus should be related to a malignant neoplasm only in a circumscribed geographical area. There is no evidence of an **exogenous modifier** of the host response such as exists in the association between malaria and Burkitt's lymphoma and one is left with the possibility that some genetic factor may be operating in the case of the nasopharyngeal carcinoma. Support for this view comes from the fact that emigration from the affected areas of Asia does not appear to lessen the risk and that clustering of HLA-A2 occurs in the people in high risk areas.

Carcinoma of the uterine cervix and herpesviruses. Epidemiological studies indicate that there is an association between carcinoma of the uterine cervix and the individual level of sexual activity. Virginity appears significantly to reduce the risk of cervical cancer and, conversely, an early start to sexual activity and a widespread distribution of favours increase the risk of the subsequent development of squamous carcinoma of the cervix.

Herpes simplex virus type 2 (HSV2) has been canvassed as a possible aetiological agent in cervical carcinoma. The frequency of HSV2 infections in patients with either frank or in situ carcinoma of the cervix is very high. Viral antigens can be identified in some of the cells in cervical cancers, and portions of the viral genome can be identified in such cells using DNA hybridization techniques (see p. 147). However, these findings should be interpreted with caution. The presence of an association between cervical cancer and HSV2 infection does not prove the existence of a causal link between them. Papilloma virus infections are also common in these women, and an oncogenic role for this virus seems highly probable.

Hepatitis B virus (HBV)

This ubiquitous virus is responsible for one of the more serious varieties of infective hepatitis. The presence of a carrier state (which can be established by identifying the surface antigen of the virus in plasma) can be found in between 10 and 20% of those who become infected with the virus. The prevalence of the carrier state varies from country to country. In the UK it is very low, but in parts of Africa and Asia it may be as high as 30% of the population. A significant positive correlation exists between the prevalence of the carrier state and the frequency with which liver cell cancer is seen. In addition, in those parts of the world where the prevalence of the tumour is high, the carrier rate is about 90% in those with liver cell cancer.

A virus resembling HBV has been found to cause hepatitis in woodchucks and liver cell carcinoma is not infrequently seen in this species. DNA hybridization techniques have revealed the presence of woodchuck virus DNA incorporated within the liver cell genome and similar observations in respect of the human virus have been made in relation to human cell lines derived from liver cell cancers. These data are strongly suggestive of an oncogenic role for the human hepatitis B virus, though, of course, it is not possible to prove this at present.

Oncogenic RNA viruses

The role of the oncogenic RNA viruses as a group is discussed in the section dealing with the **oncogene** theory (see p. 465). However, one

RNA virus does merit consideration separately — the **mouse mammary tumour virus.** A viral aetiology for breast cancer in the mouse was first proposed following the observations of Bittner in 1936, who studied strains of mice which were known to have a high prevalence of carcinoma of the breast. Bittner found that the tendency to develop breast cancer could not be ascribed wholly to the genetic make-up of the hybrid strain he was studying and that the **female parent type** was the most important factor. Furthermore, if baby mice from a high prevalence strain were delivered by caesarean section and suckled by a mother of a low prevalence strain, the young mice did not develop carcinoma of the breast to any appreciable extent when they

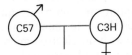

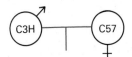

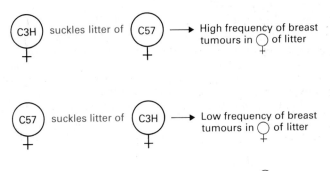

Fig. 30.6 Mouse mammary tumour virus.

grew to maturity. Conversely, when the progeny of a low prevalence strain were suckled by a high prevalence strain mother, the frequency of breast cancers in these young mice was uncharacteristically high (Fig. 30.6). These data suggested that the oncogenic agent was being **vertically** transmitted via the milk. Confirmation of this hypothesis came when viral particles were demonstrated on electron microscopy of the milk from high prevalence mothers.

In view of the commonness of breast cancer in human females, and the many recorded cases of breast cancer occurring in several members of one family, it is easy to understand why the possibility of a viral aetiology has been enthusiastically canvassed.

Some evidence which might link the data obtained from the mouse model to the human situation has come to light. Particles similar to those seen in the milk of high cancer prevalence strains of mice have been identified both in human breast milk and in breast tissue. One report suggests that such particles can be found more frequently in groups of women in whom there is a higher than expected prevalence of breast cancer, such as the Parsee community in Bombay. Sera from some patients with breast cancer have been shown to contain antibodies which bind to the virus-like particles seen with the electron microscope in breast tissue. However, these data are far from being conclusive and the case for a viral factor in carcinogenesis in the human breast is not yet proven.

Oncogenes — A Molecular Basis for Cancer

The majority of malignant neoplasms have thus far been found to be **monoclonal**, that is the cells of which any neoplasm is composed are all descended from a single 'ancestor' cell. This ancestor cell was once a normal cell but at some point it must have undergone fundamental alterations which have conferred 'immortality' on the cell line and which have released it from the normal constraints on cell proliferation and growth. Just as in the case of normal cells, the progeny of malignant cells inherit the characteristics of their parents; this suggests that the alterations mentioned above must have occurred in relation to the genome of the 'ancestor' cell. This view is strengthened by the fact that there is a high degree of correlation between the mutagenic properties of a given compound and its potential carcinogenicity.

Some insights into the type of changes that occur in the genome of normal cells which become transformed into their malignant counterparts have now become available, largely as the result of the introduction of extremely powerful new methods in molecular biology.

The realization that a relatively small number of molecular determinants may be active in malignant transformation has come from the convergence of two lines of investigation. The first of these relates to the mechanisms by which a variety of animal retroviruses can transform infected cells and induce tumours in their host species. The second has focused on the effects, largely in cell culture systems, of gene transfer from the cells of human malignant tumours not obviously viral in origin. The results of these studies suggest that there is a group of functionally heterogeneous genes which can be altered by mutation, amplified, made to overexpress their protein products, or physically moved within the genome by chromosome translocations. These genes, which are known as **cellular oncogenes**, may act individually (in certain cell culture systems) or more likely in cooperation with one another to bring about the **malignant transformation of cells**.

Oncogenic retroviruses

There is a group of RNA viruses which can produce tumours in their host species and which can also transform certain cells in culture. These are known as **oncornaviruses** or **oncogenic retroviruses**. The genome

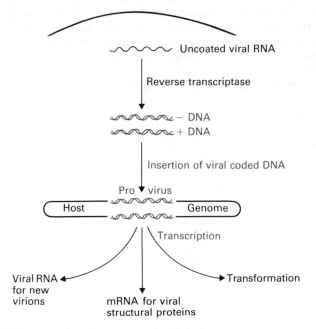

Uncoated viral RNA

Reverse transcriptase

– DNA
+ DNA

Insertion of viral coded DNA

Pro virus

Host   Genome

Transcription

Viral RNA for new virions

mRNA for viral structural proteins

Transformation

Fig. 30.7 Retrovirus (e.g. Rous sarcoma virus) infection.

of these viruses is composed of **RNA** enclosed within a capsid which is, in turn, wrapped in a glycoprotein envelope. Once this virus infects a cell, the envelope and capsid are removed and the viral RNA is copied by the viral enzyme **reverse transcriptase** into a portion of DNA which is called a **provirus** (Fig. 30.7). The provirus is incorporated into the DNA of the infected cell and by the normal processes of transcription emerges as RNA molecules identical with the original viral RNA. This new RNA can act both as mRNA for viral proteins or as RNA for the genomes of new viruses. The viral components thus synthesized can be assembled into new complete viruses, which bud off from the surface of the infected cells.

Oncogenic retroviruses can be divided into two groups. One group induces tumours very slowly. Their genome is made up of three genes:

gag, which codes for a group-specific antigen
pol, which codes for reverse transcriptase
env, which codes for envelope glycoproteins

Non-coding sequences at either end, known as **long terminal repeats** promote gene replication and expression.

These three genes contain all the information necessary for the manufacture of new viral particles within the infected cell. The group includes natural, 'wild' viruses, which typically produce malignancies of the lymphoma/leukaemia group in poultry, mice and cats.

The second group of oncogenic retroviruses can produce tumours in the appropriate host very quickly — in days or weeks. They are not common in the 'wild' state and most of them have been isolated from animal tumours. In contrast to the first group, inoculation is usually required for the viruses do not often infect animals via natural pathways. Most of these viruses lack the full complement of genes necessary for viral replication. However, there is one noteworthy exception, the **Rous sarcoma virus.** When the genome of the Rous sarcoma virus was dissected, it was found to have two distinct portions. The first contained the genes necessary for replication — gag, pol and env. The second contained a gene called **src**, which is both **necessary** and **sufficient** for the virus to cause sarcomas in animals and to transform fibroblasts cultured in a monolayer. On infection with the **src** gene, the normal orderly monolayer is lost and groups of cells pile up and form colonies which are many layers thick. This transforming gene codes for the production of a tyrosine kinase called pp60src. This viral gene (**v-src**) is now recognized as belonging to a family of about 20 transforming genes known as viral oncogenes (**v-oncs**), each of which is characteristic of a rapidly transforming virus. A number of viral oncogenes code for proteins which possess the ability to phosphorylate tyrosine in certain proteins. Another oncogene from the avian erythroblastosis virus (**erb b**) codes for a protein homologous with a portion of the cellular receptor for epidermal growth factor and yet another, **sis** from the simian sarcoma virus, codes for a protein homologous with the platelet-derived growth factor.

Viral oncogenes and cellular proto-oncogenes

With cloned DNA copied from v-onc RNA by the use of reverse transcriptase, it is possible to scan the genome of any eukaryotic cell for the presence of matching sequences. This is known as DNA **hybridization** and depends on the base-pairing relationship in double-stranded DNA. Adenine in one strand always pairs with thymine, and cytosine with guanine. Thus the sequence of bases in one strand must dictate the sequence in the other (Fig. 30.8). On this basis, it is possible to use a radioactively labelled sample of DNA as a tracer to see whether other samples of DNA contain matching sequences. If the tracer used is derived from the whole or part of a v-onc RNA, one can investigate whether DNA from normal cells contains sequences which match with those in the viral oncogene.

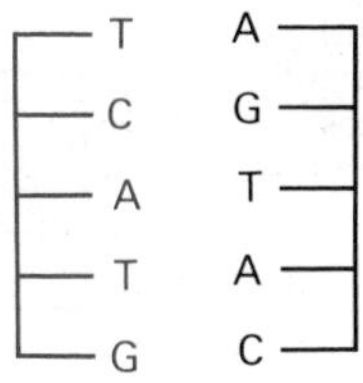

```
┌── T      A ──┐
├── C      G ──┤
├── A      T ──┤
├── T      A ──┤
└── G      C ──┘
```

Fig. 30.8 Complementarity of bases in DNA strands. T = thymine; A = adenine; C = cytosine; G = guanine.

Southern blotting

The identification of matching sequences in a DNA molecule which may contain hundreds of thousands of base pairs is made much easier by the application of a very sensitive hybridization method known as Southern blotting (Fig. 30.9). The cellular DNA is split into pieces by enzymes known as **restriction endonucleases,** which cleave DNA at specific sites defined by a base sequence which the enzyme can recognize. These portions of DNA can then be separated by electrophoresing them in an agarose gel. After such treatment human DNA may give rise to more than 100 000 such fragments. The DNA fragments are then transferred from the gel to a sheet of nitrocellulose paper (hence the term 'blotting'). A radioactively labelled sample of

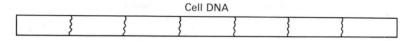

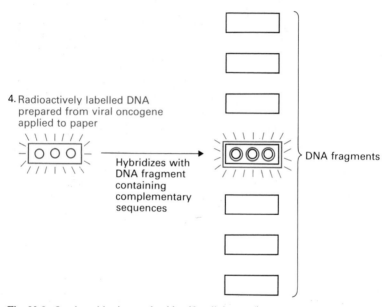

1. Cleaved by restriction endonucleases

2. Fragments electrophoresed in gel

3. Replica prepared by 'blotting' gel with nitro-cellulose paper

4. Radioactively labelled DNA
   prepared from viral oncogene
   applied to paper

Hybridizes with
DNA fragment
containing
complementary
sequences

DNA fragments

Fig. 30.9   Southern blotting used to identify cellular proto-oncogenes.

DNA (the probe) may then be applied to the paper and thus small fragments of cellular DNA containing complementary base sequences can be identified. Using this method, it has been shown that there are complementary sequences to **every single viral oncogene** in restriction fragments prepared for DNA derived from widely disparate species (e.g. human, yeast, fruit fly). These normal genes which are homologous with the viral oncogenes are known as **proto-oncogenes**, a term which implies that **these constituents of the genome of *normal* cells have the potential for being converted into active genes capable of inducing malignant transformation.**

RNA can be analysed in a similar manner by a process known as Northern blotting and this enables the level of transcription to be measured.

Viral oncogenes originate from cellular proto-oncogenes

In view of the homology between viral oncogenes and cellular proto-oncogenes, two mirror image possibilities exist to explain their relationship. Either the v-oncs are derived from cellular genes, or the reverse holds true. A number of facts suggest that the first of these suggestions is correct. Firstly, the very high degree of conservation of the cellular proto-oncogenes during evolution (from yeasts to man) supports the view that the proto-oncogenes are not derived from viruses. Secondly, the structure of the proto-oncogene differs in some respects from their v-onc homologues. In v-oncs the nucleotide sequences coding for certain proteins usually occur in a solid block. In the proto-oncogene the information is split up, portions of the protein coding sequences (exons) alternating with intervening sequences (introns). This is the characteristic structure of a vertebrate gene. After transcription of the proto-oncogene has occurred, the mRNA corresponding to the introns is stripped away leaving mRNA which is almost identical with the viral mRNA. Thirdly, cellular proto-oncogenes are not found in normal cells in association with provirus. They are also always found in the same chromosome for a given species and this argues strongly for a cellular rather than a viral origin. Lastly, some cellular proto-oncogenes code either for growth factors, growth factor receptors or enzymes concerned in the modulation of these receptors. This suggests a physiological role for the proto-oncogenes in normal cells, probably in relation to growth regulation, and hence a

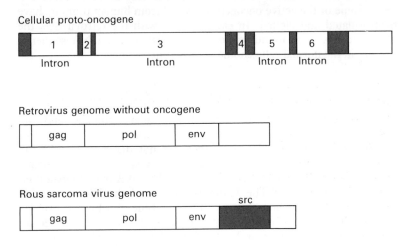

Fig. 30.10 The cellular origin of viral oncogenes. The introns are eliminated during acquisition of the cellular oncogene by the virus.

cellular rather than a viral origin. The current view, therefore, is that viral oncogenes arise as a result of transcription from a proto-oncogene, and that this cellular genetic material has been incorporated into the viral genome (Fig. 30.10).

DNA from chemically transformed cells and from some 'spontaneous' human tumours can transform cells in culture

When DNA is extracted from transformed cells and introduced into cultures of untransformed mouse fibroblasts (a technique known as **transfection**), foci of piled up transformed cells appear and these foci grow into fibrosarcomas after inoculation into young mice. Thus certain varieties of chemically transformed cells carry oncogenic sequences in their DNA.

Even more interesting was the discovery that transfected DNA from biopsies of some human tumours produced exactly the same effect. Many types of human tumour cells have now been shown to develop transforming sequences in their DNA during progression from the normal to the malignant state. They include carcinomas of the bowel, lung, bladder, pancreas, skin and breast, fibro- and rhabdomyosarcomas, glioblastomas, neuroblastoma and various haemopoietic neoplasms. In all these experiments it should be borne in mind that the recipient cell (the mouse fibroblast) differs significantly from the donor tumour cell, and it may well be that tumour-derived DNA samples which do *not* transform fibroblasts may possibly do so in other cell lines. Some of the active oncogenes derived from human tumours have been isolated and cloned. In each case, as with the retroviruses, the oncogene has been found to be closely related to a DNA sequence present in the normal cell genome (a proto-oncogene).

Is there a relationship between these two groups of cellular proto-oncogenes?

The transfection studies of DNA from human tumours and the characterization of viral oncogenes has shown that two groups of proto-oncogenes exist. However, they are not distinct. The **Ki-ras** oncogene carried by the Kirsten murine sarcoma virus is homologous with oncogenes detected by transfection of the DNA from human lung and colon carcinomas. The **Ha-ras** oncogene of the Harvey murine sarcoma virus is the homologue of the oncogene of a human bladder cancer cell line. Such relationships suggest very strongly that certain cellular proto-oncogenes can become changed into transforming genes by involvement in events that do not necessarily depend on viral mechanisms.

Interestingly enough, only two of the 18 viral-related cellular proto-oncogenes that become activated have been detected in an active form by transfection from human tumours. These are the Ha-ras and the Ki-ras genes referred to above. However, use of the Southern blotting technique has shown altered (and hence probably active) versions of the **myc** (avian myelocytomatosis), **myb** (myeloblastosis) and **abl** (Abelson murine leukaemia virus) genes in a variety of human tumours.

Other oncogenes have been detected by transfection, but these have not, so far, been shown to have counterparts among the oncogenes carried by transforming retroviruses. In human pathology these include Burkitt's lymphoma and a group of mammary carcinomas.

How do cellular proto-oncogenes (c-oncs) become activated?

Five separate mechanisms of proto-oncogene activation have been discovered so far:

1. **Over-expression of the c-onc following the acquisition of a novel transcriptional promoter.** Some proto-oncogenes can be activated by the addition of a strong transcriptional promoter. For instance, the avian leukosis virus (ALV) does not normally cause tumours but may occasionally do so after very long incubation periods. When the DNA of such rare tumours is analysed by Southern blotting, the ALV provirus sequence is found to hybridize to the same fragment as the viral oncogene **v-myc**. This suggests that the ALV provirus must have been inserted into the host cell genome very near the proto-oncogene **c-myc** and that this proximity of the normally inactive ALV had activated the c-onc, the ALV having acted as a strong transcriptional promoter.

2. **Amplification of either proto-oncogene or oncogene.** A second mechanism of activation involves over-expression due to amplification of a proto-oncogene or oncogene. In human promyelocytic leukaemia the **myc** proto-oncogene has been found to be amplified between 30 and 50 times normal. Such amplifications have also been found in relation to a number of c-oncs in several different human tumour cell lines. Once there is an increased number of copies of the gene in a single genome, it is assumed that there is a significant increase in transcription and hence in the amount of gene product; this can be demonstrated using the Northern blotting method.

3. **Alteration in the structure of the oncogene protein.** Point mutations in the oncogene proteins has been recorded in relation to the products encoded by the **ras** genes. In the case of a cell line derived from a human bladder carcinoma, a single point mutation converts the

H-ras proto-oncogene into a potent oncogene. This mutation causes the twelfth amino acid in the 21 000 dalton protein coded for by **c-ras** to be changed from glycine to valine. Some studies carried out with oncogenes of the **Ki-ras** group have also shown that alteration of the gene product at position 12 leads to oncogenic activation. A human lung carcinoma oncogene of the H-ras group carries a mutation which alters the gene product at residue 61, and it has been suggested that the codons specifying residues 12 and 61 of the gene product are critical sites which, when mutated, will often produce oncogenic alleles.

4. **'Enhancer sequences' can increase the activity of transcriptional promoters.** The level of transcription and hence the amount of gene product can be increased by the action of 'enhancer sequences', which increase the utilization of transcriptional promoters. The linked promoter may be a considerable distance from the enhancer sequence, which may be situated either up- or downstream of the promoters. Such a mechanism is believed to operate in certain avian lymphomas, where retrovirus fragments are situated downstream from the **myc** proto-oncogene.

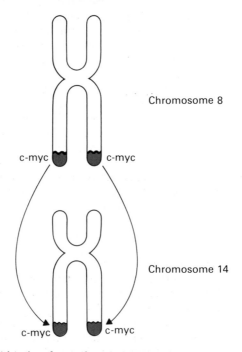

Fig. 30.11 Translocation of c-myc from the long arm of chromosome 8 to chromosome 14.

5. **Chromosome translocation.** Chromosome translocation can be associated with movement of a proto-oncogene to a different site in the genome. As a result of this change in position, the c-onc may become activated. This is believed to occur in Burkitt's lymphoma, in which translocations of material from chromosome 8 to chromosomes 2, 14 or 22 very commonly occur (the 8:14 translocation being the most frequent). The myc proto-oncogene has been located on chromosome 8 near the break point and in chromosomes 2, 14 and 22 the genes which encode immunoglobulin chains are present also near the break point. When translocation occurs, the myc gene derived from chromosome 8 and the immunoglobulin genes which are being actively transcribed in B cells become juxtaposed (Fig. 30.11). This appears in some cases to result in deregulation of the myc gene, possibly through the action of enhancer sequences contained within the immunoglobulin gene.

Oncogenes and multistep carcinogenesis

Spontaneous and chemically induced tumours are believed to arise as a result of several steps. The transformation of cultured fibroblasts of the 3T3 line by an oncogene such as Ha-ras appears to be a **single** event.

The explanation of this discrepancy seems to lie in the nature of the 3T3 cells, which are removed from their progenitors by very many generations and which have been 'immortalized' as a line. If the oncogene is applied to a line not far removed from the ordinary rat fibroblast, the complete phenotypic picture of malignant transformation is not seen to develop, though one phenotypic change, **loss of anchorage dependence**, does occur. This implies that if the recipient cell line is normal, the ras oncogene requires cooperation from some other factor or factors before transformation can take place. Put another way, it could be said that one consequence of immortalizing a line of cells, as in the case of 3T3, is the activation of cell functions that can cooperate with the ras gene to create the complete transformation phenotype.

ras can cooperate with other viral oncogenes

The changes which occur when a cell line becomes established in culture and thus 'immortalized' are poorly, if at all, understood. However, these changes can be mimicked by the action of certain DNA tumour viruses, notably polyoma and adenoviruses, which contain true viral genes capable of inducing cells to grow continuously in culture. The polyoma virus genome codes for three proteins which have been called the small, middle and large T antigens. The middle T antigen induces morphological changes in cultured cells and also loss of anchorage dependence. The large T antigen increases the lifespan of the cultured cells and also alters the dependence of these cells on certain serum factors. When large T and the ras gene are transfected into a cell line which does not transform when the ras gene alone is used, a dramatic degree of transformation occurs and inoculation of transformed foci into nude mice produces rapidly growing tumours. Thus cooperation between a viral gene and a cellular one can convert normal cells into tumour cells.

Other cellular oncogenes can cooperate with ras

The data referred to above shed no light on the possible mechanisms involved in the production of tumours where there is no obvious viral involvement. However, in some animal tumour cell lines, active **ras** oncogenes have been found to coexist with active **myc** genes. Transfection of both ras and myc into cell lines, not transformed by either when alone, again leads to a striking degree of malignant transformation. We can infer that *each* of the genes must perform some distinct function which is needed for the genesis of tumours. Such experiments may provide some explanation, at the molecular level, for the multistep nature of carcinogenesis, in that each step may involve the activation of a distinct cellular gene.

The action of oncogenes

Obviously the next step in unravelling this puzzle is to find out how the gene products of active oncogenes induce and maintain the transformed phenotype. Oncogenes encode proteins capable of acting in different parts of the cell. Some (myc is an example) are active in the nucleus and may play a part in controlling DNA replication. In normal cells, the **myc** gene is switched on, and then off, very early in the cell division cycle. This suggests that it is actively involved in switching cells from the 'resting' to the 'growing' phase. The **sis** gene, as stated earlier, encodes a protein homologous with the **platelet-derived growth factor** (PDGF), which acts as a mitogenic hormone. It is not without interest that stimulation of cells with the gene product of sis leads to an increase in the expression of two other proto-oncogenes, **myc** and **fos**. The gene product of **erb b** is homologous with the intracellular part of the epidermal growth factor receptor. **Ras** genes code for a 21 000 dalton protein situated just beneath the cell membrane which has GTPase activity; this activity is reduced in the mutated, transforming version of the gene. Such GTPase activity is thought to be related to the transduction of chemical signals bound to receptors on the cell surface. The finding that oncogenes can produce growth factors, growth factor receptors and means of transmitting signals received by receptors on cell membranes suggests that one role of proto-oncogenes is related to the control of cell growth through the interaction of growth factors and their receptors. A large family of oncogenes encode proteins with a tyrosine phosphokinase activity related to that of some hormone and growth factor receptors; this strengthens the view that proto-oncogene products are involved in generation, reception and transduction of growth factor signals. It has been suggested, therefore, that alterations in the whole system of mitogenic signals play a significant role in neoplastic transformation. Many tumours can produce growth factors which can stimulate their own growth, some produce PDGF or a molecule very like it, and others produce transforming growth factors which may be related to epidermal growth factor.

Further Reading

General

Alberts B, Bray D, Lewis J, Raff M, Roberts K & Watson JD (eds) (1983) *Molecular Biology of the Cell.* New York and London: Garland Publishing.
Anderson JR (ed) (1985) *Muir's Textbook of Pathology*, 12th edn. London: Edward Arnold.
Hill RB & La Via MF (1980) *Principles of Pathobiology.* New York and Oxford: Oxford University Press.
Robbins S, Cotran R & Kumar V (1984) *Pathologic Basis of Disease.* Philadelphia: WB Saunders.
Taussig MJ (1984) *Processes in Pathology and Microbiology.* Oxford: Blackwell Scientific.
Volk WA (1982) *Essentials of Medical Microbiology.* Philadelphia: JB Lippincott.

Cell Injury

Ciba Foundation Symposium 90 (1982) *Receptors, Antibodies and Disease.* London: Pitman.
Dixon KC (1982) *Cellular Defects in Disease.* Oxford: Blackwell Scientific.
Freeman BA & Crapo JD (1982) Free radicals and tissue injury. *Laboratory Investigation* **47**: 412.
Kerr JF, Bishop CJ & Searle J (1984) Apoptosis. In Anthony PP & Macsween RNM (eds) *Recent Advances in Histopathology 12*, pp. 1–16. Edinburgh: Churchill Livingstone.

Inflammation and Healing

Akiyama SK & Yamada KM (1983) Fibronectin in disease. In Wagner BM, Fleismejer R & Kaufman N (eds) *Connective Tissue Diseases*, p.55. Baltimore and London: Williams & Wilkins.
Babior B (1978) Oxygen-dependent microbial killing by phagocytes. *New England Journal of Medicine* **298**: 659; 721.
Fantone JC & Ward PA (1982) Role of oxygen-derived free radicals and metabolites in leucocyte-dependent inflammatory reactions. *American Journal of Pathology* **107**: 397.
Glynn LE (ed) (1981) *Tissue Repair and Regeneration. Handbook of Inflammation, Volume 3.* Amsterdam, New York and Oxford: Elsevier/North Holland Biomedical Press.
Johnston RB (1982) Defects of neutrophil function. *New England Journal of Medicine* **307**: 434.
Karnovsky ML & Bolis L (eds) (1982) *Phagocytosis—Past and Future.* New York and London: Academic Press.
Majno G (1975) *The Healing Hand: Man and Wound in the Ancient World.* Cambridge: Harvard University Press.

Majno G, Cotran RS & Kaufman N (eds) (1982) *Current Topics in Inflammation and Infection*. Baltimore and London: Williams & Wilkins.

Majno G, Shea SM & Leventhal M (1969) Endothelial contraction induced by histamine-type mediators: an electron microscopic study. *Journal of Cell Biology* **42**: 647.

Ryan GB & Hurley JV (1966) The chemotaxis of polymorphonuclear leucocytes towards damaged tissue. *British Journal of Experimental Pathology* **47**: 530.

Schiffman E, Corcoran BA & Wahl SM (1975) *N*-Formyl-methionyl peptides as chemoattractants for leucocytes. *Proceedings of the National Academy of Sciences, USA* **72**: 1059.

Segal AW (1980) Neutrophil function tests. *Hospital Update* **6**: 1043.

Segal AW, Cross AR, Garcia RC, Barregaard N, Valerius NH, Soothill JF & Jones OTG (1983) Absence of cytochrome b-245 in chronic granulomatous disease. *New England Journal of Medicine* **308**: 245.

Weissman G (ed) (1980) *The Cell Biology of Inflammation. Handbook of Inflammation, Volume 2*. Amsterdam, New York and Oxford: Elsevier/North Holland Biomedical Press.

Williams GT & Williams WJ (1983) Granulomatous inflammation—a review. *Journal of Clinical Pathology* **36**: 723.

Zigmond SH (1974) Mechanisms of sensing chemical gradients by polymorphonuclear leucocytes. *Nature* **249**: 450.

The Immune System and its Disorders

Adams DO, Johnson WJ & Mann PA (1982) Mechanisms of target recognition and destruction in macrophage-mediated tumour cytotoxicity. *Federation Proceedings* **41**: 2212.

Bodmer WF (ed) (1978) The HLA system. *British Medical Bulletin* **34**: No. 3.

Dixon FJ & Fisher DW (eds) (1983) *The Biology of Immunologic Disease*. Sunderland, Massachusetts: Sinauer Associates.

Roitt IM (1984) *Essential Immunology*. Oxford: Blackwell Scientific.

Roitt IM, Brostoff J & Male D (1985) *Immunology*. London: Churchill Livingstone/Gower Medical Publishing.

Schoenfeld Y & Schwartz RS (1984) Immunologic and genetic factors in autoimmune diseases. *New England Journal of Medicine* **311**: 1019.

Granulomatous Inflammation

Adams DO (1982) Macrophage activation and secretion. *Federation Proceedings* **41**: 2193.

Lasser A (1983) The mononuclear phagocytic system—a review. *Human Pathology* **14**: 108.

Nathan CF, Murrey HW & Cohn ZA (1980) The macrophage as an effector cell. *New England Journal of Medicine* **303**: 622.

Spector WG (1969) The granulomatous inflammatory exudate. *International Review of Experimental Pathology* **8**: 1–55.

Van Furth R (ed) (1978) *Mononuclear Phagocytes: Functional Aspects*. Proceedings of the 3rd conference on mononuclear phagocytes, London, 1978. The Hague: Martinus Nijhoff.

Amyloidosis

Durie BGM, Persky B, Soehnbein BJ, Grogan TM & Salmon SE (1982) Amyloid production in human myeloma stem-cell culture, with morphologic evidence of amyloid secretion by associated macrophages. *New England Journal of Medicine* 307: 1689.

Eriksen N & Benditt EP (1980) Isolation and characterisation of the amyloid-related apoprotein (SAA) from human high density lipoprotein. *Proceedings of the National Academy of Sciences, USA* 77: 6860.

Glenner GG (1980) Amyloid deposits and amyloidosis. *New England Journal of Medicine* 302: 1283 & 1333.

Kisilensky R (1983) Amyloidosis: a familiar problem in the light of current pathogenetic developments. *Laboratory Investigation* 49: 381.

Skinner M & Cohen AS (1983) Amyloidosis: clinical, pathologic and biochemical characteristics. In Wagner BM, Fleismajer R & Kaufman N (eds) *Connective Tissue Diseases*, p.97. Baltimore and London: Williams & Wilkins.

Viral Infections

Gadjusek CD (1977) Unconventional viruses and the origin and disappearance of kuru. *Science* 197: 943.

Jawetz E, Melnick JL & Adelberg EA (1982) *Review of Medical Microbiology.* Los Altos, California: Lange Medical Publications.

Mitra S (1980) DNA replication in viruses. *Annual Reviews of Genetics* 14: 347.

Panjvani ZFK & Hanshaw JB (1981) Cytomegalovirus in the perinatal period. *American Journal of Diseases of Childhood* 135: 56.

Preble OT & Fredman RM (1983) Interferon-mediated alterations in cells: relevance to viral and nonviral diseases. *Laboratory Investigation* 49: 4.

Snyder RL, Tyler G & Sunnas J (1982) Chronic hepatitis and hepatocellular carcinoma associated with woodchuck hepatitis virus. *American Journal of Pathology* 107: 422.

Pathological Bases of Ischaemia

Kakkar VV (ed) (1985) *Atheroma and Thrombosis.* London: Pitman Medical.

Lasslo A (ed) (1984) *Blood platelet function and medicinal chemistry.* Amsterdam and New York: Elsevier/North Holland Biomedical Press.

Miller NE (ed) (1984) *Atherosclerosis: Mechanisms and Approaches to Therapy.* New York: Raven Press.

Woolf N (1982) *Pathology of Atherosclerosis.* London: Butterworths.

Woolf N (ed) (1983) *Biology and Pathology of the Vessel Wall.* London: Praeger Scientific.

Neoplasia and Oncogenesis

Ayesh R, Idle JR, Ritchie JC, Crothers MJ & Hetzel MR (1984) Metabolic oxidation phenotypes as markers for susceptibility to lung cancers. *Nature* 312: 169.

Baserga R (1981) The cell cycle. *New England Journal of Medicine* 304: 453.

Carter RL (1982) Some aspects of the metastatic process. *Journal of Clinical Pathology* **35**: 1041.

Farber E (1982) Chemical carcinogenesis—a biologic perspective. *American Journal of Pathology* **106**: 271.

Gelboin H (1983) Carcinogens, drugs and cytochrome P-450. *New England Journal of Medicine* **309**: 105.

Hicks RM (1983) Pathological and biochemical aspects of tumour promotion. *Carcinogenesis* **4**: 1209.

Krontiris TE (1983) The emerging genetics of human cancer. *New England Journal of Medicine* **309**: 405.

Land H, Parada LF & Weinberg RA (1983) Cellular oncogenes and multistep carcinogenesis. *Science* **222**: 771.

Liotta LA, Rao CN & Barsky SH (1983) Tumour invasion and the extracellular matrix. *Laboratory Investigation* **49**: 636.

Lipsitt MB (1983) Hormones, medications and cancer. *Cancer* **51**: 2426.

Nicolson GL (1979) Cancer metastases. *Scientific American* **240**(3): 66.

Paul J (1984) Oncogenes. *Journal of Pathology* **143**: 1.

Pitot HC (1978) *Fundamentals of Oncology*. New York and Basel: Marcel Dekker.

Robertson M (1983) Paradox and paradigm: the message and meaning of myc. *Nature* **306**: 733.

Ruddon RW (1981) *Cancer Biology*. New York and Oxford: Oxford University Press.

Sporn MB & Roberts AB (1985) Autocrine growth factors and cancer. *Nature* **313**: 745.

Weinberg RA (1983) A molecular basis of cancer. *Scientific American* **249**: 102.

Weinberg RA (1983) Alteration of the genomes of tumour cells. *Cancer* **51**: 1971.

Weinstein IB (1983) Protein kinase, phospholipid and control of growth. *Nature* **302**: 146.

Wright NA (1984) Cell proliferation in health and disease. In Anthony PP & Macsween RNM (eds) *Recent Advances in Histopathology 12*, pp. 17–34. Edinburgh: Churchill Livingstone.

Index

Note: Page numbers in *italics* refer to those
pages on which illustrations or tables
appear.

abl (Abelson murine leukaemia virus) gene, 471
ABO blood group system, 107, 121, 154
    in hyperacute rejection, 188
Abscess, 69, 74–75
    cold, 216
    crypt, 102
Acanthosis nigricans, 424
Acetaldehyde–xanthine oxidase system, 53, *54*
2-Acetyl-aminofluorene, 444
Acetylcholine receptors, 168, *172–173*
N-Acetyl-glucosamine, 389
N-Acetylneuraminic acid (NANA), 242, 249
Acid fastness, 209
Acid phosphatase,
    carcinoplacental, 425
    isoenzymes, 424
Acinar atrophy, 101
Acquired immune deficiency syndrome (AIDS),
    146–148
Acromegaly, 354
Actin-myosin contraction, 52, 300
Adaptation phenomena, 379
Addison's disease, 354
Adenine trinucleotide, 270
Adenocarcinoma, *366*
    paranasal sinuses, 448
    renal, 404, 415, 417
    of vagina, 456
Adenoma, 374, 375, 413
    adrenal cortical, 419
    genesis of, 375
    parathyroid, 419, 438
    of pituitary, 413, 418, 419
Adenosine deaminase, 142
Adenosine diphosphate (ADP), 299, 301
Adenosine triphosphate, *see* ATP
Adenosis, 383
S-Adenosyl-ethionine, 24
Adenoviruses, 247
Adenylate cyclase, *3–4*, 301, 382
Adrenal glands, 354
    congenital hyperplasia, 193, *380*
    cortical adenoma, 419
    metastases in, 410
Adrenocorticotrophic hormone (ACTH), 354,
    380, 419, *420*
Aetiology, 5, 6
Aflatoxins, 446
Age,
    atherosclerosis risk, 284
    immune deficiency and, 145
    tuberculosis risk, 214
AIDS, 146–148
Air, in gaseous emboli, 319
Albinism, 353, 355
Albright's syndrome, 354

Albumin, 340
Alcohol, and lipoprotein levels, 288
Alcoholism, chronic, 23
Aldosterone, *342*, 344
Aleutian mink disease, 263
Alkylating agents, direct-acting, 446
Allergens, 123, 151, 153
Allergic individuals, 149
Allergic rhinitis, 151
Allograft, 184
    rejection, *see* Rejection, allograft
Alpha-1-antitrypsin deficiency, 78
Alpha-fetoprotein (AFP), 425
Alpha granule, 275, 298
Alpha transforming growth factors (TGF), 391
Alveoli,
    in chronic venous congestion, 349
    in pulmonary oedema, 345, 346
Ames test, 439, *441*
Amines, vasoactive, 64–65
2-Amino-1-naphthol, 444
Amplification loops, positive, 61, *62*, 63, 64
Amputation, spontaneous, 30
Amyloid, 238
    AFp, 239
    classification, 234
    identification in tissue, 233–234
    of immune origin (AL), 234, 240
    light chains, from, 235
    properties and structure, 233–234
    protein AA, 236–237
    types, other, 239
Amyloidosis, 233–240
    acquired organ-limited, 240
    acquired systemic, 234–236
    associated with multiple myelomatosis, 234
    in brain, 240
    cardiac, 236, 240
    classification, 234
    heredofamilial systemic, 239–240
    primary, 234
    reactive systemic, 236–239
    secondary, 234
Amylum, 233
Anaemia,
    chronic, fatty change in heart in, 21
    haemolytic, *see* Haemolytic anaemia
    iron-deficiency, 414, 417
    macrocytic, 417
    in malignant disease, 414, 417
Anaphylatoxins (C3a, C5a), 45, 60, 63
Anaphylaxis, 64
Anchorage dependence, 401
    loss of, 401, 473, 474
Aneurysm, 6, 7, 281
    blood stasis in, 304
    mycotic, 319
    in tertiary syphilis, 230
    ventricular, *335*, 336
Angina pectoris, 325, 326, 330
    'crescendo', *283*
Angio-neurotic oedema, hereditary, 77

492   Index